AIDS:
PRINCIPLES,
PRACTICES,
& POLITICS

AIDS:
PRINCIPLES,
PRACTICES,
& POLITICS

Edited by

Inge B. Corless, R.N., Ph.D., F.A.A.N.

Chair, Department of Secondary Care
School of Nursing
University of North Carolina
Chapel Hill, North Carolina

Mary Pittman-Lindeman, Dr.P.H.

Director of Planning and Evaluation
San Francisco Department of Public Health
San Francisco, California

● HEMISPHERE PUBLISHING CORPORATION, Washington
A subsidiary of Harper & Row, Publishers, Inc.

Cambridge   New York   Philadelphia   San Francisco
London   Mexico City   São Paulo   Singapore   Sydney

NOTICE

The publisher assumes no responsibility for any statements of fact or opinion expressed in this book. The editors and the publisher of this work have made every effort to ensure that any drug dosage schedules herein are accurate and in accord with the standards accepted at the time of publication. Readers are advised, however, to check the product information sheet included in the package of any drug to be certain that changes have not been made in the recommended dose or in the contraindications for administration. This recommendation is of particular importance in regard to new or infrequently used drugs.

This book was set in Baskerville by The Sheridan Press.
The Sheridan Press was printer and binder.

Library of Congress Cataloging in Publication Data

AIDS: principles, practices, & politics

  Includes bibliographies and index.
  1. AIDS (Disease)   2. AIDS (Disease)—Social aspects.
I. Corless, Inge B.   II. Pittman-Lindeman, Mary.
[DNLM: 1. Acquired Immunodeficiency Syndrome.
2. Politics—United States.   WD 308 A28839]
RC607.A26A3488   1988   362.1'969792   87-23656
ISBN 0-89116-772-2 (soft)
ISBN 0-89116-795-1 (hard)

This book is dedicated with affection and great respect to Calu Lester,
a contributor to this project who died prior to its completion,
and to all of the other persons with AIDS and ARC and their caregivers.

Contributors

Graham Bass, R.N., M.S.
Senior Staff Nurse, Supportive Care
    Program
St. Vincent's Hospital and Medical
    Center
New York, New York

Laurel Brodsley, R.N., Ph.D.,
    M.P.H.
Lecturer, English Department
University of California
Los Angeles, California

Rev. Bernard Brown, S.J., Ph.D.
Lecturer Medical Spirituality
Georgetown University School of
    Nursing
Washington, D.C.

Cathy Casriel, M.S.W.
Project Director
Narcotic and Drug Research, Inc.
New York, New York

Ellen C. Cooper, M.D., M.P.H.
Supervisory Medical Officer
Antiviral and AIDS Drugs
Division of Antiinfective Drug
    Products
Food and Drug Administration
Washington, D.C.

Inge B. Corless, R.N., Ph.D.,
    F.A.A.N.
Chair, Department of Secondary Care
School of Nursing
University of North Carolina
Chapel Hill, North Carolina

Don C. Des Jarlais, Ph.D.
Assistant Deputy Director
N.Y. State Division of Substance
    Abuse Services
New York, New York

Carole Donovan, R.N., M.A.
Senior Staff Nurse, Supportive Care
  Program
St. Vincent's Hospital and Medical
  Center
New York, New York

Dean F. Echenberg, M.D., Ph.D.
Director, Bureau of Communicable
  Disease Control
Department of Public Health
San Francisco, California

Michael Eller, B.A.
Research Associate
Howard Brown Memorial Clinic
Chicago, Illinois

Dianne Feinstein
Mayor of San Francisco
San Francisco, California

Jim Foster, B.A.
San Francisco Health Commissioner
San Francisco, California

Zelda Foster, M.S.W.
Chief Social Worker
Brooklyn V.A. Medical Center
Brooklyn, New York

Samuel Friedman, Ph.D.
Principal Investigator
Narcotic and Drug Research, Inc.
New York, New York

Chuck Frutchey
Assistant Director of Education
San Francisco AIDS Foundation
San Francisco, California

Robert Fulton, Ph.D.
Professor of Sociology
Director, Center for Death Education
  and Research
University of Minnesota
Minneapolis, Minnesota

Moses Grossman, M.D.
Chief of Pediatric Services
San Francisco General Hospital
San Francisco, California

Jill G. Joseph, Ph.D.
Assistant Professor of Epidemiology
University of Michigan
Ann Arbor, Michigan

C. Everett Koop, M.D.
Surgeon General of the United States
Rockville, Maryland

Elizabeth P. Lamers, M.A.
Educational Consultant
Malibu, California

Angela Lewis, R.N., M.S.N.
Assistant Director of Nursing
  Administration
Langely Porter Psychiatric Institute
San Francisco, California

Julien S. Murphy, Ph.D.
Assistant Professor
Department of Philosophy
University of Southern Maine
Portland, Maine

Sr. Patrice Murphy, R.N., M.S.
Coordinator, Supportive Care
  Program
St. Vincent's Hospital and Medical
  Center
New York, New York

David G. Ostrow, Ph.D.
Associate Professor of Psychiatry
University of Michigan
Ann Arbor, Michigan

Greg Owen, Ph.D.
Director, Office of Research and
    Statistics
The Amherst H. Wilder Foundation
St. Paul, Minnesota

Mary Pittman-Lindeman, Dr.P.H.
Director of Planning and Evaluation
San Francisco Department of Public
    Health
San Francisco, California

Judith Wilson Ross, M.A.
Associate Director UCLA Program in
    Medical Ethics
Associate, Center for Bioethics
St. Joseph's Health System
Orange, California

Michael E. Samuels, Dr.P.H.
Assistant to the Surgeon General
Rockville, Maryland

Betsy Selman, M.S.
Volunteer Coordinator and Pastoral
    Counselor
Supportive Care Program
St. Vincent's Hospital and Medical
    Center
New York, New York

Michael A. Simpson, M.D.
Director of Program Planning for
    Clinic Holdings
Pretoria, South Africa

Paul A. Volberding, M.D.
Chief, AIDS Activities Division
AIDS Outpatient Clinic
San Francisco General Hospital
San Francisco, California

Foreword

MAYOR DIANNE FEINSTEIN

AIDS is the most serious public health epidemic in this century and a crucial test of government's ability to respond effectively with prevention and treatment measures. Confusion about AIDS has been rife since its first recorded appearances in 1981. The disease continues to baffle our best medical minds, and we continue to be without medical models to help us handle a complex disease that *always* kills.

The AIDS epidemic is unique. It has required public officials to educate themselves about a deadly disease at a time when the medical community itself has been learning about its multiple dimensions. What causes AIDS? How is it transmitted? What are its effects on individuals and on whole communities? So many questions— and so few answers.

Faced with the realities of AIDS in the early 1980s San Francisco organized a broad-based response. We looked for rational programs to meet the needs created by the disease—and disavowed preconceived notions or past practices.

After quickly educating themselves, city health experts launched programs to educate others—while simultaneously organizing ways to combat an unprecedented public health crisis of unknown dimensions. Without background research, much was learned by talking directly to people with AIDS and to doctors treating them.

The general public also responded. There have been no complaints while San Francisco has spent more than $31 million to fight AIDS since 1982. In 1986, for example, the city budgeted $10.8 million for treatment and care, hospice services, community education, and counseling.

The public quickly grasped the dangers of AIDS but did not panic. Instead, the public showed compassion for victims and a willingness to help. The gay community took seriously a responsibility to change its lifestyles. Across the city, hundreds came forward and volunteered much-needed services.

San Francisco's response to the AIDS epidemic has made it a model for other cities to follow. We hope the model works and contributes to the elimination of this terrible disease.

The projected profile of the disease's development remains grim. Our resources will be challenged as demands for services escalate in the coming years—as the AIDS crisis expands into drug users, minorities, and heterosexuals. As the focus shifts from a disease striking primarily gay men, we must develop new programs culturally sensitive to diverse communities.

In this book the Editors, Inge B. Corless and Mary Pittman-Lindeman, and the authors present an overview of the history of AIDS. They trace its epidemiology in different populations and describe health, social, and political responses to the epidemic. General readers will find the book helpful in dispelling some of the fears generated by AIDS, while professionals will also gain valuable insights into how to develop practical strategies and programs to combat the disease.

This book doesn't offer instant solutions to AIDS—there simply aren't any—but it does clarify many complexities and suggests useful ways for individuals and communities to fight back. The book promises to make an important contribution to the fight against AIDS, which seems likely to preoccupy society for many years to come.

Acknowledgments

We express our appreciation for the support, guidance, and suggestions of our colleagues and contributors. Their insights and inquiries enhanced our thinking and added to the quality of this book.

In addition, we would like to thank members of our families for their patience and understanding throughout the development and completion of this project. In particular, Inge would like to thank Theresa Iola and Patricia Irene for their patience, inspiration, and support as they accompanied their mother on life's journey. She also remembers the words of James T. Corless who said, many years ago, that one day there would be two doctors Corless. Mary would like to recognize David Lindeman, her husband, whose intellectual challenge added to the development of this project and whose loving support made its completion possible.

We acknowledge the assistance of Maureen Ryan and Rebecca Hughes, whose wit and organizational skills contributed immeasurably to the progress of this work.

Introduction

INGE B. CORLESS
MARY PITTMAN-LINDEMAN

Why should *you* be concerned about AIDS? It's not your problem, or is it? AIDS, acquired immune deficiency syndrome, is a complex and far-reaching phenomenon that encompasses principles, practices, and politics. This book is an abridged version of a comprehensive approach to the subject of AIDS to be published in 1988. The chapters included in the current book address some of the most distressing issues confronting the general public. These problems are examined by experts and specialists in each area.

To understand AIDS one must begin with the retrovirus originally termed LAV, lymphadenopathy virus, by Luc Montagnier and his co-workers at the Pasteur Institute in France; HTLV-III by Robert Gallo and his colleagues at the National Institutes of Health in Washington, D.C.; and ARV, AIDS-related virus, by Jay Levy and his associates at the University of California, San Francisco. The attempt to standardize nomenclature by naming the virus human immunodeficiency virus (HIV) has been complicated subsequently by discoveries of new viruses or sets of viruses, such as LAV-II/HIV-II. Questions of scientific priority now resolved by an international accord have been overshadowed by the concern for the immense devastation in terms of human lives that the rapid spread of infection connotes. At the Third International AIDS Conference, held in Washington, D.C., in June 1987, this was expressed in a call for international cooperation and a global effort to combat AIDS.

Efforts at a cure thus far have resulted in drugs that delay progression of some of the manifestations of the disease. Simultaneously, efforts at prevention have taken two major approaches. The first is developing a vaccine, and the second is educating the public about the disease. The Surgeon General of the United States, C. Everett Koop, has taken a position based on the findings of AIDS investigators that children must be alerted to the danger of infection with HIV as a result of sexual intercourse or intravenous drug use. The potential for the virtual elimination of a generation of young people is a real and

1

present danger both in the United States and Africa. That this danger is not limited to gays and intravenous drug users is apparent from the development of AIDS in transfusion recipients and in the partners of seropositive individuals. In Africa, where AIDS appears to be largely heterosexually transmitted, problems of malnutrition, the effects of which are similar to AIDS, as well as the lack of appropriate laboratory facilities, compound the difficulty of estimating the true extent of the problem. The repeated use of needles without intermittent disinfection in some public health clinics in Africa may serve as a further source of disease transmission.

The extent to which cofactors are necessary for the development of the disease is not clear at this time. The reverse of this question is why is it that some individuals who are seropositive do not develop AIDS? The other possibility, of course, is that everyone who tests positive will eventually develop AIDS. Many feel that it is only a matter of time.

The resources required to care for those with AIDS, particularly as the number of patients increases, will have profound economic, societal, and personal impacts. The illness and death of so many persons in the prime of their working lives will have vast demographic implications not only for the current economy but also for the support of a predominantly older population.

The observation that the AIDS epidemic highlights all the weaknesses and gaps in the American health care system is significant. If there is one silver lining to the gray cloud of AIDS it may be a rationalization of the health care system with guarantees of access to all individuals. If, however, the demands for care are greater than available resources, some painful choices will be necessary. How and for whom should limited resources be utilized? And who will make such determinations? In a related issue, will national health insurance be enacted if private companies refuse to enroll clients?

Similar concerns exist regarding the ethics and decision-making process that will be used to establish public policy in the area of HIV testing and reporting. Many serious concerns are raised by the specter of a society that searches out and isolates those who are infected with the AIDS virus and restricts their civil liberties. On the other hand, the call for safety of the public's health poses a challenge that requires careful balancing between the needs of the community and the civil liberties of the individual. Thus far, the balance has been leaning toward the protection of civil liberties, but recent federal proposals for "routine" testing may indicate that the direction of public policy may be shifting.

The needs of the person with AIDS and his or her caregiver are not uniform. The medical and social needs will vary, depending not only on whether the person with AIDS is a baby, a child, an intravenous drug user, a hemophiliac, a gay man, a transfusion recipient, or the partner of a seropositive individual, but also according to the contextual and situational factors pertaining to that individual. The availability of health care and other support services as well as the political milieu and the presence of informed caregivers all affect caregiving. The presence of professional caregivers cannot be assumed. Decreases in the numbers of professionals such as nurses, combined with a fear of disease transmission, pressures by family, friends, and colleagues, and a concern with career, may decrease the availability of professional caregivers at the very time when the need is greatest.

Hospice programs face a more difficult challenge in providing care for persons with AIDS than for people with other terminal illnesses. The capacity of the hospice program to respond to the AIDS epidemic will depend in large measure on the availability of other needed resources such as housing. Unfortunately, the current Medicare reimbursement mechanism for hospice care (which emphasizes home care) may prove inadequate to the needs of persons with AIDS who lose their homes once their landlords learn of their illness; who become impoverished by their health care needs before Medicaid covers their costs; or who may or may not have family members, friends, or lovers willing to act as caregivers. This situation is not dissimilar to the Medicare recipient living alone or with a partner in frail health who has housing but no one who can assume the role of continuous caregiver.

The infrastructure of hospice programs is available in the United States, although not as broadly as needed to handle the projected number of AIDS cases. A different funding mechanism or one with different requirements for participation and agency compliance will be necessary if this resource is to be utilized. One resource that has been developed as a result of the AIDS epidemic is a volunteer buddy and support program, such as that of the Shanti Program in San Francisco. This type of resource will also need financial support to maintain the organization, even though the major portion of caregiving is provided by volunteers.

Further discussions of these principles, practices, and politics are included in the unabridged version of this book. Topics examined in that volume range from a comprehensive discussion of the virus, its manifestations, treatment, and epidemiology, to its impact on patients, family, and society. This abridged edition will provide a guide to some of the key issues important to a broad understanding of the epidemic. These issues are evolving and will profoundly affect every aspect of society. AIDS *is* a problem for you and me.

CHAPTER 1

The Surgeon General's Report on AIDS

C. EVERETT KOOP
MICHAEL E. SAMUELS

INTRODUCTION BY MICHAEL E. SAMUELS, ASSISTANT TO THE SURGEON GENERAL

On February 5, 1986, President Ronald Reagan, in an address to the U.S. Department of Health and Human Services, directed the Surgeon General of the U.S. Public Health Service to prepare a major report to the American people on AIDS. In preparing this report, Surgeon General C. Everett Koop followed two parallel lines of inquiry. He consulted with the top clinical and research experts in the field, many of whom were in the Public Health Service (e.g., Dr. Anthony S. Fauci, Director of the National Institute of Allergy and Infectious Diseases). At the same time he held private meetings with national organizations with specific interests in AIDS to listen to their concerns, share their insights, and build an informal consensus on how to inform the American people about AIDS.

Every group contacted agreed to meet with the Surgeon General and the final report contains insights and contributions from each of them. The groups were: Aids Action Council, National Coalition of Black Lesbians and Gays, National Minority AIDS Council, American Council of Life Insurance, Health Insurance Association of America, Washington Business Group on Health, National Association of Elementary School Principals, National Association of Secondary School Principals, National Association of State Boards of Education, National Education Association, National Parent Teachers Association, American Dental Association, American Hospital Association, American Medical Association, American Nurses Association, American Osteopathic Association, American Red Cross, The National Hemophilia Foundation, American Federation of Teachers, Association of State and Territorial Health Officials, National Association of County Health Officials, United

States Conference of Local Health Officers, Southern Baptist Convention, National Council of Churches, Synagogue Council of America, U.S. Catholic Conference, and Service Employees International Union.

Upon completion of the draft report, the Surgeon General had it officially cleared in record time. It was approved unanimously by these individuals or groups, in the following sequence:

Assistant Secretary for Health, Dr. Robert E. Windom
Secretary of Health and Human Services, Dr. Otis R. Bowen
The White House Working Group on Health, Dr. William L. Roper, Chairman
The Domestic Policy Council, Attorney General Edwin Meese, Chairman
President Ronald Reagan

On October 22, 1986 Dr. Koop released The Surgeon General's Report on AIDS to the American people. The report described AIDS in layman's terms and indicated that it was not communicated through casual contact. Intimate sexual contact and the sharing of intravenous needles were identified as the principal means of spreading the disease. Citing the fact that there is no vaccine to prevent AIDS and no drug to cure it, the report maintained that our only weapon is education and information to change human behavior and contain any further spread of the disease.

Dr. Koop clearly labeled the disease as a concern to everyone—heterosexual and homosexual, male and female. He also expressed concern about the disproportionate numbers of blacks and Hispanics with AIDS and the plight of children born with AIDS.

The most controversial part of The Surgeon General's Report has been the statement: "Education about AIDS should start in early elementary school and at home so that children can grow up knowing the behavior to avoid to protect themselves from exposure to the AIDS virus. The fact that AIDS is a fatal disease gives the debate on sex education a new dimension that calls for resolution."

The release of The Surgeon General's Report on AIDS on October 22, 1986 was an historic day in the history of the fight against AIDS. The nation's physician called on all Americans to educate ourselves and our children about AIDS, and to adopt the preventive behavior necessary to contain the spread of the AIDS virus. His report set off national, state, and local debates on all aspects of AIDS. These debates appear to have raised the consciousness of the American people. Only time will tell what will be the full impact of the report.

Not content with just preparing and releasing The Surgeon General's Report on AIDS, Dr. Koop took the message directly to the American people via public appearances, radio, television, and the print media. His personal efforts were temporarily halted by back surgery, but began anew in January 1987.

One of the best examples of this effort was Dr. Koop's speech before a Joint Session of the California Legislature on March 5, 1987. Rarely does a state Legislature extend an invitation to an individual to address a joint session. That the California Legislature did so shows their deep concern about AIDS and their willingness to take action. When the history of AIDS is written the pioneering efforts of Californians in many areas will be highlighted.

The Surgeon General's press release which accompanied the Surgeon General's Report on AIDS and the address to the Joint Session of the California State Legislature follow in their entirety. These two statements will give the reader a sense of both the initial phase of the Surgeon General's campaign as well as his later activities, interacting with the forces that shape our public opinion and policy.

STATEMENT* BY C. EVERETT KOOP, SURGEON GENERAL, U.S. PUBLIC HEALTH SERVICE

Ladies and Gentlemen:

Last February, President Reagan asked me to prepare a report to the American people on AIDS. The report is now completed.

In preparing this document, I consulted with the best medical and scientific experts this country can offer inside and outside the Public Health Service. I met with leaders of organizations concerned with health, education, and other aspects of our society to gain their views of the problems associated with AIDS. A list of those organizations is in your press kit. The resulting report contains information that I consider vital to the future health of this nation.

Controversial and sensitive issues are inherent in the subject of AIDS, and these issues are addressed in my report. Value judgments are absent. This is an objective health and medical report, which I would like every adult and adolescent to read. The impact of AIDS on our society is and will continue to be devastating. This epidemic has already claimed the lives of almost 15,000 Americans, and that figure is expected to increase 12-fold by the end of 1991—only five years from now.

Our best scientists are conducting intensive research into drug therapy and vaccine development for AIDS, but as yet we have no cure. Clearly this disease, which strikes men and women, children and adults, people of all races, must be stopped. It is estimated that one and a half million people are now infected with the AIDS virus. These people—the majority of whom are well and have no symptoms of disease—can spread the virus to others.

* Statement made on Wednesday, October 22, 1986 in Washington, D.C.

But new infections can be prevented if we, as individuals, take the responsibility of protecting ourselves and others from exposure to the AIDS virus. AIDS is not spread by casual, nonsexual contact. It is spread by high risk sexual and drug-related behaviors—behaviors that we can choose to avoid. Every person can reduce the risk of exposure to the AIDS virus through preventive measures that are simple, straightforward, and effective. However, if people are to follow these recommended measures—to act responsibly to protect themselves and others—they must be informed about them. That is an obvious statement, but not a simple one. Educating people about AIDS has never been easy.

From the start, this disease has evoked highly emotional and often irrational responses. Much of the reaction could be attributed to fear of the many unknowns surrounding a new and very deadly disease. This was compounded by personal feelings regarding the groups of people primarily affected—homosexual men and intravenous drug abusers. Rumors and misinformation spread rampantly and became as difficult to combat as the disease itself. It is time to put self-defeating attitudes aside and recognize that we are fighting a disease—not people. We must control the spread of AIDS, and at the same time offer the best we can to care for those who are sick.

We have made some strides in dispelling rumors and educating the public, but until every adult and adolescent is informed and knowledgeable about this disease, our job of educating will not be done. Unfortunately, some people are difficult to reach through traditional education methods, so our efforts must be redoubled. Others erroneously dismiss AIDS as a topic they need not be concerned about. They must be convinced otherwise.

Concerted education efforts must be directed to blacks and Hispanics. While blacks represent only 12 percent of the U.S. population, 25 percent of all people with AIDS are black. Another 12 percent of AIDS patients are Hispanic, while this group comprises only 6 percent of the population. Eighty percent of children with AIDS—8 out of 10—are black or Hispanic. For optimum effectiveness in reaching minority populations, educational programs must be designed specifically for these target groups.

Many people—especially our youth—are not receiving information that is vital to their future health and well-being because of our reticence in dealing with the subjects of sex, sexual practices, and homosexuality. This silence must end. We can no longer afford to sidestep frank, open discussions about sexual practices—homosexual and heterosexual. Education about AIDS should start at an early age so that children can grow up knowing the behaviors to avoid to protect themselves from exposure to the AIDS virus.

One place to begin this education is in our schools. Every school day, more than 47 million students attend 90,000 elementary and secondary schools in this nation. Our schools could provide AIDS education to 90–95 percent of our young people. As parents, educators, and community leaders we must assume our responsibility to educate our young. The need is critical and the price of neglect is high. AIDS education must start at the lowest grade possible as part of any health and hygiene program. There is now no doubt that we need sex education in schools and that it include information on sexual practices that may put our children at risk for AIDS. Teenagers often think themselves immortal, and these young people may be putting themselves at great risk as they begin to explore their own sexuality and perhaps experiment with drugs. The threat of AIDS should be sufficient to permit a sex education curriculum with a heavy emphasis on prevention of AIDS and other sexually transmitted diseases.

School education on AIDS must be reinforced at home. The role of parents as teachers—both in word and in deed—cannot be overestimated. Parents exert perhaps the strongest influence on their youngsters' developing minds, attitudes, and behaviors. We warn our children early about the dangerous consequences of playing with matches or crossing the street before checking for traffic. We have no less a responsibility to guide them in avoiding behaviors that may expose them to AIDS. The sources of danger differ, but the possibe consequences are much more deadly.

Before we can educate our children about AIDS, we must educate ourselves. The first thing we have to understand and acknowledge is that AIDS is no longer the concern of any one segment of society; it is the concern of us all. People who engage in high risk sexual behavior or who inject illicit drugs are risking infection with the AIDS virus and are endangering their lives and the lives of others, including their unborn children.

The Surgeon General's report describes high risk sexual practices between men and between men and women. I want to emphasize two points: First, the risk of infection increases with increased numbers of sexual partners—male or female. Couples who engage in freewheeling casual sex these days are playing a dangerous game. What it boils down to is—unless you know with *absolute certainty* that your sex partner is not infected with the AIDS virus—through sex or through drug use—you're taking a chance on becoming infected. Conversely, unless you are *absolutely certain* that you are not carrying the AIDS virus, you must consider the possibility that you can infect others.

Second, the best protection against infection right now—barring abstinence—is use of a condom. A condom should be used during sexual relations, from start to finish, with anyone whom you know or suspect is infected.

I'd like to comment briefly on the issues of mandatory blood testing and of quarantine of infected individuals. Ideas and opinions on how best to control the spread of AIDS vary, and these two issues have generated heated controversy and continuing debate. No one will argue that the AIDS epidemic must be contained, and any public health measure that will effectively help to accomplish this goal should be adopted. Neither quarantine nor mandatory testing for the AIDS antibody will serve that purpose.

Quarantine has no role in the management of AIDS because AIDS is not spread by casual contact. Quarantine should be considered only as a last resort by local authorities, and on a case-by-case basis, in special situations in which someone infected with the AIDS virus knowingly and willingly continues to exposure others to infection through sexual contact or sharing drug equipment.

Compulsory blood testing is unnecessary, unfeasible, and cost prohibitive. Furthermore, rather than aiding in prevention, testing could, in some instances, cause irreparable harm. A negative test result in someone who has been recently infected but not yet developed antibodies might give that person a false sense of security not only for him- or herself, but for that person's sexual partners as well. This could lessen the motivation to adhere to safe sex practices. Voluntary testing is available and useful for people who have engaged in high risk behaviors and want to learn if they are infected so that they can seek appropriate medical attention and act to protect others from infection.

You'll note that my report supports and reinforces recommendations by the Public Health Service on AIDS prevention and risk reduction. Although my involvement with AIDS is fairly recent, the Public Health Service has been deeply involved in the AIDS crisis from the start. In the past five years the PHS has made excellent progress in characterizing the disease, delineating the modes of transmission, and protecting our blood supply from contamination with the AIDS virus. Vigorous research into drug therapy and vaccine development continues, and, as you know, the drug azidothymidine—AZT —is being made available to thousands of people with AIDS who may benefit from this treatment.

Much remains to be done to stop this epidemic, and the Public Health Service will continue to work together with all elements of public and private sectors and use all our joint resources to the fullest to eradicate AIDS.

In closing, let me say that my report on AIDS is a document that people should read. It provides—in layman's terms—detailed information about AIDS, how the disease is transmitted, the relative risks of infection, and how to prevent infection. I'd like your help in letting the public know that this document is available and how they can get a copy of it. The address for requests is in your press packet. It also appears on this television public service announcement we are releasing today. I'd like to show it to you.

Thank you, and I'll take your questions now.

ADDRESS* BY C. EVERETT KOOP, SURGEON GENERAL, U.S. PUBLIC HEALTH SERVICE

Mr. President, Mr. Speaker . . . to hosts, guests, friends, . . . :

It is an honor and a great privilege for me to address this Joint Session of

* An address presented to the Joint Session on AIDS of the California Legislature, Sacramento, California, March 6, 1987.

the California Legislature. And while your invitation was addressed to me and I was pleased to accept it—I am here today—representing not just myself but also the personnel of the U.S. Public Health Service. I want very much to share the honor of this moment with them, because so much of what I have to say is the product of their hard work.

Also, the relationship between local and state public health officers in California and my colleagues in PHS is excellent. It *has* been over the years and I'm sure it will *continue* to be.

That's good for California . . . and it's good for the country.

This is an unusual event . . . an historic event . . . and I am moved by that consideration, also. However, as I stand in this chamber, I am *most* mindful of the following . . . single . . . overwhelming and profoundly tragic fact:

> That Californians were the *first* of our citizens, back in June of 1981, to be identified as being the victims of AIDS . . . They were among the first to die of the disease . . . And before the rest of our country knew about—or truly understood the nature of—this catastrophe, the people of California were already beginning to bury their dead.

I am deeply, deeply sorry that anyone—here or anywhere in the world—has had to die of this disease. And I am especially sorry that the people of this state have had to live with this grief the longest.

It hasn't been six years . . . yet, it seems like an eternity . . . since those first reports came in to our Centers for Disease Control in Atlanta. During that time . . .

> We've seen the offending virus and we've named and renamed it . . .
> We've developed a test to determine if the virus is present in someone's blood . . .
> We've been able to galvanize a large, international army of biomedical researchers, among whom, I might add, are many men and women of genius who are working on the problem in laboratories right here in California . . .
> And finally, over the past six years, we've developed a way of monitoring the spread of the disease so as to have some reasonable—although by no means perfect—basis upon which to plan the use of our resources tomorrow and for some years in the future.

That last point is a difficult one . . . especially for the elected representatives of a free people. But we know that the disease of AIDS—as it continues to spread throughout our population—will be drawing ever more heavily upon our social and political capital, as well as our medical and financial capital.

It's a difficult challenge for Americans. But we are a good people. Through 200 years of often stormy and tumultuous history, the people of the

United States have clung to this society's fundamental values of personal freedom, mutual assistance, and national unity.

Those values have withstood every test. And they are being tested again . . . right now . . . by the infiltration of this lethal disease.

But I firmly believe that those values will once more be our guides for collective action and once more we shall survive a grave threat to our health and well-being.

And right here I must recognize the leadership already demonstrated by the Legislature of the State of California, by its Governor, George Deukmejian, and by the rank-and-file public health, medical, and nursing personnel throughout this state. Like the rest of us, you've only begun what appears to be a long and fearful journey. But you've made a very commendable start.

I'm thinking in particular of your early moves to establish mandatory reporting of the disease and a statewide registry of cases.

Within a week of the approval of the blood test for AIDS, California had its own emergency regulations in place to protect the blood supply. And your network of alternative test sites ought to be a model for every other state to follow.

And throughout this time, you've been very careful to build into the law a respect for confidentiality and an understanding of the overwhelming burden it can be for a person to learn that he or she has AIDS . . . and will soon die.

I've said it many times, that we are fighting a terrible disease . . . We are *not* fighting the people who have it. And by your actions, you have made the government of this state a strong ally in the campaign to make sure that Americans know and respect the difference.

I think California has done well in the way it has expended its social and political capital so far on the issue of AIDS.

But it's only been a few years . . . and this disease will be a burden to us for the rest of this century at least.

We need, therefore, to give some thought to the way we will care for the rising toll of AIDS victims. Among them will be those with high risk behavior —homosexual and bisexual men and IV drug abusers. But more and more heterosexual victims will be identified. Many of those will have been unknowingly infected by bisexual men or promiscuous partners.

One of the spin-offs from the high profile of Nancy Reagan's anti-drug campaign will be reducing the spread of AIDS. Anything that will stop drug abuse, stops the spread of the AIDS virus.

The number of babies born with AIDS will certainly rise. Some will die within the first year or two of life. We're seeing that occur already.

But other children will carry the virus and may not exhibit any symptoms of an AIDS-related illness until they are well into their school years.

Frankly, I don't think society has yet worked out how it wants to respond to the plight of these innocent young victims. Some have had to take the brunt of the anger and resentment directed at their parents . . . Who've been better able to step out of the way.

Other children, abandoned by parents, have had to appeal through advocates for medical and social services that would have been routinely given children with any other disease.

We must generate a concern for these youngsters such as the First Lady has done with her campaign against drugs.

I do not believe that these examples will prove to be the rule. But the fact that they may have happened *at all* is reason enough for us all to feel some pain and contrition.

And the costs in dollars and cents is also going to mount. The federal contribution this year is $416 million. About $300 million of that is research . . . nearly $100 million is for public education and information . . . and about $10 million is for patient care.

As you well know, California by itself has spent nearly half the total dollars expended by all state governments on AIDS since 1983 . . . some $56 million so far, apportioned among patient care, public information, and research.

Some of our experts estimate that, by 1991, the total national bill for the care of AIDS patients will be *$16 billion* a year . . . or nearly *twice* what we're spending *this* year to support *all* the programs of the entire U.S. Public Health Service.

How will we apportion those costs? What will be the federal government's share? What share is reasonable for the states to carry? And how much can we ask the individual and his or her family to pay?

Commercial insurors—both life and health—have raised questions about coverage for persons known to be carrying the AIDS virus . . . or who are members of one or another groups practicing high risk behavior. While we can understand their concerns, from a strictly financial point of view, we need to ask ourselves how those concerns fit in with good public policy *in general*.

In other words, will our decisions regarding the way we pay to care for AIDS patients contaminate our entire social and political decision-making process *itself*? We must now allow that to happen. Such an effect on our public life would be in itself an "AIDS-related complex."

There is, of course, genuine alarm that the costs of AIDS could mushroom and bankrupt our health care economy. My advice is to take the issue seriously, but don't be frightened into taking action inconsistent with American values.

In addition, we must not let fear so paralyze us that we fail to do certain sensible and pragmatic things, such as developing alternatives to the high-cost terminal care that's given AIDS patients in our community and general hospitals.

In any case, the central question before us today . . . as it has been for over 200 years . . . is still this:

How can we live so that we may be *a humane and civilized people?*

I can't imagine this country ever becoming *financially* bankrupt. But our society—like every other society in human history—always runs the risk of becoming *morally and ethically* bankrupt.

And we must never let that happen.

Ordinarily, the Surgeon General of the United States doesn't worry about such things. He or she may be a moral and an ethical person—and certainly each of my predecessors was that kind of person and I hope I will be judged to have been one, also—but you know it's never been a requirement, as such, for holding his job.

But some things have appeared on my watch as your Surgeon General that have tested not only my understanding of medicine and health . . . but also my understanding of the nature of the American people.

Over the past five years I've had to wrestle with the ethical issues raised by "Baby Doe" and "Baby Fae" . . . by little Katie Beckett . . . by our ability to transplant organs and prolong life for the terminally ill.

My latest challenge was given to me a year ago, in February 1985, when President Reagan asked me to gather together all the information on AIDS that was then available and put it into a plain-English report to the American people.

And that's what I did for the next eight months. In the process, I met not only with doctors and nurses and public health people, I also met with representatives of concerned groups from across the spectrum of society . . .

Groups like the National Education Association and the National P.T.A. . . .

The National Council of Churches and the Christian Life Commission of the Southern Baptist Convention . . .

The Synagogue Council of America and the National Conference of Catholic Bishops . . .

The National Coalition of Black and Lesbian Gays and the Washington Business Group on Health.

I talked with the representatives of 26 groups in all. Most of them knew quite a bit about the health threat posed by AIDS. But what they were deeply troubled about were the moral and ethical issues raised by this disease.

Yes, we all agreed that the only real weapon we had to fight with at this time—since we lacked a vaccine or an effective drug—was the weapon of education.

That's where we all agreed. Where we had some differences of opinion, was the *substance* and the *direction* of that education.

Everybody had said, yes, we should teach about the dangers posed by the AIDS virus.

Most people said, well, *maybe* we should teach about the methods by which AIDS is transmitted.

And quite a few people said that, of course, we might *possibly* teach young people something about their sexuality to begin with.

I listened to everybody and took very good notes.

You may recall that my entire report is not very long. And I only devoted 92 words to the topic of education. But those 92 words have captured most of the attention of the media, of parents, of educators, and of public officials at all levels of government.

The reason is clear enough: The issue goes to the heart of each person's own system of moral and ethical values . . . or lack thereof.

I introduced the subject in a straightforward way. I said in my report that . . .

> Education about AIDS should start in early elementary school and at home so that children can grow up knowing the behavior to avoid to protect themselves from exposure to the AIDS virus. The threat of AIDS can provide an opportunity for parents to instill in their children their own moral and ethical standards.

Some people were unduly alarmed by that phrase, "early elementary school." Would that include kindergarten? I'm afraid so.

I know of good, caring approaches to sex education that can be used — and in fact *are* used — in kindergarten and first grade.

However, I recognize that it's more difficult to do and, therefore, I would be willing today, some four months after publication, to make that single change in the report . . . That is, I would agree, albeit reluctantly, to take out the word "early" and just let the sentence read . . . "Education about AIDS should start in elementary school."

I concluded the report with exactly the same thought. I said . . .

> Education concerning AIDS must start at the lowest grade possible as part of any health and hygiene program . . . There is now no doubt that we need sex education in schools and that it must include information on heterosexual and homosexual relationships. The threat of AIDS should be sufficient to permit a sex education curriculum with a heavy emphasis on prevention of AIDS and other sexually transmitted diseases.

And I would not change *any* of the words in that paragraph.

I am aware that the people of California, through their educational organizations, health organizations, and through their representatives in local and state government, have endorsed the need to begin teaching about AIDS no later than the seventh grade.

I think they're absolutely right and I applaud them for being clear-headed and public-minded on the issue.

I know, also, that many school districts in this state have adopted one or another curriculum elements that introduce human sexuality and reproductive health in a positive and caring way to children in elementary grades—generally speaking the fifth or sixth grades—and that should mean that local community standards, consistent with parental values, have been taken into account, which is as it should be.

And by the way, the School Health Task Force for Los Angeles County came to the same conclusion in January 1986, a good *10 months* before my own report was published. In *their* report, the task force members recommended the general adoption of a comprehensive school health education curriculum that routinely included sexuality right along with accident prevention, nutrition, and an understanding of the cardiovascular and gastrointestinal systems.

It's an eminently sensible recommendation. And it is an ethically positive recommendation as well. If we adults know something that could save the life of a child, then children have a right to that information. And we have the obligation to tell them.

If it makes us uncomfortable . . . If it is awkward to do . . . If it appears to conflict with other information we might have, those are problems that *we* have to resolve in a way that enables us to *nevertheless* tell our children what they *need* to know and have a *right* to know.

I'm not saying it's easy. But it's far from impossible.

For example, I gave just these two precautions in my report. The *first* one is simple enough. It advises you to . . .

> Find someone who is worthy of your respect and your love . . . Give that person both . . . And stay faithful to him or her.

In other words, short of total abstinence, the best defense against AIDS is to *maintain a faithful, monogamous relationship* in which you have only one continuing sexual partner . . . and that person is as faithful as you are.

My *second* message is for people who don't yet have a faithful monogamous relationship for whatever reason. That message is . . .

> *Caution:* It's important that you *know with absolute certainty* that neither you nor your partner is carrying the AIDS virus. If you're not absolutely certain, then you *must take precautions*. And the best one available—though far from perfect—is to use a condom from start to finish.

From my viewpoint, as a public health officer, I tell people that when they have sex with someone, they're also having sex with *everyone else* with whom *that* person has ever had sex. Naturally, if the "everyone else" is only you . . . you're very well protected from disease . . . and from a lot of other unpleasant surprises as well.

This all seems to be information that is clear enough and straightforward enough to tell children. There's nothing terribly esoteric about it. Yet, many adults—parents and teachers alike—are having trouble coming to terms with it all.

The more I've thought about this phenomenon, the more I've come to believe that the difficulty is not in the facts themselves concerning sexuality, human reproduction, and AIDS. The difficulty is in the *significance* of those facts relative to the totality of a *sensitive and affirmative* human relationship.

Such a relationship will include some fulfilling sexual activity, but it is not defined *only by* that activity. There's much more to a loving, caring, respectful, and tolerant human relationship than just "good sex." A relatio. ship devoid of love and responsibility is like a piece of pie that's all crust and no filling. And young people ought to be advised of that.

Novelists call it "true love." Sociologists call it "marital fidelity." The Surgeon General calls it "monogamy." But whatever you call it, we all want that well-rounded, balanced, loving, and fully considerate relationship . . . a relationship that's enriched by sex, not overwhelmed by it or devoid of it either.

Such a relationship is an ideal . . . But "real life" isn't always like that. It's imperfect . . . It's give-and-take.

Without a compassionate understanding of the imperfect nature of many human relationships, a child's education will be . . . itself . . . very imperfect.

So if parents are to educate their children about human relationships—sexual and otherwise—they must first understand and accept the nature of their *own*. For many, that's hard to do.

Parents—and adults in general—are not very good about talking *to each other* about their sexuality. They feel frustrated, guilty, and even angry because they are unable to do the thing that they know—intellectually and emotionally—they *should* do.

But they can't.

And for me, that's the compelling reason why our schools, churches, synagogues, and other community institutions must do whatever possible to provide our children with the best available information . . . physical, sexual, emotional, and psychological . . . to help them negotiate their own way through the human condition.

You, as responsible legislators, are being called upon to contribute to that process, also. And I know that this legislature is indeed writing such a record in the indelible inks of compassion and duty.

I've delivered this message—and variations of it—many times in the past few months. But it doesn't get any easier.

It's essentially a grim message and I guess I'm something of a grim courier.

My only hope is that every American who hears or reads my message, will believe it and do his or her part to stop the spread of AIDS . . . to protect and save the lives of people at risk, including and especially our unsuspecting young people . . . and that they will help return sexuality back to its rightful place in the spectrum of human experience: Have it again be a *part* of the total complex of human, caring, interpersonal relations.

Such relations, in my book anyway, are known as "true love."

Which leads me to my final word. It's not mine really. It's the last sentence of *The Bridge of San Luis Rey*, the little novel written by the late Thornton Wilder, one of our greatest novelists and playwrights. Wilder concluded that novel by observing . . .

> There is a land of the living and a land of the dead and the only bridge is love . . .
> the only survival, the only meaning.

Thank you.

CHAPTER 2

Epidemic Control Measures for AIDS: A Psychosocial and Historical Discussion of Policy Alternatives

DAVID G. OSTROW
MICHAEL ELLER
JILL G. JOSEPH

INTRODUCTION

The epidemic of acquired immune deficiency syndrome (AIDS) is unprecedented in recent medical history. The increasing incidence of the typically fatal syndrome, its transmissibility through sexual and blood contact, and the continuing lack of either an effective vaccine or cure have created a broad series of challenges.[1] Despite the relatively rapid isolation of the etiologic agent, human immunodeficiency virus (HIV, formerly referred to as HTLV-III/LAV), and the development of antibody detection assays,[2,3] many of these challenges are predominantly psychosocial in nature. Some are well recognized; for example, increasing attention is being paid to the extent and determinants of behavioral changes required to reduce HIV infection[4,5] and to the complex social and psychological needs of those diagnosed with AIDS or who are HIV seropositive.[6,7] Another set of issues, largely unrecognized in the medical or social science literature, deals with the relationship of those at risk for AIDS to the broader social and political environment. As the majority of AIDS cases have occurred in socially stigmatized groups—homosexually active men, intravenous drug users, and immigrants—it is not surprising that there have been attributions of blame and countercharges of discrimination. There has been little scientific discussion of this phenomenon, its origins, and possible consequences.

We will examine ways in which the attitudes and activities of the majority, heterosexual culture may impede or facilitate the adaptation of homosexual/bisexual men to the crisis of AIDS. Although specific to this particular risk group, comments offered here may be more broadly applicable to others at risk. These impressions are based upon a systematic review of qualitative data collected across a period of two and one-half years in a cohort of approximately 1000 homosexual or bisexual men at risk for AIDS. This discussion will be prefaced by a more general historical description of social responses to epidemic disease and will be followed by comments on the potential for responsible and positive choices by all of us confronting the problem of AIDS.

HISTORICAL CONTEXT

Epidemics and their psychosocial consequences are not new; furthermore, there is a predictable series of events which can occur as epidemics threaten the sense of control and mastery implicit in most forms of social organization. By examining historical parallels it may be possible to better understand our current situation, thus minimizing the fear and discrimination that subvert the formulation of effective public health policy. In the discussion that follows, special attention is paid to the ways in which "epidemic control" measures (such as quarantine) may arise more from a need to blame or to control than from an accurate epidemiologic assessment of risk.

The potential threat produced by epidemic disease can be profound, particularly when the existing social order appears impotent to provide the protection it implicitly promises. Such implicit promises may arise from the theological bases of a feudal system or from the assumed biomedical-technological hegemony of our own society. The extreme social reaction to epidemic disease in such a context will only be exacerbated by the well-described phenomenon of misestimating health risks.[8,9] Research evidence suggests that we optimistically underestimate risk that arises from our own behavior,[10,11] while the opposite is true of external threat. External risk is frequently misperceived as more threatening and serious than is factually accurate. Therefore, when the epidemic is seen to originate from infected "others" (some stigmatized and easily identifiable subgroup), the sense of risk or threat is likely to be further increased, thus intensifying the need for more stringent "control" measures. Three historical antecedents illustrating these points are discussed below.[12]

The Plague in Medieval Europe

Beginning in the fourteenth century, pandemics of plague afflicted Medieval Europe, reoccurring at regular intervals until well into the seventeenth century. Although estimates of the proportion of the population that died vary, it is apparent that this epidemic was devastating. The profound effects on the religious, political, economic, and social order have been well documented.

For example, dramatic decreases in the supply of local labor had the potential to shift economic organization toward the concept of wage rather than servitude. Of greater interest for our purpose, however, were the complex and largely abortive attempts to control dissemination of the disease. Attempts to quarantine affected villages have been carefully described, as has the frequent neglect of those stricken. While these mesures likely increased the suffering of those taken ill, there is no evidence that they slowed or halted the spread of plague in Europe. Such efforts were based on an understandable but inaccurate assessment of the mode of transmission of plague. Except for the pneumonic form of the disease, transmission was from fleas carried by the commonly occurring brown rat. Thus, the isolation of individuals or communities was largely ineffectual. Similarly, the reaction of some physicians was both exaggerated and unnecessary. For instance, physicians in parts of France wore full-length leather cloaks, wide-brimmed hats, and used pointers to avoid close contact with plague victims. Quite by coincidence, the only value of such practices may have been to avoid close contact with fleas.

By the fifteenth century yet more distressing social phenomena were apparent. As the epidemic continued to take its toll erratically but largely unabated, more extreme measures were used to preserve the prevalent theistic world view. Bands of devout pilgrims appeared in large numbers, moving through the major population centers of Europe, stripped to the waist and publicly whipping themselves. These flagellants, perceiving plague as punishment for previously unrecognized sin, sought relief in their mortifications. By voluntarily submitting to self-imposed pain and suffering, they believed that the wrathful God punishing them could be propitiated. Simultaneously, they turned on the vulnerable and stigmatized Jewish population. Although fundamentally inconsistent with the concept of plague as divine retribution, flagellant groups simultaneously held Jews to be responsible for transmission of the disease. Flamed by an inability to control the epidemic even through penance, rumors of well-poisoning and other malicious activities by Jews spread rapidly. Flagellants therefore felt further justified in systematically seeking out and murdering large Jewish populations. In Brussels, for example, following a procession by flagellants, the entire Jewish population was massacred. Indeed, within a decade there were virtually no Jews left alive in either Germany or what later became Belgium.

In spite of desperate "control measures," largely based on a misunderstanding of disease transmission or a theology of retribution, epidemics of the plague continued at irregular intervals. Ultimately, by the late seventeenth century, they abated, for reasons which remain largely unexplained.

Cholera

In August 1817 an epidemic was documented in the British possession of India, in a district approximately 70 miles from Calcutta. Whether previously endemic in the Indian subcontinent or not, it is certainly true that the modern history of cholera begins with this episode. Carried both overland and by sea, the disease soon penetrated Russia and the Austro-Hungarian Empire. The rapid dissemination of this new and lethal affliction again prompted the search for those who could be blamed for its occurrence. In central Europe rumors spread that the rich were deliberately infecting peasants or poisoning their water supply. More commonly, however, it was the poor themselves who were seen as the source of disease. Writing in 1832, an English physician described the reasons he believed his locality was susceptible to an epidemic of cholera. ". . . Our population may be described as vicious, immoral, and miserable; a full half being liable to the vice of all others the most destructive to religion and morals—I mean drunkenness."[13] He went on to suggest that not only drunkenness but Catholic emancipation in 1829 might further explain why cholera was inevitable. The dual notions of moral and physical filth placing a group at risk were also expressed in the United States where it was reported regarding cholera, "drunkards and filthy, wicked people of all descriptions, are swept away in heat, as if the Holy God could no longer bear their wickedness, just as we sweep away a mass of filth when it has become so corrupt that we cannot bear it."[14]

In addition to general notions regarding classes of people who were responsible for or susceptible to the epidemic, there was a consistent attempt to identify specific individuals who brought the disease to a previously unaffected location. Three shoemakers were reportedly responsible for the introduction of cholera to Scotland. Similarly, a woman known to be a public drunkard was blamed for bringing the disease to the Isle of Bute off the coast of Scotland. A young woman who traveled, although desperately ill with cholera, to the home of her mother was dragged from her bed for fear she would bring cholera to the rest of the community, and sent in a cart to a foundry where she died. (Her mother was subsequently forced out of her home which was burned with all its contents.)

In the United States a general pattern of response to the threat of cholera emerged. First, attempts were made to prevent transmission of the disease, usually including the institution of a quarantine. Although medical opinion of the time held that no disease was contagious and that therefore such measures were unnecessary, popular opinion generally supported their adoption. Second, there was an attempt to clean towns of the accumulated waste and garbage typically littering the streets. Often the garbage was deposited in local rivers or simply left outside city limits to rot. Finally, medical facilities and personnel were generally made available for the poor who became ill. Although there was general agreement that such facilities were necessary, there was often a similar agreement that they should be made available in someone else's neighborhood. Measures as innocuous as petitions and as lethal as arson were used to dissuade the establishment of cholera hospitals. These attitudes arose not only from a fear of disease but from the prevalent attitude well described in the words of one observer who reported, "The visitor finds few others in those receptacles than the inpenitent sot and debauchee."[14] Finally, because personal habits were believed to be an important cause of cholera, it became the duty of public officials to protect the community from perceived human excesses. Connecticut physicians demanded that the Board of Health should have "the power to change the habits of the sensual, the vicious, the intemperate."[14] In addition, in most communities affected by cholera, the sale of certain foods were forbidden, including unripe fruits, cucumbers, and corn in New York. These, as well as alcohol, were held to increase the likelihood of cholera.

Syphilis

With the discovery of the *S. pallida* in 1905, the Wasserman test in 1906, and arsphenamine (Salvarsan or "606") in 1909, the way was paved in the United States for public health control programs aimed at controlling syphilis. Persons with syphilis were frequently viewed as unclean and deserving of their affliction because they had chosen illicit sexual behaviors despite the threat of disease. While men with syphilis were rarely quarantined, females accused of "solicitation" were forced to undergo Wasserman testing and, if positive, were detained and treated until considered noncontagious. The use of preventive measures such as condoms and urethral disinfectants were opposed by moralists, who believed they promoted promiscuity. It was only during wartime, with increasing morbidity in soldiers due to syphilis and gonorrhea, that the military began to widely promote prophylactic measures. Nonetheless, prevention was also linked to chastity and American soldiers were urged to "discipline" their sexual urges. This was illustrated in an extreme form by the government order issued in July 1917, which made contraction of venereal disease by soldiers a punishable offense.

Between 1935 and 1938, 26 states passed laws requiring premarital syphilis testing and prohibiting seropositive persons from marrying. Despite evidence against nonsexual transmission of syphilis, ordinances requiring food handlers and domestics to be tested were commonplace. Quarantine of prostitutes, although substantially abandoned earlier, was reimposed. Employment restrictions were not effectively ended until penicillin became available in the late 1930s. Nonetheless, such ordinances from the 1920s and 1930s regulating control of sexually transmitted diseases remain, and are often referred to, as the basis for AIDS control measures. Recently, bills have been introduced in many state legislatures that would mandate premarital HIV serotesting and prohibit seropositive individuals from marrying.[15] Similarly, state and federal proposals for mandatory reporting on HIV seropositivity and contact-tracing of partners of seropositive individuals are based on the methods used in the 1930s and 1940s for syphilis control.

These measures of mandatory reporting and contact-tracing to control venereal disease had been avoided by those who were able to use private physicians. Such physicians were less likely to report patients by name to public health authorities, resulting in underreporting of STD (sexually transmitted disease) statistics. With the development of effective treatment for syphilis, the emphasis switched from reporting and contact-tracing to ensuring effective treatment of persons suspected of exposure.

In the 1970s and 1980s, there was a significant increase in the proportion of syphilis reported due to homosexual transmission and renewed attempts to apply contact-tracing and prophylactic treatment to this population. However, the anonymous nature of many homosexual contacts, as well as the reluctance of gay men to have their names or those of their partners reported to public health authorities, rendered such measures generally ineffective as they sought care from private practitioners willing to protect their identity.[16] There were some exceptions. This was only untrue where local health authorities worked cooperatively with the homosexual community, establishing trust in their ability to provide both confidentiality and needed medical treatment.

It is apparent that many of the current proposals for "controlling" the AIDS epidemic recapitulate earlier, unsuccessful experiences. Adequate control of transmission must inevitably take into account both the characteristics of the pathogen and the social context within which it is appearing. A misunderstanding of the vector for transmission of plague led to inappropriate control measures that increased human suffering while still failing to halt the spread of the epidemic. This failure, in turn, fueled the need to identify a group who could be blamed and punished. The emerging consensus about HIV transmission must influence the development of public policy as well as provide the impetus for further scientific investigations. This virus is comparatively difficult to transmit since it is usually spread by either sharing blood or sexual activity.

The early attempts to control cholera mentioned previously are also instructive. Illness and contagion reinforced existing, moralistic stereotypes regarding the poor, the alcoholic, and the immigrant. The emerging concern for the indigent ill competed sharply with the desire to protect one's own neighborhood from the perceived threat of epidemic illness. Once again, basic facts about transmission were unavailable and in this vacuum, preexisting world views became the basis for social and political responses to the epidemic. Currently misguided attempts to exclude children with AIDS from schools or to prevent the establishment of hospices have been documented, demonstrating that knowledge of transmission may not be well-assimilated and/or heeded and that panic can lead to actions that conflict with pervasive norms of compassion for the young and the dying. The homosexual male is undoubtedly at great risk for "scapegoating" in this milieu and such social responses make attempts to control the epidemic only more difficult. Efforts to develop effective public health policy must take into account these extreme and often morally derived reactions. It is essential for scientists and health care providers to join the policy debate; failure to recognize the social reactions to this epidemic, to take such reactions seriously, and to counter inappropriate policies will have as adverse consequences as ignorance of basic biomedical data.

Finally, the history of syphilis should sharpen awareness of the need to think clearly about the presumed effectiveness of proposed policies. When test-reporting and contact-tracing is mandated, those with the means to do so will avoid using public services.[16] Accurate reporting of sexual contacts will decline in an atmosphere of repression, especially when no definitive prevention or cure is available. For example, there is already excellent anecdotal evidence that use of alternative test sites decreases dramatically when mandatory reporting and contact-tracing are instituted or even rumored.

Control measures based on other transmission models may be ineffective and perhaps damaging. They can distract from the real work of education in high risk groups and can alienate those in need of such educational programs. All proposed measures short of quarantine, but including contact-tracing, mandatory testing, or even tattooing the seropositive individual, do not obviate the need for effective educational efforts. Education is necessary to understand what it means if oneself or a partner is seropositive and how to regulate relevant behaviors. Unfortunately, no evidence is yet available demonstrating that knowledge of one's serologic test results decreases the likelihood of risk-related behavior. This is an issue urgently requiring further investigation because it *is* known that *all* of those at risk ought to avoid behaviors linked to HIV transmission.

These brief historical discussions highlight the ways in which periods of epidemic are psychological, social, and political events as well as biomedical phenomena. Inappropriate and ineffectual efforts to control an epidemic are often derived from the sense of disease as deserved punishment along with an extreme, exaggerated fear of personal harm. This produces a social climate in which certain vulnerable groups, ranging from Jews to prostitutes to homosexuals, become targets for scapegoating. In addition, attending appropriately to the needs of those who are already ill becomes difficult in the moralized environment where illness is perceived as punishment. Many of these themes have reemerged during the AIDS epidemic. In the next section we discuss ways in which such social reactions impinge upon the ability of at-risk gay men to adapt to the current crisis.

ADAPTATION AND FEAR

Data used in this section were obtained from a cohort of 950 homosexual/bisexual men in Chicago participating in both a biomedical[17] and a psychosocial[4] study of AIDS risk. On a semiannual basis, participants are seen for an extensive medical-epidemiological-virological evaluation, and given a self-administered psychosocial questionnaire to complete approximately two weeks following this evaluation. The delay between the clinic visit and completion of the questionnaire was established in order to obtain a more accurate assessment of psychosocial functioning. (Pretesting suggested biomedical evaluations often heightened concerns about AIDS, and could transiently increase psychological distress.) The structured questionnaire examines behavioral, social, and psychological responses to the threat of AIDS. It also documents the perceived need for, and impact of, community support programs, personality, and interpersonal dynamics on coping and change. At the time of enrollment, April 1984 to March 1985, the cohort was 92% white, with a mean age of 36 years, and with an average of 16.4 years of education.

In addition to the structured closed-form questions, an open-ended question asks: "Is there anything else you would like to tell us about yourself or about AIDS?" Approximately 250 men in each of the first four waves of the study responded to this question, and all responses have been reviewed and analyzed by the authors. In addition, participants are given the opportunity to express any concerns of distress to the on-site Research Associate. Participants with significant distress or who request help are evaluated, and appropriate intervention or referral is then provided. Both written comments at the conclusion of the questionnaire and notes of discussions with participants provide the basis for comments offered in this report.

We have previously characterized the phenomenology of AIDS as including extreme threat, uncertainty, and stigmatization.[18] Major stressors experienced by persons at high risk of AIDS include the fear of transmitting and developing a fatal illness, the loss of friends or partners with associated grief, and the strain of making radical lifestyle changes, while questioning the effectiveness of such changes. Motivation for effective behavioral risk reduction necessitates perceiving one's vulnerability, yet such perceptions are often distressing. Participants must struggle to maintain a balanced, positive adaptation that includes appropriately altered behaviors, psychological well-being, and solid social networks.

Furthermore, although there were few reported incidents of obvious discrimination or ill-treatment, there were consistent increased fears of anticipated discrimination, anti-gay violence, and employment or health care difficulties because of AIDS. In mid-1985, for example, 39% of the cohort reported fears of police harassment, 41% cited concerns about workplace hostilities, and 56% were worried that heterosexuals generally perceived gay men as diseased. Over one-third of the participants (38%) reported worries that their families were uncomfortable because they were gay. These specific concerns were paralleled by reports of general AIDS-related worries. The cohort described these concerns as often intruding on their thinking (47.3%), and as interfering with their ability to relax (20.2%) or to feel comfortable with other gay men (22%). Between one-quarter and one-half of all participants reported feeling tense (26.6%), angry (31.6%), or worried (46.1%) because of AIDS.[19]

When open-ended responses were analyzed for all four waves, it was apparent that many participants attempt to discern some positive effect of this devastating epidemic. In the words of one participant, "AIDS has become a modern day plague which has affected all of us in some way . . . The only thing positive about AIDS [is that] people are becoming more aware of the disease and wanting to learn and educate others. It has brought more caring and concern among the gay community." Similarly, many develop an altruistic attitude, reporting volunteer activities in the community or among those already affected with AIDS. One participant typically commented, "I am trying to do whatever I can to make someone's life a little more happy, to be there for others."

There is also considerable sadness and anger expressed by participants. This was perhaps best explained by the participant who wrote, "Living with AIDS is living with a time bomb. You can only hope it doesn't explode inside you." Another stated, "I have always believed that love created life and that love sustains and nurtures life. Now I see a dilemma where love destroys life." Some subjects have developed clinically significant depression, often related to the death of friends or lovers due to AIDS or a sense of mortal threat to their own lives. In perhaps its most ironic form, the psychological distress is experienced as an internalized, self-directed homophobia. One participant wrote, "The thought of getting AIDS sets off my guilt at being homosexual. In a way, I guess I almost do view it as 'God's punishment' since I was taught that being gay is bad."

The complex process of adaptation to the AIDS crisis by gay men is constantly being disrupted by negative events in the broader social environment. One participant wrote, "To be gay and have to read day after day about AIDS only adds stress and fear to an already difficult life." Another commented, "After Rock Hudson died rumors circulated at work that I have AIDS. One coworker even addressed me with, 'Hi Rock.'" As the media discussed proposals regarding mandatory HIV antibody testing, one participant responded, "I am very scared that the availability of the test could open up a crisis where forced testing for jobs, insurance, housing, etc. would be required." Another participant suggested during the same time period, "Lately, with talk of quarantine, I have a fear of concentration camps. It's scary and anger-provoking; I want to both run and to fight." Another reported, ". . . These fears of discrimination definitely take their toll on one's emotional well-being." There were dramatic increases during late 1985 in comments expressing fear or anger over society's responses to AIDS. This increase in hostile or fearful responses corresponded to increased media coverage in Chicago of proposals for mandatory AIDS testing, reporting, and quarantine during that same period.

We believe that the reactions reported by our participants highlight a progressively evolving set of social stressors and their negative psychological consequences. We chose to call this phenomenon "fear of holocaust" to differentiate it from previously reported sources of AIDS-related stress in gay men. It seems likely that our subjects are responding to a wide-ranging set of legislative, corporate, and social activities that are currently occurring or being publicly debated. Such actions or proposals can clearly create a negative social milieu which adds significantly to the already identified chronic stress experienced by gay men.

This social milieu might be expected to lead to increased psychological distress in our participants through at least two mechanisms. By directly adding to the burden of fear experienced by persons at high risk of AIDS, "fear of holocaust" would significantly increase the intensity and extent of AIDS-related chronic stress. In addition, this new form of stress frequently indicates rejection of the person at risk from the "general society"; therefore, an individual perceiving himself to be the subject of these proposals may feel more isolated and vulnerable, with less access to medical and psychological care. Unless effective interventions are found for both society's ill-informed anxiety and our subjects' sense of social isolation, increasingly extreme psychological responses can be expected. Whether or not actual physical quarantine or other equally repressive responses to AIDS do occur in the United States, the perception of their plausability by an increasing proportion of the general public and by at-risk populations significantly intensifies the negative psychosocial consequences of the AIDS epidemic.

Although quarantine generally did not contain the transmission of the diseases discussed earlier, it nonetheless offered an illusory sense of protection from a perceived external threat. It is, however, consistent and well-validated epidemiologic data regarding HIV transmission which should be used to formulate public health policy. In particular, as we have already emphasized, because only blood exchange and certain sexual behaviors (whether homosexual or heterosexual) serve as effective routes of HIV transmission, anyone can effectively eliminate their risk of AIDS by regulating their own behavior rather than that of others. Unfortunately, misguided and unnecessary policies continue to be discussed. Inevitably, these have a negative impact on the men attempting to adapt to this crisis. One respondent expressed this clearly and dramatically when he wrote, "I remember the Jews who were shot in World War II. They wore a yellow star. I also remember the gays who were shot in World War II. They wore a pink triangle. Last week in the [Chicago] Tribune they talked about quarantine for gays. That is the third article that I have seen in two weeks. Next, we will all have to wear pink triangles as in WW II and be shot." There can be little doubt that however inappropriate are such policies as quarantine, merely discussing them can increase the distress of gay men.

FUTURE PROSPECTS: RESPONSIBILITY AND CHOICE

Clearly, the solution to the AIDS epidemic is currently behavioral. Given that HIV can insert into human DNA, probably for a lifetime, such behavioral changes will need to be extremely long range. Therefore, it is in the interest of all that we encourage and facilitate appropriate behavioral changes. There is already good evidence that gay men are reducing the sexual behaviors which transmit HIV.[20,21] The salient question is how both those who are at risk and those who are not can work together, to produce a society in which a positive adaptation to the crisis of AIDS is possible. We discuss this issue in this final section of the chapter.

In many ways the present AIDS crisis recapitulates past experiences of epidemic disease. Currently defined risk groups are seen as diseased, dirty, and morally destitute;[22] collectively, they are perceived as a source of danger not only to health, but to the existing social order. These stereotypes, rather than available and accurate epidemiologic information, provide the basis for the extreme "epidemic control measures" being proposed. Paradoxically, such measures are not only unnecessary but may actually impede control of this epidemic. The fragile coalition between the majority (and often medical) culture and the currently defined at-risk populations is disrupted by such proposals. Furthermore, they create added burdens of distrust, anxiety, and anger that are potentially disruptive to the process of establishing safer life-styles. At their worst, they have the potential for alienating gay men from those services and the care-providers whose help may be so essential to them. For instance, an individual who believes that HIV antibody testing is personally valuable may avoid such testing if the potential legal and financial consequences seem excessive and outweigh any personal gain. In other words, if society takes punitive measures to "control" AIDS, the epidemic will be driven "underground" and once it is "underground" it will be even more difficult to control.

What role then, might those who are not members of at-risk groups play? We would argue that all of us are confronted with the necessity of making responsible choices which may alter the course of this epidemic. For at-risk gay men these choices have been well discussed, and focus on the alteration of sexual behavior. For too long, our society, the dominant culture, has seen its task as control of the "other"—the homosexual, the intravenous drug user, the immigrant. This external focus might more appropriately be turned inward, with a careful examination of our personal attitudes and behaviors. By mastering our own sense of impotence and futility we may be less inclined to support or even to give credence to the politically extreme and epidemiologically naive proposals for control of AIDS. Our own experiences in working with groups as diverse as school administrators, prison guards, health care providers, and major employers suggest that this is indeed the case. Understanding basic biomedical and epidemiologic information is within everyone's grasp and can provide the foundation for a more appropriate approach to the issues surrounding AIDS. Unions, employers, and workplace supervisors need not only to have access to such information, but also to institute appropriate policies to reinforce acceptable behavior. Hospitals have found that the combination of information, supportive counseling when required, and clear behavioral guidelines has done much to mitigate workplace anxiety and discrimination.

It may also be possible that the majority culture is able to change equally important attitudes. There has been considerable censure of gay men for their sexual behavior, which has been perceived as "promiscuous" or "fast-track." Less attention has been paid to the ways in which the dominant society may contribute to certain components of such homosexual behavior. It has been suggested in cross-cultural research that a society's homophobic attitudes are correlated with increased numbers of homosexual partners and decreases in long-term, stable coupling.[23] A society that condemns the open, social, and sensual bonds between gay couples, may encourage men to turn to closeted, clandestine, and brief sexual encounters. For example, it is ironic that those who condemn sexual activity outside of traditional marriage may be even more distressed by the prospect of sanctioning gay marriages. Although it is obvious that the determinants of both heterosexual and homosexual behavior are complex, this factor may provide an important opportunity for dealing with one aspect of the AIDS epidemic.

Change is possible. In general, staffs of hospitals, particularly intensive care units and specialized AIDS-treatment facilities, have come to accept and support gay relationships. The value of this acceptance is observed readily in these circumstances and needs to be extended outside the hospital environment. Perhaps instead of focusing upon the "other" and the imperative for change elsewhere, it is time that we each examine and, if necessary, change our own attitudes and priorities. This lesson, too, has been learned—however reluctantly and late—in other epidemics. It is precisely such lessons which may facilitate rather than impede effective control of the AIDS epidemic.

This work was supported by research funding from the National Institute of Mental Health (2 R01 MH3936-02A1) and the University of Michigan.

The authors wish to express their thanks to the men in the Coping and Change Study whose participation makes this research possible.

NOTES

1. Curran, J. W. The epidemiology and prevention of AIDS. *Annals of Internal Medicine* 103:657–662 (1985).
2. Barre-Sinoussi, F., et al. Isolation of a T-lymphotropic retrovirus from a patient at risk of acquired immunodeficiency syndrome (AIDS). *Science* 222:861–871 (1985).
3. Popovic, M.; Sardgadharan, M.; Read, E.; Gallo, R. Detection, isolation and continuous production of cytopathic retroviruses (HTLV-III) from patients with AIDS and pre-AIDS. *Science* 224:497–500 (1984).
4. Emmons, C. A.; Joseph, J. G.; Kessler, R. C.; Wortman, C. B.; Montgomery, S. B.; Ostrow, D. G. Psychosocial predictors of reported behavior change in homosexual men at risk for AIDS. *Health Education Quarterly* 13:331–345 (1986).
5. Martin, J. L. AIDS risk reduction recommendations and sexual behavior patterns among gay men: A multifactorial categorical approach to assessing change. *Health Education Quarterly* 13:347–358 (1986).

 6. Deuchan, N. AIDS in New York City with particular reference to the psycho-social aspects. *British Journal Psychiatry* 145:612–619 (1984).
 7. Nichols, S. E. Psychosocial reactions of persons with the acquired immunodeficiency syndrome. *Annals of Internal Medicine* 103:765–767 (1985).
 8. Kirscht, J.; Haefner, D.; Kegels, S.; Rosenstock, I. A national study of health beliefs. *Journal of Healthy Human Behavior* 7:248–254 (1966).
 9. Harris, D., and Guten, S. Health protective behavior: An exploratory study. *Journal Healthy Society Behavior* 20:17–29 (1979).
10. Weinstein, N. Why it won't happen to me: Perception of risk factors and susceptibility. *Health Psychology* 3:431–457 (1984).
11. Kasper, R. G. Perceptions of risk and their effects on decision-making. In *Societal Risk Assessment: How Safe Is Safe Enough?* R. C. Schwing and W. A. Albers, eds. New York: Plenum, 1980.
12. Material for the historical section was taken from a limited number of major sources. Rather than repetitively citing each, the interested reader is referred to: Brandt, A. M. *No Magic Bullet: A Social History of Venereal Disease in the United States Since 1880.* New York: Oxford Univ. Press, 1985; Cipolla, C. M. *Cristofano and the Plague: A Study in the History of Public Health in the Age of Galileo.* Berkeley: Univ. of California Press, 1973; Delaporte, F. *Disease and Civilization: The Cholera in Paris, 1832.* Cambridge, MA: MIT Press (English translation, 1986); Longmate, N. *King Cholera: The Biography of a Disease.* London: Honish Hamilton, 1966; Nohl, J. *The Black Death: A Chronicle of the Plague.* New York: Harper & Row (English translation, 1969); Rosenberg, C. E. *The Cholera Years: The United States in 1832, 1849, and 1866.* Chicago: University of Chicago Press, 1962.
13. Longmate, N. *King Cholera: The Biography of a Disease.* London: Hamish Hamilton, 1966.
14. Rosenberg, C. E. *The Cholera Years: The United States in 1832, 1849, and 1866.* Chicago: University of Chicago Press, 1962.
15. Gostin, L., and Curran, W. J. Legal control measures for AIDS: Reporting requirements, surveillance, quarantine, and regulation of public meeting places. *American Journal of Public Health* 77:214–218 (1987).
16. Darrow, W. W. Social and psychologic aspects of the sexually transmitted diseases: A different view. *Cutis* 27:307–311 (1981).
17. Kaslow, R. A.; Ostrow, D. G.; Detels, R.; Phair, J. P.; Polk, B. F.; Rinaldo, C. R. The Multicenter AIDS Cohort Study: Rationale, organization, and selected characteristics of the participants. *American Journal of Epidemiology* 126:310–316 (1987).
18. Joseph, J. G., and Ostrow, D. G. The crisis of AIDS: Implications for health care providers. In *Biobehavioral Control of AIDS.* D. G. Ostrow, ed. New York: Irvington Publishers, 1987.
19. Ostrow, D. G.; Eller, M.; Joseph, J. G. Fears of a new holocaust: Emerging AIDS-related psychosocial issues. Paper presented at the Second International Conference on AIDS, Paris, France (June 1986).
20. McKusick, L.; Horstman, W.; Coates, T. J. AIDS and sexual behavior reported by gay men in San Francisco. *American Journal of Public Health* 75:493–496 (1986).
21. Martin, J. L. Sexual behavior patterns, behavior change, and occurrence of antibody to LAV/HTLV-III among New York City gay men. Paper presented at the Second International Conference on AIDS, Paris, France (June 1986).
22. Hastings, G. B.; Leather, D. S.; Scott, A. C. AIDS publicity: Some experiences from Scotland. *British Medical Journal* 294:48–49 (1987).
23. Ross, M. W. Predictors of partner numbers in homosexual men: Psychosocial factors in four societies. *Sexually Transmitted Diseases* 11:119–122 (1984).

CHAPTER 3

The Treatment of People with AIDS: Psychosocial Considerations

ZELDA FOSTER

INTRODUCTION

The impact of AIDS in our society is a continuing personal and social tragedy that is still unfolding. Never before in the history of a disease have so many physical and social forces collided with such a catastrophic outcome. The threatening personal and social context of this disease creates multiple dynamics which determine who becomes infected, how the disease is spread, the extent of its influence on the larger population, and societal responses. Thus, psychosocial considerations are of major consequence, playing a pivotal role in the treatment of persons with AIDS, the effects on their families and social networks, as well as on the health care providers who themselves are affected participants. The psychosocial considerations are complex but readily identifiable and can help determine meaningful psychosocial treatment approaches. The challenge for health care providers and relevant health and social organizations is to generate the strength, direction, and determination required to respond to these encompassing needs and demands.

Psychosocial considerations for individuals who have a diagnosis of AIDS or ARC, for their loved ones, and for those who have the responsibility for providing social and health care are extremely profound. Much has been written describing themes which pervade the experiences of each risk group and these provide meaningful generalizations about psychosocial issues and treatment implications.[1-3] The anguish, the physical and emotional devastation, and the frequent collapse of economic and social supports of people with AIDS are prevailing themes. There are also, however, examples of remarkable efforts to cope with these agonizing changes and threats to survival. These include using the experience of having AIDS or being closely associated with people who have AIDS in a positive manner by advancing new programs and trying to change the public's attitudes.[4]

The current and anticipated impact of the AIDS crisis on individuals, families and loved ones, social networks, the general community, and the health care system is almost immeasurable due to a number of key factors characterizing this disease. People who develop AIDS at this time in medical history have a debilitating, often fatal illness. Most of these people are relatively young and are members of stigmatized populations—homosexuals and intravenous drug users. AIDS was contracted in the great majority of cases either by sexual transmission or by the sharing of infected needles. At risk therefore, are sexual partners as well as babies who may be infected perinatally. The lack of full knowledge about the etiology, incubation, transmission, possible changes in the virus itself, and treatment makes AIDS a mysterious and extremely threatening disease.

This chapter will focus on both the problem-specific and the more universal psychosocial issues and psychosocial treatment considerations for members of population groups who are facing a possible diagnosis of AIDS. The risk groups considered are homosexuals, IV drug users, families and their children diagnosed with AIDS, and people who received contaminated blood products. Although these groups may have a number of overlapping members, there are major differences which warrant each respective group's distinct concerns to be addressed separately.

Two important phenomena must be considered in any discussion of the psychosocial impact of AIDS: one is the very real concern about the ever-increasing spread of AIDS and the second is the stigmatizing and stereotyping of people with AIDS.

There are forecasts in the mass media and the professional literature of anticipated growth in the number of people who will develop AIDS to epidemic proportions.[5] There also will be simultaneous shifts in the population groups at risk for contracting and spreading this disease.[6,7] The resultant psychosocial considerations have monumental implications for individuals, families, friends, and for all of our social institutions. The projections of the sheer numbers and the populations at risk highlight a critical and dramatic need for a massive and comprehensive public health campaign which must deal with community education, prevention, and global and specific changes in our health care delivery system. The potential for ill-considered and inadequate social health policy development threatens the quality of our lives and the communities in which we live. Continuing negative public reaction to AIDS can have serious consequences by discouraging people to come forward for testing, educational, and preventive help. Repressive and retaliatory public policy toward those with AIDS or in high risk groups is a possible future negative outcome.

The second phenomenon is the negative impact of stereotyping and stigmatizing persons with AIDS. Stereotypes and deep-seated prejudices about homosexuals and IV drug users have allowed the general population to be detached and unempathic. These stereotypes are extremely destructive. The wish on the part of the "unaffected" population is for protection and separation from groups whose behavior and practices will ultimately "ravage innocent people." It is easier, for example, to view the IV drug user as a heroin addict who was infected by using dirty needles in an anonymous shooting gallery, rather than as a possible past drug user who is part of a family, a parent to young children. Similarly, the homosexual can be seen as a person involved in promiscuous, compulsive sexual activity in bathhouses rather than as a creative, useful member of society. Certain ethnic and racial groups also have strong indictments against homosexual practices. For example, there are prohibitions in some segments of black and Hispanic cultures against homosexuality.

Other strong social prejudices are prevalent in perceptions of the "AIDS threat." IV drug abuse is closely associated with black and Hispanic populations; therefore, already existing negative feelings toward these populations may be further heightened. It is crucial that individuals in each risk group not be stereotyped. The Gay Men's Health Crisis, AIDS Institute, AIDS task forces, social agencies, and self-help networks are working hard to eradicate, or to at least modify, stereotypes, deal with discrimination, and provide necessary services to all affected groups.[8]

There is neither a monolithic population at risk nor a monolithic disease. Who gets it, how it develops and progresses, and the response to biopsychosocial treatment must be looked at in each individual set of conditions.

The following discussion should not have as its outcome a universalizing of "truths" but is presented instead as a guide and focal point for a deepened grasp of the meaning of the behaviors, needs, and helping conditions relevant to the community of people personally and professionally touched by AIDS.

COMMON CONCERNS

People with AIDS experience common concerns and face a multitude of obstacles which can severely damage their coping capacities. The diagnosis of AIDS immediately threatens long-term survival and predicts a remaining quality of life jeopardized by severe debilitation, extreme susceptibility to infections, hospitalizations, disfigurement (in the case of Kaposi's sarcoma), and multiple and staggering personal losses. These losses are intensified by feelings of rejection and self-blame. The anticipated decline and fear of loss of life evident in patients with incurable cancer is not nearly as overwhelming as the stigmatization faced by AIDS patients who are associated with being part of a group whose promiscuous behavior or drug abusing practices has brought this disease upon themselves and who may in turn transmit it to the general public. There is also increasing clinical evidence of AIDS patients who are exhibiting signs of dementia as a result of direct effects of the virus on the central nervous system.[9] The staggering management and care problems of this patient group create additional burdens on social support and health care delivery systems. This situation of limited resources for an infected and stigmatized population facing debility and death and causing transmission to others is the general climate surrounding the live of persons with AIDS. Members of each risk group have distinct and specific characteristics which influence their care and treatment. These will be discussed below.

IV DRUG USERS WITH AIDS

Intravenous (IV) drug users are a major risk group with far-reaching implications for effective and productive psychosocial treatment. Personality as well as behavioral and social patterns severely obstruct how help is sought and accepted in this group.[10] Most health and social agencies have not yet embraced this population in outreach efforts and have not forged relationships in ways which are sufficiently responsive. Public health issues emerge as a particularly serious aspect of treatment. Most IV drug users are seropositive (at least 62%) and 30% are women who are largely of childbearing age.[11] Additionally, a portion of these reportedly are prostitutes. The transmission of AIDS through the use of infected needles and heterosexual sexual activity increases the probability that members of this population will develop AIDS and also infect others.

Women who are IV drug users, prostitutes, or who are associated with men who are IV drug users, are not only at risk themselves but also risk giving birth to babies infected with AIDS. The increasing number of babies born with AIDS to infected mothers is a cause for alarm. The mother may be asymptomatic (not manifest signs of AIDS or ARC) but may be a carrier and, possibly, susceptible to future illness.

IV drug users, whether male or female, are clearly carriers of the virus and are often ill and at extreme risk. A population of probable disease carriers presents agonizing dilemmas in terms of social policy (for example, mandatory testing). It also presents enormously difficult ethical and treatment issues since the IV drug user may refuse to consider using safe practices to protect partners and children yet to be born. Health care treatment teams need to emphasize this responsibility to partners; they must also know how to offer help to partners who have developed AIDS or become seropositive.

This population of drug users—who are likely to be carriers and who may be facing serious debilitation and death—are characterized by alienation, antisocial behavior, poor economic situations, inadequate social supports, severed personal bonds, and chaotic and sometimes criminal lifestyles. Consequently, there are substantive questions regarding how to effectively engage and offer this population treatment. Difficulties in trust, in forming relationships, in expressing feelings, and in recognizing anxiety would be a barrier to productive treatment under most circumstances.[12] In these situations, heightened anxiety and immobility makes patterns of avoidance and denial less achievable but desperately sought by patients as they try to cope with intolerable feelings of pain and anxiety. The likelihood of ongoing opportunistic infections and a rapid physical decline further compromises the time available and the capacity to work on problem resolution.[13] Increased demanding and manipulative behavior, and the creation of chaos and crisis are often present in these treatment situations. Many health care workers are not accustomed to such behaviors and may react in ways which increase the potential for negative interaction.

Effective psychosocial treatment strategies require addressing both the internal and external influences on patients as well as how the reactions of the health care providers influence the success or failure of treatment. The central issue in each individual situation is how a person can be sustained, nurtured, and offered medical and psychosocial treatment while facing the extreme likelihood of severe incapacity and death. Of critical importance is the strengthening of social supports including a place to live, home care, financial management and income from entitlement programs, care management services, a consistent treatment team with follow-up responsibilities, and an alternative to hospitalization programs (hospices, residential drug programs, half-way houses, supportive housing, hospital-based home care). It is advised to involve the IV drug user in a drug treatment program whether the person is drug-free, on methadone maintenance, or a current user. The person who is drug-free may be at great risk to return to drugs and may be considered for methadone at this crisis point or for a referral to a drug-free program.[14] Whichever specific program is chosen is perhaps less important than connecting the person with AIDS to programs that offer clear, consistent, and firm structures while providing supportive help. However, some drug treatment programs will need special consultation to learn more about dealing with the physical decline and the emotional issues for both staff and patient which are stirred up by this overwhelming disease.[15]

Infectious disease staffs and primary health care staffs also need consultation from the drug treatment programs to better grasp how to engage and manage patients with these personality/behavioral characteristics. This points to the value of a strong investment in "sharing" patients, in interdisciplinary teams in collaboration rather than functioning as fragmented or competitive providers. There is a convergence of unique and usually separated factors and of health care providers who are usually not closely related to one another in practice. New teams may be designed which encompass skill in responding to death and dying concerns, drug use/behavior, infectious disease, and primary care. Coordination and communication is an essential dimension in offering care. These new resources and partnerships will take work, investment, and a lack of territoriality to establish and nurture. While a most intensive and concerted thrust is needed for educational and preventive services, there will be a growing population of seriously ill and dying people.

There is much to learn from hospice and death and dying conceptual frameworks. How people face their remaining days and death, how families might be reconciled, and what settings offer the best opportunities for care are known. Relevant for treatment of the former or current drug user is the professional obligation to conceptually spell out effective treatment interventions for this population. Approaching the emotional life of drug users is not easy. How does one and should one deepen relationships, open up anxious and conflicting feelings, seach for opportunities for reconciliation with family, and explore for meaning and purpose in the face of death? The past or present drug user with AIDS who is viewed as having a fatal disease will present a dilemma for staff. The wish to be nurturing and all-giving might be best tempered and balanced by limits and holding to guidelines. The patient's struggle with trust and involvement may test the limits of the program. There are many questions. The patient may need anxiety reduction drugs but will this induce a flight back into drug dependency? When is methadone a treatment of choice? How do you involve the patient in considering safe sexual practices, birth control, and possibly abortion? How might these patients become more active in political advocacy for increased services and also in establishing more self-help networks? Do Vietnam Era veterans with AIDS have additional needs and other networks to draw on? How does one deal with low frustration tolerance, need for immediate gratification, and manipulative behavior while attempting to maintain the patient in treatment? What help do family members and patients need as they feel regret and bitterness for a troubled past, a difficult present, and a sorrowful future? Discussions with health care providers report a wide spectrum of experiences. These must be evaluated, considered theoretically, and incorporated into treatment concepts and approaches which can be disseminated among the interdisciplinary professionals working in this area.

HOMOSEXUALS WITH AIDS

This disease has had devastating impact on a community of people tied together by lifestyle and social networks. Drawn by the anonymity, opportunities, and acceptance permitted in a number of major U.S. cities, many gay people have gathered together and established their own separate communities within them. This has led to the simultaneous consequence of significant numbers of members of these communities either having died of AIDS, being ill with AIDS or ARC, being seropositive for the AIDS virus, or being at future risk. Bereavement overload and heightened anxiety are evident. There has been a monumental effort made for collective action to stem the transmission of the disease by practicing "safe sex" and to develop services for people with AIDS regardless of risk group. Services developed by the Gay Men's Health Crisis in New York City, and many other networks and task forces cover a wide range of needs, including companion help, support groups, and legal action to deal with discriminatory acts.[16]

Irrational fear and reaction to homosexuality existed prior to the occurrence of AIDS and was then intensified when AIDS, initially thought to affect only homosexuals, appeared. The existence of AIDS accentuated and deepened the rage toward and fear of homosexuals. Societal blame, attacks, and terror create an environment which holds danger for homosexuals with AIDS in the form of abandonment, social ostracism, isolation, and damaging discriminatory behavior. Homosexuals themselves are experiencing self-blame, fear, loss of social networks, and changed lifestyle patterns.[17] They are confronted daily by the death of loved ones and other members of their community. Self-hatred, guilt, and loss of self-esteem are concomitant reactions to these societal judgments. Self-help organizations and groups act as counterforces to the internalization of perjorative and condemnatory reactions. Further complexity is created for some by the secret of their homosexuality hidden from families and/or irreconcilable differences in life patterns causing estrangement and conflict between family members and partners. Families, even when reconciled to the knowledge, may live far away. Other families are confronted with their son's (brother's) homosexuality and dying at the same time.

Many situations have been reported where the parents have been summoned to a major city to learn that their son is dying and they must then simultaneously cope with the diagnosis of AIDS, the secret homosexual lifestyle, and a kinship circle of loved ones (partner, friends) who are alien to the parents. For the patient, the parent, and the partner, there are disturbing and powerful feelings which need resolution. Sometimes it's possible for parents to provide care, for parents to join with partners, or for current partners to assume major responsibility. Current partners may have varied abilities to assume responsibility. For other patients there is no one available and they are alone and isolated except for the limited help of support networks and health care systems.[17,18] For these, housing, financial management, and supportive housing services are required.

Other situations have been reported where bisexual men involved in current marriages or other heterosexual relationships have developed AIDS. This is an especially traumatic event when the partner did not know of the past or present homosexual practice and now is at risk herself. If she remains emotionally and physically involved in the continuing relationship, there are many decisions which need to be made and there is much with which to cope. Some women have contracted AIDS as a result of sexual relationships with bisexual men. For them, there is the reality of the disease as well as the feelings of betrayal, rage, and shame.

Treatment considerations must be encompassing, reaching inner feelings while offering practical and comprehensive help with the management of the illness and current existence.[19] All related networks must be included and encouraged to work cooperatively on behalf of the patients who are torn further apart by conflict and guilt. This requires a high level of skill and sophistication on the part of the health care providers responsible for psychosocial treatment. For many patients, there is a struggle to cope with multiple losses, fear of dying, exposure of homosexuality, self-recrimination, family conflicts, and changing relationships with loved ones.[20] These are issues which can be meaningfully helped with counseling. Psychosocial treatment must begin at the point of the diagnosis and continue throughout the course of the diseases and in bereavement help to the survivors.

How people face terminal illness and what are effective helping interventions are well documented.[21] The nature of AIDS and its social context influence the number, intensity, and complexity of the issues. The feelings of self-blame, rage, lowered self-esteem, loss of status, sense of expendability, alienation, discriminatory acts, knowledge of one's infectiousness, and the existence of two separate kin networks (family and partners/friends) change the scope and dimensions of the dynamics involved. Unresolved conflicts around homosexuality, one's role in causing the disease because of lifestyle, and the impact of exposure of homosexuality to employers/family and others are areas with which counseling can be effective, helping provide a greater sense of peace and acceptance. Treatment considerations must encompass and integrate these additional dynamics while relating to the struggle to cope with decline and dying. Intensive therapy is indicated to encourage sharing of feelings, decision-making, working through of denial, and processing of critical life events. Each physical and emotional phase during the course of the illness will require specific address. Patients evidencing signs of dementia will benefit from early assessment, clear guidance, and therapy. Liaison psychiatry must have an ongoing role in treating these neuropsychiatric manifestations. Psychiatric consultation will also be valuable in offering diagnostic help and treatment regimens including prescribing psychotrophic medication. Hypnosis, positive imaging, relaxation techniques, diet, rest, holistic medicine, and spiritual help are all possibilities worthy of being offered at relevant times to appropriate patients. Needed services and connections to peer support groups can be sought with the patient's participation in both establishing treatment directions and in problem-solving efforts. It is vital for patients to find new ways to socialize, deal with sexuality, and maintain relationships.

This disease strikes relatively young people who have in the main been financially independent, vocationally productive, and contributors to their environments. Losses in every sphere, unrelenting psychosocial stressors, and confrontations with one's severe debility and mortality create struggles for treatment staff as well, as they attempt to cope with their own feelings of distress, grief, and vulnerability.

THE IMPACT OF AIDS ON FAMILIES AND THEIR CHILDREN

The ratio of people with AIDS who are or were IV drug users is increasing as compared with the homosexual population. A significant portion are women IV drug users with some accounts claiming a 30% ratio of women among IV drug users.[22] Other women with AIDS, ARC, or seropositivity have been infected by heterosexual contact, most often by men who are IV drug users. The risk to themselves, to the babies born to them, and to their current and future male partners presents at this juncture a major public health concern.

The psychosocial implications are anguishing. Most mothers and their families are poor and black or Hispanic. They often live in inadequate housing, have had poor access to health care, and rely on marginal and stressed social supports. Entitlement programs are fragmented and are unable to provide a comprehensive scope of services. Each mother who has a baby with AIDS is herself at risk. Either she has AIDS, ARC, or at the very least, is seropositive. The mother will need to consider issues relating to her own sexuality, fertility, and infectiousness. Cultural factors are relevant to feelings and decision making in these areas. These mothers may be experiencing their own illness either full-blown or in beginning signs. There certainly is an ever-present fear of developing the illness which results in living day to day with uncertainty and fear.

There are hundreds of cases of infants left in hospitals when the mothers because of illness, death, or lifestyle patterns (addicts, prostitutes) cannot care for their children. These children are virtually abandoned and receive care from either hospital staffs or the foster care system. Children who do go home live with mothers and in families beset with overwhelming problems in everyday management. In some families a number of the family members are ill, there is poverty, and multiple sociocultural barriers exist to going outside to obtain needed resources, for example, hospital, clinics, schools. There is a reliance on social service and home care agencies which do not resolve the terrible living conditions or traumatic family relationships. There are examples of extended families, neighbors, and helpful social agencies but the totality of the problems encountered in the care of a sick, often dying, child living in poor, inadequate conditions and frequently with other ill family members speaks to the scope of counseling and practical help which must be made more totally and readily available.

The illness of the child is directly related to the mother's transmission of the disease. This dynamic is added to the horror of coping with the illness and anticipated death of one's child. The care and management of the child is complex as problems in physical and psychological growth emerge, as dependency on educational, health, and social agencies increases, and as the family unit tries to function against what seem to be unsurmountable attacks on it.

There are examples of health care agencies behaving responsively, of entitlement programs devising specific and earmarked services, and of the young mother's parents, partner, and neighbors rallying. Yet, for many this help is insufficient or not available. The social and emotional cost to these mothers is infinite. If there is an involved father or a current partner, this relationship has a most significant role in treatment and planning.

Psychosocial treatment has focused on the provision of services including public assistance, home care, and support groups. To be fully effective, each situation must be assessed so that help is directed to the entire network of concerned members including grandparents, siblings, and extended family. The impact of current drug use, the capacity to provide care, and how the mother and child are coping can be assessed while practical services are being made available. Feelings of unbearable grief, self-blame, helplessness, and rage may be expressed. At the same time, the mother may be able to provide some care and to give love to her child, and in this giving of love, some hope and restoration may be possible. Bereavement help is vital to the mother and other family members to encourage a more successful working through of grief in its acute and long-term forms. The pain and grief attached to the loss of a child always remains and although never fully resolved, can be made less damaging to functioning and present relationships.[23]

In situations where the mother cannot cope, where the mother is ill or has died, or where the child is abandoned, another set of problems emerges. Boarder babies in hospitals, difficulties in finding foster homes, and children not thriving and in obvious great peril, are the victims and social consequences of this disease. The development of safe and caring environments where children can thrive as best as is possible is one of the greatest challenges facing the social welfare system and the humanity of our social organizations.

AIDS AND CONTAMINATED BLOOD PRODUCTS

People who become seropositive or develop ARC or AIDS due to receipt of contaminated blood products consider themselves unaware and innocent victims of an evil and cruel fate. They also, in the role of carrier pose a great threat to partners, spouses, and infants born to infected mothers. They may be developing or have developed a disease to which great stigma is attached and which threatens current existence and survival. Their loved ones also may be in jeopardy. Dealing with a blow of this nature and facing the course of an illness so devastating and incomprehensible without rage and despair is not possible. The skill of solid and well-developed psychosocial treatment services is key with this population as well as with the previously described ones.

Although the reported number of hemophilia-related AIDS cases is not presently increasing, the high degree of seroprevalence is cause for concern.[24] It is no doubt a population at risk for developing AIDS, as possible carriers may be jeopardizing those with whom they are in sexual contact. Educational assistance and therapeutically directed counseling is essential to reach those affected to help deepen coping and problem-solving abilities and to enlist available resources to enable the most positive emotional adaptive outcome possible.

FURTHER TREATMENT IMPLICATIONS

The pressure to offer effective psychosocial treatment to increasing numbers of people in need is mounting. Extreme stress is being placed on health providers as they become part of the lives of this young, stigmatized, and often dying population. The likelihood of health care providers feeling overwhelmed, guilty, and helpless, suggests the value of instituting planned and ongoing staff support services. Hospice experiences has shown that recognizing the needs of staff has important application to staff effectiveness. The work and treatment environments for most professional caregivers is either in acute hospitals or home care agencies. Both environments have unique sets of stressors and large numbers of health care staffs who are not prepared for the extent of death and dying issues confronting patients and themselves.

The form of supportive help for staff can take many shapes. Opportunities to increase self-awareness and knowledge, share reactions and disturbing feelings, seek mutual help from peers, obtain ongoing supervision and consultation, and have respite periods away from the work are possible ways for recognizing needs and helping staff to better cope. The role of hospice also must be evaluated as a resource which can be expanded but which will require an investment in careful training, resource development, and a program balance between cancer patients who are the usual candidates for hospice,[25] and persons with AIDS (who also have an especially limited life span). Hospice philosophy values the role of the caregiver and promotes caregiver support through groups, volunteers, and respite services. Caregivers of patients with AIDS face difficult symptoms and concerns regarding infectiousness and encounter stress on every level.

The focus on practical and psychotherapeutic help needs to be balanced so that community resources are developed which meet the wide range of services needed to maintain an ill population while recognizing that enhancing coping abilities go beyond the provision of concrete services. Help to multiple networks of involved relatives, lovers, and friends, recognizing the value of and providing support group and bereavement services are important aspects of a treatment program.

There is an imperative to provide preventive and educational services, especially as one considers the vast numbers of people who are seropositive and therefore contagious. At the same time, persons with AIDS will continue to require extensive, intensive helping services. Advocacy work in changing health care delivery systems and in responding to discriminatory acts becomes an important part of the professional role.

Coordination is necessary to promote the development of inpatient and outpatient comprehensive interdisciplinary teams and also for the integration between hospital and community services. Hospitals which are designated AIDS centers may be able to accomplish this more easily but sound planning, program development, and communication to assure more effective service delivery remain as challenges.

Well-organized interdisciplinary teams can lend strength to its members and to those treated. Multidisciplinary physician specialists, nurses, and social workers have core roles in providing treatment, ongoing care management, and psychosocial coordination.[26] Chaplains, dieticians, psychologists, and other health professionals must join in offering their expertise. Drug programs, task forces, self-help groups, social agencies, and AIDS service/research/educational institutes all have key roles to play.

Health care providers will have a major voice in how AIDS as the major biopsychosocial problem of these times is treated. They will bear witness to suffering beyond comprehension and will participate in shaping how care is offered. To be effective, health care providers need to speak with a voice which is unified, well organized, and powerful in its leadership. AIDS is one disease which requires response on individual, institutional, and societal levels. All in health care will be called upon to find a commitment to service never before asked. AIDS will test the systems in which we live and work and ultimately, each individual's values and capacities.

REFERENCES

1. Furstenbert, A., and Olson, M. Social work and AIDS. In *Social Work in Health Care*. New York: The Haworth Press, Inc., 1984:45–61.
2. Christ, G., and Wiener, L. Psychosocial Issues in AIDS. In *AIDS: Etiology, Diagnosis, Treatment, Prevention*. Philadelphia: Lippincott Co., 1985:275–297.
3. Lehman, V., and Russell, N. Psychological and Social Issues of AIDS and Strategies for Survival. In *Understanding AIDS: A Comprehensive Guide*. New Brunswick, NJ: Rutgers University Press.
4. Health Letter/5. Gay Mens Health Crisis Inc., May 1985.
5. World Drive on an AIDS Pandemic. *The New York Times*, November 23, 1986.
6. The AIDS Epidemic. Future Shock. *Newsweek*, November 24, 1986.
7. Heterosexuality and AIDS: The Concern Keeps Growing. *The New York Times*, October 28, 1986.
8. Persons with AIDS Coalition. *Newsline*, December 1986.
9. Perry, S., and Jacobsen, P. Neuropsychiatric Manifestations of AIDS-Spectrum Disorders. *Hospital and Community Psychiatry*, (February 1986):135–141.
10. Angel, S. From Action to Reflection, New Depth in Psychotherapy with Drug Addicts. *Clinical Social Work Journal* :151.

11. Drucker, E. AIDS and Addiction in New York City. *American Journal of Drug and Alcohol Abuse* 12(1 and 2) (1986):165–181.
12. Cohen, M., and Weisman, H. A Biopsychosocial Approach to AIDS. *Psychosomatics* 27(4) (April 1986).
13. Maayan, S., et al. Acquired Immunodeficiency Syndrome (AIDS) in an Economically Disadvantaged Population. *Archives Internal Medicine* 145 (September 1985):1607–1612.
14. Personal communications with Melodye Schoonmaker, Chief of Counseling, U.S. Navy Family Service Center, Roosevelt Rd., Puerto Rico (Formerly AIDS Coordinator, VAMC, Bronx, NY); and Rose Jacobs, Supervisory Social Worker, VAMC, Bronx, N.Y.
15. Editorial. AIDS and the Substance Abuse Treatment Clinician. *Journal of Substance Abuse* 2 (1985).
16. Violence vs. Homosexuals, Rising Groups Seeking Wider Protection. *The New York Times,* November 23, 1986.
17. Nochols, S., et al. *Acquired Immune Deficiency Syndrome.* Washington, DC: American Psychiatric Press, Inc., 1984.
18. Merin, S.; Charles, K.; Malyan, A. The Psychological Impact of AIDS on Gay Men. *American Psychologist* 39 (November 1984):1288–1293.
19. World Drive on an AIDS Pandemic. *The New York Times.*
20. Health Letter/5.
21. Furstenbert, A., et al. Social Work and AIDS.
22. Drucker, E. AIDS and Addiction in New York City.
23. Arnold, J., and Buschman, P. *A Child Dies: A Portrait of Family Grief.* Rockville, MD: Aspen Systems Corp., 1983.
24. Surveillance Maintained on Hemophilia–Associated AIDS. *Oncology Times,* January 15, 1987.
25. National Hospice Organization Policy Statement—AIDS.
26. Psychosocial Treatment of Patients with Acquired Immune Deficiency Syndrome (AIDS). VA Clinical Affairs Letter IL 11-86-15. September 1986.

CHAPTER 4

Development of AIDS Awareness: A Personal History

ANGELA LEWIS

"I heard about the strangest disease today. It's a rare skin cancer that usually happens in old men, but I understand they are beginning to find it in young gay men. A doctor from New York talked about it and the information was so new that he used hand-drawn slides!" I remember the conversation so well. I also remember the day. It was a beautiful Saturday afternoon in June 1981, and as a friend and I chatted, driving over the Golden Gate Bridge, we never thought that within five years this disease would attract the attention and concern of the entire world.

Later that summer, I attended two medical rounds on "Kaposi's Sarcoma in Gay Men" that were presented where I work, the Medical Center at the University of California, San Francisco. I was one of a very few women, and perhaps the only nurse, in the audience. As I sat and tried to listen to the clinical discussion, my thoughts were occupied with a deep concern for the men experiencing this condition. In particular, I thought about how difficult it would be to be gay and terminally ill. I am a lesbian, and I know what it is like to be closeted. I remembered the emotional turmoil I experienced during two hospitalizations, especially the one in the small hospital where I worked in Florida during the mid-sixties. At that time I was literally terrified that someone would guess I was "queer." I didn't want my lover to be around when I went to the operating room because I felt it would look unusual; I was so preoccupied with that concern that I didn't stop and realize that many people have a friend visit before they leave for the operating room. I was careful about how we addressed each other, even when talking on the phone, and holding hands was reserved for times when the door was closed and bed curtain drawn. I was deep in my secret closet and felt I could only trust or confide in others whom I knew were in the same situation.

A man with KS (as Kaposi's sarcoma was being termed) didn't have the choice of staying in the closet—not with those purple marks—he was out; he was a homosexual. What would it be like to be young (most patients were in

47

their twenties or thirties), reaching that time in life which should be the most productive, and then to be diagnosed and openly identified? In a society obsessed with physical attractiveness, how would it feel to begin developing ugly purple spots? Already the prognosis was grim and the media were beginning to discuss a "gay plague". If you haven't come out to your family, or your friends, or on the job, what must it be like to do so under these circumstances?

After the second lecture on KS, I introduced myself to the speaker, explaining that I was both a Nurse Educator in Nursing Education and Research and a lesbian who would be willing to visit patients and/or provide a perspective of and connection to the gay/lesbian community. In retrospect, that quite political act was very atypical of me. I certainly never considered myself an activist nor was I "connected" to the San Francisco gay community. But I had been a lesbian and a nurse for over 15 years and I knew firsthand the isolation that the health care system could impose on people who didn't "fit."

I was invited to join the physicians who had recently formed the "KS Study Group." There I met and talked with many individuals whose personal and professional lives would be changed by the epidemic. Immediately after the initial meeting, one of the physicians asked me to visit the first U.C.S.F. patient who had been hospitalized with KS. When I went to the oncology unit, I wasn't sure how I would be received; it wasn't one of my assigned units, and Nurse Educators in our setting usually don't have direct patient contact. I initially met with the Administrative Nurse and had the first of many "coming out" talks I would have with professional colleagues over the ensuing years. I had been gradually coming out in social situations since Harvey Milk's death in 1978, but professionally, only in very limited situations. Although I worked at one of the few institutions in the United States where my job was protected regardless of sexual orientation, I was concerned about what people would think. However, I believed then, and still do today, that it is very important for persons with AIDS to know some of their caregivers provide a positive affirmation of their shared lifestyle. I have also come to believe that to fight stereotypes of gay and lesbian people, it is critical that as many of us as possible come out and make our presence known. My personal fear in this process was I might lose the respect and/or peer support of my colleagues, but in reality, it was their support and love which made the process so enriching. Positive self-affirmation was healing. For someone who had spent much of her life hiding from others, being open allowed me to finally be in control of my own life; by sharing my personal perspectives, I made a unique contribution to both patients and staff.

The first time I saw Juan, he was lying quietly in bed. From my discussion with the Administrative Nurse, I knew he was an illegal alien who spoke broken English even though he had been in the United States many years. He was a very private, intensely religious man who had no visitors other than the hospital priest and his brother who came every afternoon. I put on the requisite isolation gown, went in his room and pulled a chair close to his bed. All visible parts of his body—face, hands, and arms—were covered with large, ugly purple lesions. "Juan, my name is Angie Lewis. I am a nurse here and I'm also part of a campus association of gay and lesbian people. I want you to know that we are concerned about you and would like to provide any support we can." That statement was the first and last time the words "gay," or "lesbian," or anything similar, were ever mentioned between us. With his agreement, I began a pattern of brief daily visits, most often just 10 or 15 minutes long. I would sit quietly by the bed holding his hand or massaging his feet. Touching is very important for patients who feel so untouchable. I made a conscious decision to not wear gloves, although I always washed my hands very carefully after each meeting. Occasionally he would ask for something— a deck of cards or a magazine—but mostly we just sat quietly. The unit staff was very accepting and supportive of my visits to Juan. As the weeks passed, they began to ask questions about the study group and include me in discussions on Juan's care plan.

By this time I was also visiting a second patient, who presented a distinct contrast to Juan. Patrick was an openly gay white man diagnosed with Pneumocystis carinii pneumonia (PCP). A very articulate individual, he was actively involved in the San Francisco music community and had so many visitors that limits were set so he could rest. Additionally, he had very supportive and loving parents who came from the Midwest to stay with him. When I first met Patrick, he had just been discharged from the Intensive Care Unit where he had required intubation for several days. When I introduced myself to him, his face lit up; he smiled and clasped my hand, saying that although he had several caregivers whom he felt were gay or lesbian, I was the first to acknowledge it. He was obviously pleased and touched by my visit, but because he had strong support systems we both agreed frequent visits were not needed. Also, since we did not yet know how the diseases were spread, I was concerned with possible transmission of infection between Patrick and Juan.

After a brief trip home at Thanksgiving, Juan returned to the hospital for his final stay. With his life and his death, he left a legacy of quiet dignity that remains with those who knew him. He also helped remind many of us that our role as caregiver is to meet the emotional needs of patients as they perceive them, not as we think they should be. Juan had chosen not to talk with his family about his lifestyle. Some staff members felt this reflected "unfinished business," and they wanted to encourage Juan to deal with this issue. Several intense multidisciplinary conferences centered on this topic as staff confronted their fears and feelings related to homosexuality and death. For some staff members who themselves were gay men or lesbians, the dialogue reflected basic questions with which they were struggling. Crucial to the resolution of the situation was the support which was apparent among all of the staff, and their acceptance of a diversity of lifestyles. Their recognition of each person's right to make his or her own choices led to their final decision to not persuade Juan to reveal his lifestyle choices to his family and/or priest. This allowed Juan to die peacefully, content with his decision. Patrick's choices, on the other hand, served a different purpose. For the last few months of his life, he struggled against his disability to complete his musical works and raise AIDS awareness in the musical community. His legacy was the impact he made on others through his music and his willingness to be a "public" person with AIDS.

I was involved in a variety of AIDS activities over the following months. The social work department called asking if the gay/lesbian community had resources for assisting those in need. I made over 50 phone calls in a vain attempt to locate a single lesbian/gay-identified organization that worked with sick persons. In the winter of 1981–'82 few, if any, of the people with whom I spoke had even heard about this new problem! We soon realized that for the time being the traditional agencies, for example, visiting nurses, home health, and so on, would have to suffice. Shortly thereafter, a small group of individuals in the gay/lesbian community, most of whom were involved in health care, held the first meeting of what would evolve into the San Francisco AIDS Foundation. I remember sitting in a school cafeteria leading a small group discussion on provision of patient care services. From that tiny beginning has evolved an organization with over 47 employees and a budget of $2.7 million.

Another major organization, Shanti, which provides counseling and support services, evolved from an agency that had been in quiet existence for many years. In the past, their counseling services were provided to patients and families dealing with cancer, but as needs related to AIDS escalated, they found themselves caring for more and more AIDS patients. Ultimately, they decided to focus all their resources on AIDS patients. As these organizations were evolving, the San Francisco Department of Public Health recognized the need for a coordinated effort to confront the problem, and I became a member of their KS Advisory Committee. In reality, many members of this committee were a core group of people who were providing direct care, developing the community agencies, and generally devoting much of their time to the issue of AIDS. The committee facilitated the development of networks among public and private agencies. All of us involved during the early months tried to avoid duplication of services. We attempted to identify the services which were then or would eventually be needed and then determine which organization(s) could logically provide them. We also made very deliberate efforts to include people with AIDS as active participants in all AIDS-related organizations.

As a Nurse Educator, I presented several in-service programs at U.C.S.F. and elsewhere. At the same time, I was also aware of the need to present a broader program for nurses and other health care providers in the community. With the cooperation and hard work of a small, dedicated group of nurses, social workers, respiratory therapists, and nutritionists from U.C.S.F., a multidisciplinary conference entitled, "Kaposi's Sarcoma and Pneumocystis pneumonia: New Phenomena Among Gay Men," was presented in June 1982. We believe this conference, attended by almost 100 participants, was the first all-day program in the nation designed for providers other than physicians. Since then, many other agencies have joined in supporting a series of similar programs addressing the needs of health care providers and community agencies. These programs have now been attended by over 3000 participants.

During the late summer of 1982 I attended, for the first time, the Lesbian and Gay Health Workers National Conference, which was held in Houston. Several sessions were devoted to AIDS, and providers from across the country shared their personal experiences of giving care to persons with AIDS. We spoke of our frustrations in securing not only funding, but basic recognition of the seriousness of the problem. At this point, the term in use was GRID, or Gay-Related Immune Disorder, and at this conference I heard the term AIDS for the first time. One of my most vivid memories from this meeting was helping a friend edit her presentation, and discussing with her our fears and feelings about transmissibility. At that time, no one knew for sure how it was spread; irrational as it seems now, we both hid silent, dark feelings that maybe as lesbians, we were vulnerable. Maybe just because we were one of "THEM," we were destined to get it. I shared with her my experience of awaking with a fever one night, and lying in bed convinced that I was experiencing the first symptoms. Only later was it recognized that while it is possible for AIDS to be transmitted during sexual contact between women, the possibility is far less than for individuals who engage in other types of sexual activity. To date, only two possible cases of sexual transmission between women have been reported in the literature.[1,2]

The early months of AIDS work formed the pattern which I and many others were to follow for several years; AIDS became a driving force in our lives, frequently overshadowing other aspects of our personal and professional responsibilities. Looking back, I can now see that while the work we did was necessary and important, it also dominated my life, sometimes in a negative way. Further, it became the focus of concern for my community; money, time, and energy which previously might have been allocated for other gay or lesbian health issues were often directed only to AIDS. Study into less dramatic, but still important health problems such as the Epstein-Barr virus or alcoholism, slowed to a virtual standstill. As the number of those ill or dead increased, funds allocated for lesbian/gay health care from both the public and private sectors excluded other important health areas, especially those related to women. Although each of us realized the crucial significance of the fight against AIDS, there were and still are feelings of frustration. Some lesbians and gay men have expressed anger at the drain on limited resources in order to fight the epidemic. When I consider the future expenditure of America's health care dollars necessary to care for persons with AIDS/ARC, I envision similar anger and frustration in the general society.

Another correlate can be found in the current controversy on sex education in schools and advertising for condoms. In the early years of the epidemic, heated debate in the gay/lesbian community centered on public education and how it should be accomplished. Questions of how much should be revealed publicly about gay sexual activity, how explicit the language should be, and exactly what messages should be given were gradually resolved, although minor areas of disagreement do remain. Some of the experiences of my community during the past five years have served as a portent of what might be ahead for the broader society. What started as a problem perceived to belong only to the gay community has become the nation's number one health concern; every sexually active person is at risk, and all of us who work in health care will feel the effects.

In my AIDS work, I was meeting new friends and colleagues whose support and friendship I continue to treasure, but I also saw and experienced the destruction of other relationships and/or friendships because of my "AIDS obsession." This obsession was heightened as the disease spread; it began to affect each of us more personally as we saw both old and new friends get sick and die. The man with whom I had my longest friendship died from PCP; another friend of over 10 years acquired KS and after 4 years of struggling each day to survive, he passed away last month, just 17 days after his lover died; a nurse I hired and supported in his career died during his first hospitalization. Bobbi Campbell, the "AIDS Poster Boy," as he called himself, a new and cherished friend, became an important part of my life; to this day I remember the lapel button he always wore, "I Will Survive." At times it seems it will never end. And regardless of when it does end, I and most people I know will never be the same. Our lives have been profoundly changed not only by the friends and professional colleagues we have met, but most particularly by having experienced the courage and dignity shown by so many of the people with AIDS.

Nursing has played a crucial role in the evolution of a care system for patients with AIDS. Given the fact that no definitive treatment is known, the care required is *nursing care*. It is nurses who offer supportive interventions that improve the quality of life for persons with AIDS and their families, friends, and loved ones. It has often been nurses who have played an instrumental leadership role in the development of educational programs, home care programs, and other creative approaches to provision of care and service. At the bedside, it is the nurse who has been and will be there through the long hours. It is important that we recognize that each of us can make a difference—we can help others look at how "family" is defined in relation to visiting rules; we can be supportive of a diversity of lifestyles; we can be vigilant in relation to confidentiality; and most importantly, we can decrease fear and hysteria by imparting knowledge to others and can help stem the spread of the disease by supporting AIDS education on our jobs, in our community, and in our schools.

REFERENCES

1. Sabatini, M. T.; Patel, K.; Hirschman, R. "Kaposi's Sarcoma and T-Cell Lymphoma In An Immunodeficient Woman: A Case Report." *AIDS Research* 1:135–7 (1984).
2. Marmor, M.; Weiss, L.; Lyden, M.; et al. "Possible Female-to-Female Transmission of Human Immunodeficiency Virus" (Letter). *Annals of Internal Medicine* 105(6):969 (December 1986).

CHAPTER 5

Literature and AIDS: The Varieties of Love

LAUREL BRODSLEY

INTRODUCTION

AIDS is a frequently lethal disease, usually sexually transmitted. By its very nature, it raises a fundamental question. When the most intimate act of sexual expression becomes deadly, how can people, using our common phrase, "Make love"?

Recently, a series of stage, television, and film dramatizations have helped us understand how our definitions of love are challenged by AIDS. In *An Early Frost,* parents reestablish loving support of their son suffering from AIDS. In *As Is,* an infected man confronts the loss of his promiscuous sexuality and learns to accept a monogamous and nurturing relationship. *The Normal Heart* portrays a leader in the battle against AIDS who loves truth but lacks political tact. In *Parting Glances,* the AIDS patient weighs his love for life against the inevitable anguish of a miserable death. In the Los Angeles-based theater-piece, *Aids/Us,* AIDS patients, their partners, parents, children, and counselors, voice their individual responses to the nature of love under the challenge of this condition. Through these and other works, authors are sharing with all of us the special nuances of love among people suffering from AIDS.

We also have another source to help us understand our feelings, behavior, and alternatives when faced with this terrible disease. Our legacy of great literature offers examples of delicate and insightful explorations of every parameter of human relationships. While the original topics could not be AIDS, throughout history people have battled terminal illness, confronted handicaps, withstood terrible plagues, and come together to weep and to celebrate.

Literature can offer immense comfort. Dr. Gerald Friedland, the leader of the AIDS treatment team at the Montefiore Medical Center in New York, mounted on his office wall a quotation from Camus' great novel, *The Plague.*

So that he should not be one of those who hold their peace but should bear witness in favor of those plague-stricken people; so that some memorial of the injustice and outrage done them might endure; and to state quite simply what we learn in a time of pestilence: that there are more things to admire in men than to despise. He knew that the tale he had to tell could not be one of a final victory. It could be only the record of what had had to be done, and what assuredly would have to be done again . . . by all who, while unable to be saints but refusing to bow down to pestilences, strive their utmost to be healers.

Dr. Friedland placed it near his desk, he told reporters from *Newsweek*, as a credo, "a rationale for carrying on a struggle whose only outcome for doctors was burying the dead" (Goldman and Beachy 1986). The journalists' description of Dr. Friedland's work, his patients, and his staff, is permeated with echoes from Camus, whose great work can give shape and meaning to our responses to AIDS.

I will discuss how three works of art portray love under tragic circumstances analogous to those of AIDS. In Shakespeare's sonnet #71, "That Time of Year . . . ," a dying man enjoins his lover to see his illness and death clearly, and through this process of honest perception, enhance their love. John Milton's religious poem, "When I Consider How My Light Is Spent," addresses the crisis of a sudden and devastating loss of physical function and its effects on his secular commitments and his love for God. Camus' *The Plague* demonstrates, among so many other insights, how men can express love for each other, their community, and God, through their dedication to conquering disease. Great literature can help us understand the meaning of relationships when our sexuality and our very survival are threatened by AIDS.

WILLIAM SHAKESPEARE'S SONNET #71, "THAT TIME OF YEAR"

Shakespeare's sonnet, "That Time of Year," is a love poem spoken by a dying man physically ravaged by disease. Terminally ill, yet possibly quite young, he addresses his beloved, a woman or a man, who has known his past glory and stands by him at his final demise. Aware of his condition, the speaker expects no pity; instead, he simply requests that his beloved accept and understand his condition, and through this act of perception, their love will be increased.

SONNET #71 (ca. 1595)

That time of year thou mayst in me behold
When yellow leaves, or none, or few, do hang
Upon those boughs which shake against the cold,
Bare ruined choirs where late the sweet birds sang.
In me thou see'st the twilight of such day
As after sunset fadeth in the west,
Which by-and-by black night doth take away,

Death's second self that seals up all in rest.
In me thou see'st the glowing of such fire
That on the ashes of his youth doth lie,
As the deathbed whereon it must expire,
Consumed with that which it was nourished by.
  This thou perceiv'st, which makes thy love more strong,
  To love that well which thou must leave ere long.

This poem, in itself, is especially poignant for AIDS victims and loved ones. The speaker, like so many victims, is a man of talent and accomplishment, for his body, now a "bare ruined choir" was one "where late the sweet birds sang." His time on earth has been reduced from the promise of a full life to one of a season, or a night, or the last moments of a brief and dying fire. Yet, in the midst of his disease and its inevitable conclusion, his beloved has remained at his side, a witness to both his earlier glory and his present decay. The poem's mood radiates a sense of tenderness, beauty, and compassion, as the two partners mutually accept their terrible plight and comfort each other through the power of their love.

The reader is immediately moved by the poet's evocation of visual beauty, even while describing illness and decay. The opening four lines, with their description of autumnal trees, has an elegance not unlike a Japanese print. The bough, the few, lightly tinted leaves, the entwining patterns of the bare branches, create a pattern which is permeated with light and space. The analogy of ruined choirs evokes a glimpse of historical ruins with their rich suggestion of past civilization and glory. The sweet birds who once sang recall the poet's earlier productivity and art. Thus even as his illness wastes his frame, it also reveals more ancient, and essential, contours of his body and spirit, through space and time.

The poet then compares death to sleep, his passing to a sunset. Yet the sunset which fades in the west points to the black night which will come, reminding us also of the day we enjoyed. Death itself, while sealing us off from life, also brings rest.

In the comparison of life to a fire, the speaker delineates the paradox of death-in-life and life-in-death. The fire, even as it consumes him, glows with vitality. The ashes which now snuff out his life were the product of his former glory. His very illness, like that of AIDS, was a product of his youthful energy, vigor, and love.

The final couplet reaffirms the poet's relationship with his partner. Their love grows in inverse proportion to the decay of his flesh, almost as if it were purified through the falling away of the dying man's earthly existence.

Shakespeare's sonnet exquisitely transforms the agony of decay into an intensity of love, through the power of perception, understanding, and truth. As such, it can act as an inspiration and model for AIDS patients and their companions, for they too seek to understand, accept, and maintain their love through the ravages of this disease.

Shakespeare also hints at another aspect to this relationship. The speaker, with his emaciated body, fragile flesh, and shaking limbs, is a dying man. The beloved, who sees, perceives, and finally, must leave, is intact. Together, they are maintaining a bond within the constraints of this tragedy. The beloved is staying by his lover, nurturing him, caring for him until the end when he must relinquish him to death. In this tender relationship between the weak, dependent patient and his strong, able caretaker, both accept the harmony and appropriateness of this bond—the dying man without shame, the beloved, without qualms. Hence this poem offers a model for loving care by those confronted with AIDS. The beloved honestly perceives the frailty and needs of his or her partner; the partner, in truthful assessment of this disease, welcomes the concern, care, and compassion of the companion.

Shakespeare's theme of nurturance is being explored anew by contemporary writers on AIDS. *As Is* portrays the challenge of two lovers renegotiating their relationship from one of sexuality to nurturance. In *AIDS/US* one speaker describes his loving care for his partner and how, a year later, a vision of this bond formed during his caretaking becomes a spiritual epiphany which helps him to accept this disease.

Thus, as we see in both Shakespeare's poem and many patients with AIDS, partners are accepting the responsibilities of a nurturing kind of love. They maintain an unconditional acceptance of their weakened partners. And the patients learn to accept this care, without resentment or shame. As Shakespeare reveals through his verse, honesty, autonomy, and maturity are possible even within a physically unequal relationship. It is not sexuality, but compassionate perception and acceptance of the truth of the disease, "which makes thy love more strong."

JOHN MILTON'S "WHEN I CONSIDER HOW MY LIGHT IS SPENT"

Shakespeare speaks of the loving companionship between partners, even as one of them is dying. Milton, in his religious sonnet "When I Consider How My Light Is Spent," questions the personal meaning of an illness and its devastating psychological, political, and spiritual effects. Reason and logic cannot provide meaning for such a catastrophe, but an understanding of God's love for all men, including those stricken by disease, can help us accept our condition and survive.

WHEN I CONSIDER HOW MY LIGHT IS SPENT (1655)

When I consider how my light is spent
  Ere half my days, in this dark world and wide,
  And that one talent which is death to hide,
  Lodged in me useless, though my soul more bent

To serve therewith my Maker, and present
  My true account, lest he returning chide;
  "Doth God exact day-labor, light denied?"
I fondly ask; but Patience to prevent

That murmur, soon replies, "God doth not need
  Either man's work or his own gifts; who best
  Bear his mild yoke, they serve him best. His state

Is kingly. Thousands at his bidding speed
  And post o'er land and ocean without rest:
  They also serve who only stand and wait."

As the poem opens, Milton attempts to comprehend, through the use of logic, the meaning of his terrible disease. Yet as he "considers" his predicament, he faces a paradox. His worth, as an individual and within the scheme of God and his country, resides in his capacity to share his talents with the world. Without sight, unable to read or write, his life seems devoid of meaning. How could God both demand that he express his genius, yet deny him the health to do so?

Milton's question is shared by most patients suddenly overwhelmed by a catastrophic accident or disease: "Why did I get this disease?" For many AIDS patients, the answer is painfully clear: they engaged in "unsafe" practices which transmitted the HIV virus. But for others—wives of hemophiliacs, partners of IV drug users or bisexuals—their only "fault" was to "make love." Logic and reason cannot bring meaning to Milton's blindness nor to the disease of AIDS.

As the poet refers to his own life, a deeper significance is suggested. For Milton, the foremost spokesman for a revolutionary government, the question "Why me?" refers not only to his personal but his public achievements. He had devoted his life to defending a political and ethical system which was anathema to other nations. If his work was curtailed by his blindness, all that was gained by his efforts might be destroyed and his society might return to its previous oppressive practices. Handicapped by disease, his work would stop, and the promise of his achievements would come to naught.

The analogy between Milton and leaders in the AIDS support community is painfully apt. So many have devoted years to freeing homosexuality from cultural and legal restraints and are now dedicating their lives to battling AIDS. This virus is killing some of its most prominent and talented members, and as more and more people die, both the individual achievements of gay leaders and the acceptance of the gay community itself are threatened.

In his poem, Milton perceives that reason alone is impotent. Through the intervention of Patience he turns to the wonder of faith. God does not value men only for their work or their talents; people have worth simply by being themselves. Milton accepts God's love, which he will receive even if he cannot live according to the tasks God had decreed for him. Likewise, he must learn that God accepts all men, no matter what kind of life they have led.

Similarly, some AIDS patients are realizing that their lives are not valuable only because they do important work or serve a fine cause. Merely being human is good enough. Many are learning to accept themselves, even with their disease. And others, empowered through the ordeal of their illness, are discovering a higher power which sanctifies their lives.

Milton reveals a man confronting the personal, political, and spiritual consequences of his unexpected and devastating disease. He found solace through his acceptance of God and his faith that patience and love would be sufficient. He coped successfully with his blindness, and years later produced one of the greatest poems in English canon, the religious epic, *Paradise Lost.*

At this point in the AIDS crisis, the homosexual community as well as the nation at large cannot know the outcome to this terrible epidemic. Milton reminds us, however, that the group, if not the individual, has the power to survive. New leaders will arise: some will defend homosexual rights, others will develop new treatments or perhaps discover a vacine or cure for AIDS-related disorders. As Milton says, there are thousands who will accomplish the necessary tasks. For those who cannot, "They also serve who only stand and wait." We must have faith in our love for God and in His love for us. Strengthened by this spiritual relationship, we can overcome the challenge of AIDS.

ALBERT CAMUS' *THE PLAGUE*

Camus' *The Plague* (1947) portrays a world devoid of Shakespeare's initimate love or Milton's spiritual commitment. The town of Oran is ugly and materialistic, concerned only with the immediate gratifications of money and pleasure. Its citizens lack any values that would give meaning to illness and death. For Camus, the plague, as horrible as it is, will offer this community an opportunity to transcend its petty existence. Through men's honesty in the face of terror, their compassionate moral choices, and, finally, their commitment to their fellow men, they will achieve a new awareness of the meaning of life and of love.

In a curious way, the havoc wrought by our modern-day plague, AIDS, is forcing our culture also to redefine its values, behaviors, and ethics. Oran is not unlike our own towns and cities. We also have refused to face the devastations of sickness or the trauma of death. Camus' plague-ridden world speaks directly to us.

The abrupt quarantine of Oran initiates the process of the citizens' redefinition of love. Husbands are separated from wives, parents from children, lovers from their partners. In a chapter of exquisite lyricism, Camus describes how the townspeople suffer with their terrible sense of loss. As the support and comfort normally available through family and intimate friends are withdrawn, the people are left desolate and alone. As the memories of their beloveds fade, their sense of the past, their hopes for the future, and their very identities wither and die. Bereft of intimate relationships, they feel like the living dead. Some even welcome infection by the plague as a reprieve from their meaningless lives.

Although we do not have a formal quarantine system in America, we do have intense, informal pressures which isolate people with AIDS from the support normally granted to people with handicaps, illness, or terminal disease. Despite the fact that AIDS is not generally contagious, except through the exchange of body fluids, its victims may be shunned as if they were pariahs, denied the rights of education or employment, armed service or the sacrament. Our culture has not yet come to understand how isolation affects our capacity as individuals or as a community to love.

In the circumstances of a plague, people must create new patterns of love. For Camus, alternative forms are neither religious, as for Milton, nor private, as for Shakespeare. Instead, Camus suggests a more abstract kind of devotion: a commitment to truth, compassion, and moral action. Camus' words for these types of love, "abstraction" and "friendship," refer to the love of truth and love for one's fellow man. They do not relate to individual benefit but to public good.

Our American culture, with its focus on individual rights and repressive moralistic policies, inhibits the development of programs to serve the greater community. Educational programs on AIDS transmission and prevention, which must reach a broad spectrum of our citizens, are attacked by clergy and politicians for their content, values, and advocacy of the use of condoms. Mass screening for AIDS is seen as a violation of individual rights of privacy. Distribution of sterile needles is rejected because this may seem to "condone" illegal intravenous drug abuse.

Our model of private health care and insurance, which is dependent upon the individual or his employer's ability to pay, is threatened by the growing number of AIDS/ARC patients. When people who are seropositive are denied coverage and public health care funding is tight, AIDS/ARC patients may find that—in a country which prides itself on its health care—they cannot receive medical services at all (Oppenheimer and Padgug 1986).

The process of shifting health care from individual patients to the group is a difficult task. In *The Plague,* when Dr. Rioux identifies the obscure disease as the plague and suggests public health measures, he is faced with general denial and rage. Recognition of the disease and implementation of essential measures would bring severe economic and political consequences for the town. In the face of this criticism, Dr. Rioux insists that public officials must sacrifice private needs and act out of a love for truth to best serve the needs of the town.

Similarly, the homosexual community was initially reluctant to face the truth of AIDS, its mode of sexual transmission, and the identification of gays as the primary high risk group. In both Oran and our own cities, only after intimate friends had died from the disease did people accept the necessity of public, rather than private, responses. Ironically, as AIDS now moves into the IV drug user and heterosexual communities, we are again resisting what needs to be done.

An honest perception of the truth is only the first step in our confrontation with a plague. Camus demands that individuals must next make a moral decision to act. In his novel, each character, finally acknowledging the lethal nature of the disease, nevertheless dedicates himself to serving his community. As individuals, they do not even consider themselves heroes. Dr. Rioux narrates, "It's a matter of common decency . . . It consists of doing my job." This commitment to acting for the common good is even more powerful than the ties of romance. Rambert, who must choose between his mistress and the town, discovers that men may not be capable of dying for love, but can be fully prepared to die for an idea. Panaloux, the priest who initially preached that the plague was God's punishment for the town's sins, now has a vision of God's love, and dies, dedicating himself to helping his fellow man.

Camus insists that love demands a total surrender to the service of others in the face of this terrible disease. Cottard, the only "villain" in the book, seeks selfish rather than communal ends. His behavior is presented not as evil, but as lacking Camus' moral values of "abstraction" and "friendship." Cottard had "an ignorant, that is to say, a lonely, heart."

In America, we are coming to recognize the importance of community services for AIDS. In the major cities, men and women are creating humane educational, support, and treatment programs to serve the needs of seropositives, ARC and AIDS patients, and their loved ones. Some medical centers are shifting from expensive and private health care plans to ones which can satisfy both individual and community needs. AIDS patients themselves are sacrificing their precarious health status to work on hot-lines, serve on counseling groups, give public performances, and participate in medical experiments, so they can help others who may now or in the future have AIDS. Slowly, policies based on love rather than fear are helping AIDS sufferers, homosexual and heterosexual alike.

Camus, like Shakespeare, also demonstrates that "Agape," love for our fellow man, as well as "Eros," or sexual desire, can be expressed through individual and communal relationships. Dr. Rioux and his helper Tarrou, through their discussions and actions, demonstrate their love for the truth and for their community. As they combat the plague together, they also become intimate friends. Near the end of the story they take a few hours off from their work. Together, they wander to the beach, then, wordlessly, swim into the sea. Here, in a passage of lyric beauty, Camus portrays the loving intimacy of the two men. Soon afterwards, Tarrou succumbs to the plague and Dr. Rioux nurses him throughout his illness and stands by him at his death. His grief for Tarrou is intense: the loss of a true friend is irreparable.

Dr. Rioux's and Tarrou's model for intimacy was not a romantic, sexual, or sacred union, although their vision of peace touched upon spiritual revelation. In its quiet intensity, their love is closest to the acceptance and comfort a mother gives her child, or in Shakespeare's sense, a beloved gives his partner. True friendship transcends the fear of personal death. It supports the partner through every ordeal, nurturing him when he is sick and comforting him in his dying. This love is beyond words; it is a silent devotion.

From Camus, we can learn that in the crisis of a fatal disease like the plague or AIDS, romantic and sexual love become less relevant. Instead, an opportunity arises allowing men and women to achieve a higher kind of intimacy and meaning through their selfless commitment to the welfare of others. From this communal interaction comes a love for the truth, for moral action, and for spiritual peace that directs and enriches our lives shattered by crisis, disease, and death. Of all actions, the most exquisite, intense, intimate, and painful, is the loving care of a dying friend.

BIBLIOGRAPHY

Camus, Albert. *The Plague* (1947). Translated by Stuart Gilbert. New York: Vintage Books, 1972.

Goldman, Peter, and Beachy, Lucille. "One Against the Plague." *Newsweek* 115:3, July 21, 1986, pp. 38–50.

Hoffman, William A. *As Is*. New York: Vintage Books, 1985.

Katz, Michael. *AIDS/US*. Unpublished play, Los Angeles, 1986.

Kramer, Larry. *The Normal Heart*. New York: New American Library, 1985.

Oppenheimer, Gerald M., and Padgug, Robert A. "AIDS: The Risks to Insurers, The Threat to Equity." *Hastings Center Report* 16:5, October 1986, pp. 18–22.

CHAPTER 6

Women with AIDS: Sexual Ethics in an Epidemic

JULIEN S. MURPHY

As the number of AIDS cases in the United States approaches 30,000, the threat of AIDS to the public health becomes more ominous.[1] Concern with fighting the spread of AIDS has been shaped by a notion of "public health" entangled in social biases. For instance, "public health" has been historically skewed toward heterosexuality, as indicated by the initial slow responses to the homosexual and bisexual men first diagnosed with AIDS. The concept of "public health" in relation to the AIDS epidemic, however, has initially been biased more toward gay men, exhibiting a gender bias against women as well. That women too are afflicted with AIDS is rarely mentioned. Many people are not even aware that women can be infected with AIDS, and very few know that women with AIDS are not a recent phenomenon, but rather, that women have been afflicted with AIDS since the very beginning of the epidemic.

In the years 1979–1981, when AIDS was called the Gay-Related-Immune-Disorder (GRID), there were 27 cases reported in women. Currently, there have been 1993 cases of women with AIDS in this country with a projection of 18,900 cases in women by 1991.[2] Seventy percent of the current cases of women with AIDS have been diagnosed in the past two years. In addition, there are two classifications in which even more women have been affected: (1) 105,000 asymptomatic women carriers of the AIDS retrovirus; (2) 14,000 women with AIDS-related complex (ARC).[3]

Homophobia and sexism contribute to the lack of public awareness about women with AIDS because the more the disease is stigmatized as a "gay male disease" the more unthinkable it becomes to consider that women may be at risk for AIDS. It has been an invisible fact that women have consistently comprised 7% of the U.S. AIDS cases (9% in Europe,[4] 50% in Central Africa). Women are frequently omitted from AIDS brochures and media coverage, and eclipsed in medical research. Some public health officials would like to hold prostitutes responsible for AIDS in the United States and elsewhere—

an unsubstantiated and sexist claim.[5] Even children, who comprise only 1% of U.S. AIDS cases have gotten more media coverage, albeit controversial, and more research attention than women—despite the fact that 75% of pediatric AIDS cases are acquired in pregnancies among infected women.

In general, women with AIDS are made to fit into a male-AIDS-profile which cannot address the central physiological and sociopolitical differences between the sexes, namely, that AIDS, like many sexually transmitted diseases, immerses women in complex fertility and reproductive decisions. As the number of women with AIDS continues to rise, discussion of the ethical dilemmas of fertility and reproduction will become all the more important. It is not known exactly how many asymptomatic HIV carriers and persons with ARC will develop full-blown AIDS or the manifold immune disorders that will be identified before the epidemic is over. In the meantime, we need to shape a notion of public health appropriate to meet the special problems of women with AIDS, a notion that neither regards women and fertility as a disease nor ignores the needs of infected women and their possible offspring.

Ethical discussion of women with AIDS begins with the awareness that, by and large, these women represent the least advantaged groups in society. Women with AIDS are predominantly black (53%), and engaged in the illegal practices of intravenous drug use (51%) and sometimes prostitution.[6] Small wonder, then, that their plight has received so little attention. Nonetheless, women can protect themselves against AIDS. Most women with AIDS (78%) fall into two primary risk categories, both of which can be altered by behavior changes: intravenous drug use (51%) and heterosexual contact with an infected partner (27%).[7] Many of the remaining (22%) cases of women having no known risk factor may be cases of sexual contact with an asymptomatic carrier. Hence, education and behavior changes could greatly diminish the increase in new cases in women and also curb pediatric AIDS. Four major ethical concerns that specifically relate to women with AIDS are the implications of AIDS transmission by intravenous drug use, by heterosexual contact, by prostitution, and by pregnancy.

AIDS AND WOMEN DRUG USERS

One way to curtail the highest risk factor for women with AIDS (intravenous drug use) is instituting a needle exchange program that provides addicts with legal access to sterile drug injection equipment. Such programs are already in successful operation in Amsterdam and Sydney.[8] The first U.S. program is being instituted in New Jersey[9] where one of the largest group of AIDS-infected IV drug users has been found. Although the sterile needle program would, in theory, eliminate AIDS transmission by the sharing of dirty needles among drug users, it has been seen by some as an implicit approval of abusive drug behavior—supplying drug addicts with the means to their illegal habits.

However, the punitive attitude towards addicts, presuming that they get the diseases they deserve, cannot be morally justified because the AIDS-infected drug addicts endanger not only their own health but health of their sexual partners and offspring. A needle exchange program with follow-up checks and counseling not only provides a humane attitude toward drug addiction but also an effective AIDS-prevention measure for women drug abusers, their infants, and the women partners of male addicts.

AIDS AND HETEROSEXUAL CONTACT

The major ethical issues of the AIDS epidemic for women concern AIDS transmission by heterosexual contact, the second highest risk factor for women. A discussion of these issues will be useful as well for exploring the implications for fertility and reproduction in sexually transmitted diseases in general. So far, AIDS has not commonly been a bi-directional sexually transmitted disease in the United States. It is highly controversial whether female-to-male transmission of AIDS is anything but an extremely rare route of transmission.[10-14] Of the 566 heterosexual transmission cases in males, 474 of the men's cases are considered heterosexual transmission cases not as a result of direct evidence but because these men had no other identified risks, and were born in countries with high rates of heterosexual transmission. By contrast, 430 of the 545 heterosexual transmission cases in females occurred with women who had heterosexual contact with a man infected with or at risk for AIDS. It has been well-documented that women can be infected by sexual contact with a male partner who has AIDS, ARC, or is an asymptomatic sero-positive.[15] Particularly at high risk are women partners of gay or bisexual men, IV drug users, and hemophiliacs. Although the presence of AIDS infection has been found in the vaginal secretions of women with AIDS[16] and seropositive women,[17] there are no documented cases of AIDS transmission between gay or bisexual women.

To safeguard the blood supply, it has been recommended that wives of hemophiliacs should refrain from donating blood.[18] The same recommendation could extend to sexual partners of all high risk men. Along with protecting the blood supply from contamination by women donors with heterosexually acquired AIDS, we should be concerned with protecting the health of women partners of high risk males.

The ethical issues concerning AIDS are particularly exigent because AIDS is usually a terminal disease. For instance, what are the implications of sexual intimacy when it involves the risk of death? Is there an ethical principle by which women can justifiably refuse unprotected sexual contact with an infected or even a dying partner to whom she has pledged her love "in sickness and in health until death"? Will some women be tempted to ignore the health risks of sexual intercourse with an infected partner just as they neglect contraceptive use? If so, can this choice be justified, or is it irresponsible be-havior, or perhaps is it indicative of a larger social ill—namely, that women are socialized to believe they cannot control their own sexual practices for the sake of their own health or desires?

An ethical principle for safe sex would provide justification for women to refuse unprotected sexual contact with an infected or high risk partner. An ethical principle for safe sex claims that: *Any act of sex that undermines the respect and autonomy of oneself or one's partner by endangering the health and livelihood of either or both persons treats persons as mere instruments of but not the proper ends of sexual pleasure.* Hence, to violate the ethical principle for safe sex is to choose to place one's own or one's partner's sexual pleasure above one's own or one's partner's health and well-being. Acts of violent or demeaning sex, as well as unprotected sexual contact with a person infected with or at risk for sexually transmitted diseases including AIDS, would be incompatible with this ethical principle. Similarly, it would be unethical for a woman to knowingly place herself at high risk for AIDS by heterosexual contact even though her love for her partner might be very significant.

A sexual act in violation of this Safe Sex Principle might require a woman to demonstrate her love for her partner by sacrificing her own health as a romantic symbol of commitment. Such an act would be highly exploit-ative, undermining the woman's integrity and her right to her own life inde-pendent of her partner's life. Admittedly, the desire for sexual contact—safe or unsafe—with an infected, at risk, or dying AIDS partner presents an ex-tremely tragic and stressful context for an intimate relationship. Given that women are socialized to self-sacrificing behavior in our culture, the Safe Sex Principle is necessary to protect women's own interests and health. It would be unnecessary and horrific if women were to place themselves knowingly at risk for AIDS out of a blind allegiance to their partners. Such a choice, amidst a growing epidemic, could come to epitomize an AIDS suttee—adapting the Indian ritual by which widows willingly were cremated on their husbands fu-neral pyres to the AIDS epidemic.

The Safe Sex Principle also addresses situations in which a woman feels coerced into sexual contact with an infected or at-risk partner. Such cases combine the act of rape with possible exposure to a terminal disease, posing a double threat to a woman's well-being. There may be other situations that do not qualify as rapes but involve the deliberate failure of an infected or at-risk partner to honor precautions agreed upon in advance of a sexual encounter which both partners desire. Such failure is especially serious in AIDS cases, since the negligent partner, in breaking his agreement, jeopardizes the health of his partner. Slightly less serious is the act of breaking an agreement about contraception—particularly when a pregnancy results. Once again the broken agreement has major implications for the health of the woman partner but does not pose the threat of death that AIDS might. Although it would be unfortunate if it became popular to officially contract out the conditions of sexual contact, what is needed is an increased awareness about risks and responsibilities to one's own health and the health of one's partner, particularly in the AIDS era.

How far should sexual responsibility extend? It is clearly unethical for someone to knowingly infect a sexual partner through deception about one's risk potential or status of health. For instance, the fact that a person is seropositive is no longer a private matter when one is proposing a sexual encounter that would place someone else at risk. But to what extent is the information about AIDS infection a matter of confidentiality? Consider a hypothetical example. If person A knows that person B has AIDS and is not telling sexual partner C while engaging or intending to engage in unsafe sex with C, does A have an ethical responsibility to tell C that B is infected with AIDS? Does it matter if A is B's physician, clergyperson, therapist, grocer, sister, or colleague? Does it matter if that information could have punitive or legal ramifications? In this example, the ethical need for B's sexual responsibility is in conflict with B's right to privacy. Similarly, A's duty to respect the confidentiality of B conflicts with A's duty to protect an innocent person from harm. What are the parameters of respecting information conveyed in confidence when the information is life-threatening to someone else? Clearly, it is not the responsibility of A to correct each and every untruth that B may use in his sexual relationships. Assume B tells A that he lets C believe that he loves her, although he admits he really doesn't. If A were to give C this information, it would be inappropriate, for it would violate B's right to confidentiality and C's right to make sense of her sexual relationships on her own terms. For the sake of C's autonomy and self-respect, it may be appropriate neither to encourage C in her love for B, nor to dash her hopes by divulging a truth held in confidence. However, when information is life-threatening (B is infected with AIDS), B's deception of C places her health and her life at stake without C's awareness. B's right to confidentiality is superceded by C's right to know the state of B's health since C could be infected with a fatal disease.

Particularly because AIDS is a new disease and people are either unaccustomed to or reluctant to incorporate safe sexual practices into their normal sexual behaviors, the obligation to inform someone who might be at risk for AIDS by heterosexual contact is especially crucial. Ideally, B should inform all of his sexual partners of his disease or refrain from activities that would place them at risk. Other people's knowledge of B's health status should not be a "well-kept secret" when there is good reason to believe that B is failing in his responsibility to inform his sexual partners himself. This obligation does not, however, grant people the right to inform anyone besides B's sexual partners. Some proposals to inform persons through premarital blood testing programs are based on this principle.

The obligation to inform sexual partners of people with or at risk for AIDS is most pertinent for safeguarding women from AIDS, since many women simply do not know about all their partner's sexual activities. Also, some AIDS-infected men may practice unsafe sex as a form of denial—rejecting the painful truth of being terminally ill. In any epidemic, and AIDS is no exception, fear runs rampant and along with fear comes denial. Identifying responsible actions that might protect the health of people not yet exposed to AIDS will counter this denial and circumvent the implications of self-deception on the part of the infected.

In many ways, the obligation to inform an unsuspecting sexual partner of an infected or at-risk person makes sex a public matter. Sexual freedom cannot be an absolute right when epidemics of severe sexually transmitted diseases, such as AIDS, are possible. Likewise, the right to privacy about one's sexual contacts cannot be an absolute right, since certain sexual acts may threaten the health of others. Hence public health officials should seek out the sexual contacts of AIDS-infected persons and offer testing and counseling while protecting the confidentiality of all persons involved. Because AIDS is a rapidly spreading disease, it is important that possible exposure to AIDS exposure by sexual contact not be completely reliant on the "honor system." However, at the same time, there are justifiable fears that such measures could stigmatize infected men and women in ways that might threaten their professional and private lives. That is why it is imperative that public health policy vigorously promote the rights of persons with AIDS while also ensuring confidentiality in identifying sexual contacts.

Some might argue that the right to privacy in sexual behavior supercedes all other concerns, for it safeguards the freedom of persons to live as they wish. This position opposes state intervention, even in matters of health, and holds each individual completely responsible for his or her own health and for learning about any new health risks. Yet, our society does not really encourage such individual responsibility nor do we have in place the necessary resources that would make self-education possible. The argument assumes that individual freedom, without state intervention in sexual behavior, is more important than the prevention of deaths of people unaware of their exposure to AIDS. In short, it implies that it is better to die free than live with state intervention. Without private education facilities widely available, such a position undervalues the health of persons most vulnerable to AIDS exposure, and is therefore unjustifiable.

An argument may be made that the attempt to diligently inform women who are at risk through heterosexual contact is futile since it has not been established precisely what precautions offer enough protection, nor what the relationship is between being infected and being infectious. In addition, some might fear that assiduous efforts to inform women who are at risk would promote greater sexual panic, perhaps leading to quarantine, and further stigmatization of people with AIDS. These concerns must be addressed in any prevention education campaign. Yet, since certain precautions are indeed possible to reduce the risk of AIDS exposure in sexual contact, this alone

merits the identification of sexual partners at risk. Further, there is a larger
social end involved—namely, the containment of the AIDS virus.

Although the sexual contact discussion has focused on heterosexual
women, lesbians, too, can acquire AIDS through sexual contact, though the
risk is much smaller. Some of the 7% of U.S. AIDS cases that are women
are lesbians who acquired the AIDS infection through IV drug use, blood
transfusions, or prior heterosexual contact. Although no cases of lesbian
sexual transmission have been reported in the United States, it is completely
feasible that a woman infectious with the AIDS virus could transmit the virus
to her female partner by sexual acts that involve blood-to-blood or vaginal
secretions-to-blood contact. As the cases of AIDS in women increase, it is
likely that lesbian sexual contact cases will appear, which could constitute a
new AIDS risk group. Hence, lesbians, who are not accustomed to deliber-
ating about contraceptive or other precautions before engaging in sex, need
to take safe sex seriously by endorsing the Safe Sex Principle so that their
health and the health of their partners may be preserved.

Can a sexual ethics in the AIDS epidemic stop short of a sexual moratorium? In cases of AIDS transmission by heterosexual contact would a sexual
moratorium be perhaps the "safest" possibility for women with infected
partners? It has indeed been suggested that sexual contact with anyone who is
at risk or who is infectious should be avoided. However, since it is not known
how long an infected person might be infectious, and since more and more
people are developing the virus, such a suggestion might bring about the
undesirable classification of people into two groups: the uninfected, sexually
active, and the infected, sexually forbidden. This could encourage a desexua-
lization of persons with AIDS, denying these persons one of the most essential
expressions of human life.

A more humane response might be to revise the notion of sexual responsibility to include concern for protecting one's own health and the health of
one's partner, and to broaden forms of sexual expression so that the most
"exciting" sexual acts are not also acts that put one at high risk for AIDS.
Sexual activity ought to be in part, a celebration of one's existence, not an
endangering of one's health. The right to sexual expressions, assuming they
are not health-endangering or exploitive, is a human right and especially necessary in times of epidemic where life seems frail and death pervasive. More
than simply limiting current sexual practices to safe sex requirements, we
need to discover new sexual practices that can serve as passionate forms of
intimacy without the risk of developing AIDS.

AIDS AND PROSTITUTION

A woman's chances of exposure to AIDS are greatly increased by prostitution
since prostitution requires frequent sexual encounters with multiple

partners.[19] Prostitutes have been considered "reservoirs" for AIDS infection by some AIDS researchers.[20,21] This image of prostitutes as "AIDS reservoirs" suggests that women's bodies are infectious pools of AIDS viruses, storing large quantities of infected liquids, and the source of disease for many. It also implies that men are unsuspecting transmitters of sexual diseases, moving infection from one woman (a prostitute) to another (female sexual partner). The sex bias in this metaphor is apparent. Women are not the originating cause of sexually transmitted diseases. In the case of AIDS, prostitutes may be an infected pool but not necessarily an infectious pool of disease. As many as 40% of prostitutes in some U.S. cities are infected with the AIDS virus,[22] with high rates among prostitutes abroad as well (in Nairobi,[23] Greece,[24] Rwanda,[25] Zaire,[26] Brussels[27]).

It is perhaps idealistic to argue for safe sex measures in prostitution in the United States when prostitution is for the most part illegal and prostitutes subject to arrest. Prostitution continues to be, as Marx stated, an explicit instance of body-enslavement, of "the worker only as a working animal—as a beast reduced to the strictest bodily needs."[28] Even where prostitution is legal, such as in Nevada, bordello operators are more concerned with the amount of business a prostitute can produce than with her health. Bordello operators recommend that prostitutes be regularly tested for the AIDS antibody so their customers will be assured the prostitute is "AIDS-free." The same operators do not require screening of clients for AIDS infection, mandatory condom use, nor do they prohibit unsafe sex acts. Some are quick to insist that an infected or seropositive woman be barred from her job without any financial provision for medical care or other needs. The complete expendability of a prostitute's health is made most apparent in the AIDS epidemic where little effort is made to safeguard prostitutes from AIDS.

Given that few economic alternatives exist for women in prostitution, and that prostitution is related to deeper social issues concerning the marketing of sexuality and female bodies, it is difficult to accept the view held by some that prostitutes deserve the diseases they get. It is just as unethical to expose a prostitute to AIDS as it is to expose any person. Simply because the prostitute receives payment for sexual acts does not mean that she warrants less respect or human concern than a person who does not demand payment. Of course, the act of procuring a prostitute is already an act of sexual exploitation and is unethical. The inhumane nature of prostitution suggests that there may be some forms of labor that are neither necessary to society nor consistent with the preservation of human dignity. It might be argued that legalizing prostitution would ensure better health care for prostitutes as well as encourage AIDS prevention measures. Yet, legalization of prostitution would also imply a social endorsement of this form of labor. The most effective approach to ending prostitution would be to institute viable economic alternatives, including job training for the (former) prostitutes and for women who might otherwise resort to prostitution. At the same time, it is necessary is to educate both prostitutes and their customers about safe sex practices.

AIDS AND PREGNANT WOMEN

The problems of women with AIDS sometimes affect not only themselves but also their fetuses. AIDS infection in pregnancy decreases the chances for a healthy infant, and increases the likelihood of the mother developing AIDS symptoms. About two-thirds of the pregnancies of AIDS-infected women result in infected infants, and half of those infants will be affected with disease within two years.[29] It is possible for the AIDS infection in the fetus to be greater than the level of AIDS infection in the mother. It is not only women with AIDS that give birth to infants with AIDS, but also women with ARC,[30] and even asymptomatic carriers.[31] AIDS in pregnancy is not only detrimental to the fetus, but there is reason to believe that seropositive and ARC women's chances of developing AIDS are increased by the state of being pregnant. Pregnancy seems to accelerate the development of AIDS in seropositive women,[32] and a second pregnancy is even more likely to provoke the presentation of AIDS in seropositive women.[33]

Pregnancy by artificial insemination (AI) can also be a risk for women if the semen donor is infected. Four women have been infected this way.[34] Although little attention is given to births by AI, there are over 10,000 per year in the United States. Hence a large number of women could be at risk for AIDS by AI. Protective measures are needed which would require the systematic screening of all semen donors similar to screening of blood donors.

A key ethical question that arises concerning pregnancies in women with AIDS concerns the right to be pregnant. Does a woman who is seropositive, or has ARC or AIDS have the moral right to choose to be pregnant? Does she have the right to maintain a pregnancy once her disease is diagnosed? Is the right to begin and sustain pregnancy part of women's right to control their bodies, or is the right to pregnancy contingent in part on whether or not it harms the health of the mother and/or the infant? One researcher suggests automatic HIV screening on all antenatal women, irrespective of their consent to such testing.[35] Another suggests that serological testing for AIDS virus antibody prior to issuing marriage licenses.[36] Testing for marriage licenses would give people information concerning the antibody status of their partners only at the time of marriage. However, should marriage licenses be refused to those who test positive on the grounds that refusal would be an effective prohibition against AIDS pregnancies, particularly when it is estimated that there may be as many as 3000 infants and children with AIDS in the United States by 1991? Clearly a measure prohibiting marriage licenses for seropositive individuals would be invasive, especially since not all people marry in order to have children. But if this measure is rejected because it violates the basic human freedom to wed independent of procreation, does a woman have the right to begin pregnancy if she knows her husband is sero-positive?

Given that the odds are against a healthy pregnancy, and that pregnancy poses a threat to accelerating AIDS infection in the mother, several re-searchers have recommended abortion of all pregnancies among infected women for health reasons alone, and advised against infected women begin-ning pregnancy.[37-39] There may be moral grounds as well to prohibit preg-nancy when, most likely, the fetus will have a severely damaged immune system and will die within the first two years of life. Given the severity of AIDS, the fact that mothers themselves often die prior to the deaths of their diseased infants, and given the further risk to women's health that pregnancy presents, one might justifiably abort a fetus if one is infected with AIDS pro-vided one believes that every woman has a responsibility, first, to her own health, and secondly, to the health of the fetus, and that the abortion protects the health of the mother and spares the infant AIDS by terminating the fetus. Abortion in this case would not only be consistent with a woman's right to control her body, but would be ethical on the additional grounds of pro-tecting a woman's autonomy through preserving her health and sparing a fetus needless pain and suffering.

Conservatives might argue that every fetus, even a fetus with AIDS, has a right to life, and presumably, a right to an AIDS death. Liberals cite the tremendous drain on medical resources that AIDS infants present, particu-larly as the numbers increase, and hence, liberals may find abortion of fetuses in AIDS-infected pregnancies warranted. It might be argued that advising against pregnancy and promoting abortion in AIDS-infected pregnancies is a racist tactic since many of the AIDS mothers are women of color. Yet, the appropriate way to address any such racist implications is not to insist that black or brown women with AIDS any more than white women with AIDS terminate their pregnancies, but rather to insist that there be equal access to medical and economic resources for blacks and other minorities.

Perhaps the strongest objection to mandatory abortion measures and ad-vising against pregnancy in cases where women are infected with AIDS is that such measures are a step toward mandatory abortion practices for a wide range of "defective" fetuses: is the fear of a widescale eugenics program. However, there is a major difference in recommending abortion in AIDS pregnancies and recommending abortion for other diseases such as cerebral palsy, or Downs Syndrome—namely, that in AIDS pregnancies the mother herself is already infected with the virus and needs to take every precaution to protect herself from further development of AIDS. Mothers with AIDS might spend their own remaining months of life sustaining a pregnancy that may very well produce an infected infant. One of the dilemmas facing the pregnant woman is the uncertainty of whether the fetus is or is not infected. This is not to say that abortion for pregnancies in which the fetus but not the mother is infected with severe disease would not be morally permissible. It is merely to make the claim that the two situations are quite distinct. Moreover, there may be additional reasons for justifying abortion in AIDS-infected pregnancies including the right not to be pregnant if one doesn't choose to be, as well as the right to end a pregnancy because of the psychological stress involved. The constant awareness of a possibly terminally ill fetus in the womb might be a difficult reality to face, especially for a woman who is herself infected. The awareness that the disease might be taking over her body and that her body could be the vehicle by which AIDS is carried into the next generation might be unbearable as well.

The above grounds may justify abortion when a woman has AIDS or ARC, is seropositive, or even is merely exposed to AIDS. But does a woman have ethical grounds, on the other hand, to *maintain* a pregnancy if she is infected with the AIDS virus? The refusal of abortion by infected women could be seen as not only not a "right" but rather an act of cruelty for it could result in the suffering of another human entity. What end is being served by bringing an infant into existence that most likely will live in continual pain and suffering? A woman may choose to sustain her pregnancy in hopes that she might still produce offspring, which might give her life meaning. For example, perhaps the woman is asymptomatic and her husband is dying of AIDS. This pregnancy would be their last chance to have a child together, a tangible way for a part of him to live on. A pregnant woman with AIDS might choose to sustain pregnancy as an act of giving life when her own impending death is crowding life out of her.

However understandable these reasons may be, an ethical justification for sustaining pregnancy when it could result in injury and harm to a new human entity must carefully weigh both the mother's right to reproduce and the possibility of an infant born into suffering, disease, and most likely iminent death. In choosing to continue pregnancy, an infected woman is also choosing to further endanger her own health in order to give birth to an infant who might or might not be free of the AIDS virus. She is not choosing to consciously inflict pain and suffering. But, it is very possible that the infant will be born severely infected, and with no legal precedent of infanticide or active euthanasia, the infant would be destined to suffer for as much as two years. This is not to say that choosing to play the odds and go against current medical advice, despite the risk of a negative outcome for herself and her infant, could never be morally justified. But rather, an infected woman should carefully determine if there are any responsibilities she has first to her own body-in-disease.

Clearly everyone owes this to themselves: a meaningful life, and a meaningful death. But how one achieves both amidst a state of bodily infection with perhaps terminal illness must be left to the individual. If an infected woman decides to maintain her pregnancy while fully understanding that it might cause her seropositivity to begin to manifest itself with AIDS symptoms and shortly bring about her death by AIDS, a death that might otherwise not have occurred, she is entitled to respect as a moral decision maker. Conversely, if a woman chooses abortion to avoid becoming an AIDS casualty herself and to avoid giving birth to an infant with AIDS she should not be judged harshly for not self-sacrificing. To seek to enjoy life ever more intensely as AIDS threatens a premature death is also a valid choice—one which is particularly within the moral rights of infected people.

WOMEN AND THE FUTURE OF AIDS

The effects of AIDS on drug use, sexual activity, and pregnancy are the central but not the only implications of AIDS for women. Women will also suffer sex discrimination in access to medical resources and may even suffer a higher rate of incorrect diagnoses.[40] Moreover, given the economic disparity between men and women and the racial biases of our society, women with AIDS will most likely have less access to information and services relevant to their specific needs.

The gender bias of our notion of "public health" needs to be eradicated and the AIDS epidemic could provide the impetus. Public health policy needs to effect the following changes to protect women from AIDS: a broad-based education program on intravenous drug use and drug rehabilitation, including counseling and sterile needle exchange services; the dissemination of safe sex information, an outreach program for testing and counseling prostitutes with a task force for creating alternative income options for them; counseling and medical services for women considering pregnancy or who are already pregnant; free access to abortion for all women; assistance programs for seropositive women who are unemployed; medical insurance for infected women; child care facilities and mother-assistance services for infected women; visitation rights for infected women who may have placed their children in foster care; the adaptation of hospice programs to accommodate women with facilities that would enable them to be connected with their children as much as possible if they so choose.

Meanwhile, more of the over 100,000 seropositive women in this country will go on to manifest ARC or AIDS symptoms. More and more relationships, including lesbian or bisexual relationships, will include a seropositive partner and require special care in maintaining the health of each of the partners. There will be more AIDS pregnancies, and more infected infants as well. The hope of a vaccine for AIDS remains a dream. The grim reality of the epidemic is depicted with projections of more than 18,000 women with AIDS in the United States within five years. By 1991, the number of women with AIDS will nearly equal the number of men who have currently been diagnosed with AIDS. It is crucial that the awareness of AIDS and precautions against AIDS be taken seriously now for much can be done. By 1991, AIDS will no longer be some strange virus out of nowhere. Neither pleas of ignorance nor lack of action will ease the burden of the rising AIDS count. Short of a cure for AIDS, our strongest weapons are education and public policies that seek to preserve the health of all in the community—including women —and compassion in our responses to the epidemic.

We are just now beginning to confront the bleak realities of women dying of AIDS—the multitude of worries they may have about their fate; the children they leave behind; their loss of sexual partners and friends; the anger they may feel toward a sexual partner who may have infected them; the shock and frustration of being pregnant while being gravely ill; the grief at perhaps ending a pregnancy they might have otherwise wanted. Although every death from AIDS is a particularly sad death, women's deaths from AIDS have tragic qualities all their own. Women with AIDS are, in many ways, a spin-off effect of the larger epidemic which has affected predominantly men (93%). Women with AIDS present a new social and ethical dilemma at the intersection of issues regarding sex, fertility, reproductive rights, and economics.

We cannot hope to improve the situations of women with AIDS without openly addressing these issues and thereby formulating policy which will improve the conditions of women in general, and in particular poor women and women of color. We might do well to prepare for these policy discussions by calculating projections for the spread of AIDS in women and to use this devastating information as a motivating force for development of the resources necessary to meet the challenge of AIDS in women.

I would like to thank Alison Deming for her many helpful comments on this paper and John Corcoran for his research and computer assistance.

NOTES

1. All statistics unless otherwise indicated are from the *AIDS Weekly Surveillance Report, Jan. 26, 1987,* Centers for Disease Control, and refer to U.S. AIDS cases only.
2. Projected estimate assumes that 7% of the 270,000 projected U.S. AIDS cases in 1991 will be women.
3. Estimates assume that at least 7% of the estimated 1.5 million seropositive cases and of the estimated 200,000 ARC cases are women.
4. World Health Organization, Geneva, Weekly Epidemiological Record. "AIDS: Report on the Situation in Europe." 60:305–312 (1985).
5. See Cohen, Judith B.; Hauer, Laurie B.; Cracchiolo, Bernadette, et al., "A.W.A.R.E. A Community Study of AIDS Antibody Prevalence among High Risk Women in San Francisco." Paper delivered at the Annual Meeting of American Public Health Association, Washington, D.C., November 17–21, 1985.
6. CDC *AIDS Weekly Surveillance Report.* op. cit.
7. Ibid.
8. "Jersey 'Willing' to Give Addicts Clean Needles." *The New York Times,* July 24, 1986. See also Buning, E. C., et al. "Preventing AIDS in Drug Addicts in Amsterdam." *Lancet* I(8495):1435 (June 21, 1986).

9. Ibid.

10. Polk, F. B. "Female-to-Male Transmission of AIDS" (Letter). *JAMA* 254(22):3177–3178 (December 13, 1985).

11. Haverkos, J. W., and Edelman, R. "Female-to-Male Transmission of AIDS" (Letter). *JAMA* 254(8):1035–1036 (August 23, 1985).

12. Schultz, S.; Milberg, J. A.; Kirstal, A. R.; Stoneburner, R. L. "Female-to-Male Transmission of HTLV-III" (Letter). *JAMA* 255(13):1703–1704 (April 4, 1986).

13. Wykoff, R. F. "Female-to-Male Transmission of HTLV-III" (Letter). *JAMA* 255(13):1703–1705.

14. Redfield, R. R.; Markham, P. D.; Salahuddin, S. E., et al. "Heterosexually Acquired HTLV-III/LAV Disease (AIDS-Related Complex and AIDS): Epidemiologic Evidence for Female-to-Male Transmission." *JAMA* 254(15):2094–2096 (Oct. 18, 1985). See also Redfield, R. R.; Wright, D. C.; Markham, P. D. "Female-to-Male Transmission of HTLV-III" (Letter). *JAMA* 255(13):1705–1706.

15. Vogt, M. W.; Craven, D. E.; Crawford, D. F., et al. "Isolation of HTLV-III/LAV from Cervical Secretions of Women at Risk for AIDS." *Lancet* I(8480):525–527 (March 8, 1986).

16. Wofsky, C. B.; Hauer, L. B.; Michaelis, B. A., et al. "Isolation of AIDS-Associated Retrovirus from Genital Secretions of Women with Antibodies to the Virus." *Lancet* I(8480):527–529 (March 8, 1986).

17. Harris, C.; Small, C. B.; Klein, R. S.; Griedland, G. H., et al. "Immunodeficiency in Female Sexual Partners of Men with the Acquired Immunodeficiency Syndrome." *New England Journal of Medicine* 308:1181–1184 (1983).

18. Ragni, J. V.; Rinaldo, C. R.; Kingsley, L., et al. "Heterosexual Partners of Haemophiliacs Must Refrain From Blood Donations." *Lancet* I:(8488):1033 (May 3, 1986). See also Jason, J. M.; McDougal, J. S.; Dixon, G., et al. "HTLV-III/LAV Antibody and Immune Status of Household Contacts and Sexual Partners of Persons with Hemophilia." *JAMA* 255(2):212–215 (Jan. 10, 1986).

19. Polk, F. B. "Female-to-Male Transmission of AIDS" (Letter).

20. D'Costa, L. J.; Plummer, F. A.; Bowmer, I., et al. "Prostitutes are a Major Reservoir of Sexually Transmitted Diseases in Nairobi, Kenya." *Sexually Transmitted Diseases* 12:64–67 (1985).

21. Redfield, R. R.; Markham, P. D.; Salahuddin, S. Z., et al. "Heterosexually Acquired HTLV-III/LAV Disease (AIDS-Related Complex and AIDS).

22. Vogt, M. W.; Craven, D. E.; Crawford, D. F.; Hirsch, M. S., et al. "Isolation of HTLV-III/LAV from Cervical Secretions of Women at Risk for AIDS.

23. Kreiss, J. K.; Koech, D.; Plummer, F. A.; Holmes, K. K.; Lightfoote, M.; Piot, P., et al. "AIDS Virus Infection in Nairobi Prostitutes," *New England Journal of Medicine:*414–418 (Feb. 13, 1986).

24. Papaevangelou, G.; Roumeliotou-Karayannis, A.; Kallinikos, G.; Papoutsakis, B. "LAV/HTLV-III Infection in Female Prostitutes." *Lancet* II:(8462):1018–1019 (Nov. 2, 1985).

25. Van DePerre, P.; Carael, M.; Robert-Guroff, M.; Freyens, P.; Gallo, R. C., et al. "Female Prostitutes: A Risk Group for Infection with Human T-Cell Lymphotropic Virus Type III." *Lancet* II(8454):524–52 (Sept. 7, 1985).

26. Piot, P.; Quinn, T. C.; Taelman, H., et al. "Acquired Immunodeficiency Syndrome in a Heterosexual Population in Zaire." *Lancet* II(8394):65–69 (1984).

27. Clumeck, N.; Carael, M.; Rouvroy, D.; Nzaramba, D. "Heterosexual Promiscuity Among African Patients with AIDS." *New England Journal of Medicine* 313(3):182 (July 18, 1985).

28. Marx, Karl. *The Economic and Philosophic Manuscripts of 1844.* International Publishers, 1964, 74.

29. Pinching, Anthony, J. and Jeffries, Donald J. "AIDS and HTLV-III/LAV Infection: Consequences for Obstetrics and Perinatal Medicine." *British Journal of Obstetrics and Gynecology* 92:1211–1217 (1985).

30. Rubinstein, A.; Sicklick, M.; Gupta, A., et al. "Acquired Immunodeficiency with Reversed T4/T8 Ratios in Infants Born to Promiscuous and Drug-Addicted Mothers. *JAMA* 249:2350–2356 (1983).

31. Joshi, W.; Path, M. R. C.; Oleske, J. M.; Minnefor, A. B., et al. "Pathology of Suspected AIDS in Children: A Study of Eight Cases." *Pediatric Pathology* 2:71–87 (1984).

32. Gilmer, E.; Fischer, A.; Griscelli, C., et al. "Possible Transmission of a Human Lymphotropic Retrovirus (LAV) from Mother to Infant with AIDS." *Lancet* 1:229–230.

33. Pinching, op. cit.

34. Stewart, G. J.; Cunningham, A. L.; Driscoll, G. L.; Tyler, J. P. P., et al. "Transmission of Human T-Cell Lymphotropic Virus Type III (HTLV-III) by Artificial Insemination by Donor." *Lancet* II(8455):581–584 (Sept. 14, 1985).

35. Entwistle, C. C. "Prevention of AIDS." *Lancet*:1364 (Dec. 14, 1985).

36. Lundberg, George D. "The Age of AIDS: A Great Time for Defensive Living" (Editorial). *JAMA* 253(23):3440–3441 (June 21, 1985).

37. Pinching, op. cit.

38. Ancelle, R.; Asaad, F.; Borgucci, P. V., et al. *Bulletin of the World Health Organization* 63(4):667–672 (1985).

39. Luzi, G.; Ensoli, B.; Turbessi, G., et al. "Transmission of HTLV-III Infection by Heterosexual Contact." *Lancet* II(8462):1018 (Nov. 2, 1985).

40. Masur, H.; Michelis, M. A.; Wromser, G. P., et al. "Opportunistic Infection in Previously Healthy Women: Initial Manifestations of a Community Acquired Cellular Immunodeficiency." *Annals Internal Medicine* 97:533–539 (1982).

CHAPTER 7

An Ethics of Compassion, A Language of Division: Working out the AIDS Metaphors

JUDITH WILSON ROSS

THE AIDS METAPHORS

Each new issue in medical ethics produces a near avalanche of journal articles, newspaper editorials, and television appearances by medical ethics specialists, replete with detailed arguments about the right and wrong way to think as well as to act. This hasn't happened with AIDS. There has been much scientific writing and considerable editorial page pontificating, but, until very recently, not much serious ethical analysis, especially from the bioethics community.[1] This reluctance suggests the thorny nature of the ethical problems related to AIDS, particularly those concerning justice and fairness.

What have been proposed, however, are punitive and hostile actions where all the burdens would be borne by one group of people and all the benefits accrue to another group. William F. Buckley's proposal to tattoo all people with AIDS as well as all asymptomatic individuals infected with the human immunodeficiency virus (HIV)[2] is but one example of this kind of thinking.[3] Public opinion polls have reported that a majority of respondents believe that quarantine—even if lifelong—is appropriate for those who have been infected with HIV.[4] This, too, exemplifies an acceptance of actions that are neither just or fair. The extremity of these proposals—given what is known about the disease and its means of transmission—suggests that the general attitude about AIDS is irrational and not based on ordinary concerns with right and wrong.

Most people receive their information about this disease from the popular literature—TV, newspapers, and the general-circulation weekly and monthly magazines—not from academic journals, CDC (Centers for Disease Control) reports, physicians with practical experience, AIDS education groups, or the AIDS research community. The academic and policy-making communities are both publicly silent about the ethical implications of various actions. Only gay community representatives have consistently addressed ethical issues, but these writers are often seen to be acting solely from self-interest. For the most part, the popular media are setting the terms by which the public perceives this disease.

One need not look at popular media, however, to realize that much of what is increasingly being termed "the AIDS hysteria" is born of fear. Originally, the fear was produced in part from the fact that large numbers of people were dying from an infectious disease that medical science was so powerless to halt. Each year more people die from other diseases than from AIDS. Fifty-four thousand people die in automobile accidents annually—a risk everyone takes each time he or she climbs into a car—but no hysteria drives a public demand for safer cars or lower speed limits. The hysteria generated by AIDS is not just a fear of death. It is also a fear of the unknown.

AIDS is a new disease, at first inexplicable and thus strange. The immediately suggested parallels are historic ones (bubonic plague, influenza epidemics, leprosy). There is no place in our personal memories for these diseases (not, at least, for most Americans under the age of 70) and these historical realities leave little mark beyond linguistic relics ("I'd avoid him like he had leprosy" or "I'd avoid it like the plague"). As a result, AIDS presents itself to this culture as a new phenomenon, not just another difficult disease in a long line of difficult diseases.[5] Its newness means that we have to find a way to conceptualize it. Like the Cargo Cult people who had to create a narrative to explain the existence of World War II planes that dropped industrial world goods into a primitive culture, we need to create a story that explains AIDS to us.[6]

The narrative of a new event is not developed consciously, but coalesces over time as connections (whether accurate or not) are made between known phenomena and the new incident. With AIDS, parallels were promptly drawn in journalistic coverage to plague and leprosy. Beyond this, however, writers frequently adopted a metaphorical style of writing that showed the AIDS phenomenon as part of a more familiar story: AIDS as death, AIDS as punishment for sin, AIDS as crime, AIDS as an enemy occasioning a war, and AIDS as otherness (i.e., a means of dividing the world into two entirely separate segments). Some writers used a single metaphor, others used several, even within one article. The metaphors were common enough and frequent enough to create a single narrative in which AIDS is both a crime against others, a crime deserving punishment, and also a punishment, by death, for those who have divided the civic unity by violating social rules. As Lakoff and Johnson have pointed out, "language is an important source of evidence for what [our conceptual] system is like."[7] In the case of AIDS, these metaphors tell us a great deal about how AIDS fits into our world picture. Within the metaphors lies a fuller justification for many of the actions and policies that have been reported or proposed.[8]

When Susan Sontag analyzed social attitudes toward tuberculosis and cancer in *Illness as Metaphor,* she claimed that discovering the cause of tuberculosis had stripped the disease of its metaphoric existence, with the implication that cancer, too, would lose its metaphors if we understood it better as a physiological phenomenon.[9] This implication has not been borne out for AIDS. Despite the remarkably rapid discovery of the viral etiology and modes of transmission, the metaphors of AIDS have persisted, suggesting an extremely powerful underlying narrative that facts alone will be unlikely to dispel.

It has long been recognized that metaphor is a powerful tool of rhetoric. Metaphor is used to highlight similarities between two otherwise different objects, events, individuals, and so on. Thus, to say that AIDS is a plague or that the person with AIDS is a modern-day leper is to make a statement based on a limited number of parallels between the two. Unfortunately, the metaphor does not include an elaboration of which specific aspects of the two are the same nor how many similar aspects there are. Although the speaker and the audience may agree that AIDS is a modern-day plague, the statement probably has many different meanings to different members of the audience. To illustrate this, let us look briefly at some commonly known and salient characteristics of plague: it is a disease with a very high death rate; death often occurs very quickly after exposure to the disease; it can spread rapidly —within weeks—throughout a population; because of its contagiousness through casual contact, those with the disease should be avoided; it has existed throughout recorded history, appearing and then disappearing without any explanation for its sudden outbreaks; those with the disease along with their families have been locked up in houses (quarantine and isolation); and its transmission includes insect and animal vectors (rodents, fleas). When the speaker says that AIDS is a modern-day plague, which (if any) of these characteristics does he have in mind? Strictly speaking none is necessarily accurate; the death rate from HIV infection (which is the disease) is high (20–30%, perhaps), but not uniformly fatal, as is often claimed and as pneumonic plague is still likely to be. Death, if it occurs at all, does not occur rapidly. Those with full-blown AIDS live about one to two years after diagnosis.[10] It does not spread very rapidly within a population because it is not spread by casual contact as is plague. Thus, there is no reason to avoid ordinary contact with those who have the infection nor to lock them away in quarantine or isolation. It is apparently a brand new virus and does not appear to involve animal or insect vectors.

When metaphor is used in this unadorned fashion (i.e., without any further clarification as to which aspects of the metaphor source are being isolated and asserted as parallels), the audience is invited to "fill in the blanks," as it were, making as many parallels as seem useful to their personal psychology without concern for factual accuracy. Herein lies the great danger of the metaphor: used casually, as it almost always is, it easily becomes (or, more accurately, is perceived to be) an analogue or a model. The plague, as a metaphor for AIDS, suggests that the two diseases have one or more important things in common. When plague becomes an analogue for AIDS, it is seen as having many, even most characteristics in common. When it is perceived as a model, it is perceived as sharing all relevant features.

AIDS shares a very few important characteristics with the plague or with leprosy, yet both are used so commonly as metaphors and as implicit analogies that it is difficult to recall their many differences. The characteristic that unites the three most strongly is the fear people have of all of them, but the truth of that commonality lies more in human psychology than in the essential nature of the diseases.

When more complex metaphors are used to characterize AIDS, the possibility of more far-reaching misstatements about the disease arises. Thus, although identifying AIDS with plague or leprosy permits a limited number of erroneous implications about the nature of the disease, a metaphor like death, sin, or crime is much more pervasive and much more dangerous.

The metaphor of AIDS as personified death is evoked by those who say they "lost" friends or lovers to AIDS, by those with the disease who ask, "Why did it get me?", by writers who characterize the disease as "striking entire families." This methaphor shows AIDS as a powerful and independent figure choosing its victims. AIDS as death includes a sense of immediateness. As a matter of fact, many people with AIDS live for months and even years, for the most part outside the hospital. Those who are infected by the virus may never be ill or may develop chronic illness that is not fatal. Yet to have AIDS or to have the AIDS virus are equally to be claimed by death within this metaphor. The metaphor of AIDS as death permits us to dismiss all of those who have been infected by HIV, whether they have AIDS, ARC, or are asymptomatic presumed carriers; they are dead to us. When this metaphor is filled out, it tells us that we need not worry about the feelings of those with AIDS or HIV when deciding how to act toward them because they are effectively, if not actually, dead.

The metaphor of AIDS as death contributes to and coexists happily with the metaphor of AIDS as punishment for sin. When Death comes to look for victims, it must have some principle of choice. We are uncomfortable with death as a random event. Those whom death has chosen to visit (or their families, or even perfect strangers) may ask "Why was I (or he/she) chosen? What have I (or he/she) done to deserve this?" The personified death that chooses its victims is seen within this metaphor/narrative as a punisher. The punishment is Death's choice itself: death is the punishment for sin. Those who are chosen look to see what sin they have committed that justifies this selection; those who have not been chosen look to see what they have *not* done in order to understand why they have been spared. The metaphor does not permit a description of death from disease as an individual-neutral event. It does not encompass the notion that a virus will flourish if it finds itself in conditions that permit it to do so. HIV does not flourish because it finds itself in homosexual relationships, in multiple sexual partnerships, in IV drug users, or in illegal activities. It is simply a virus doing its job. Because it is a virus doing its job, anyone who comes into contact with the virus may find him/herself suffering the effects of the virus's "job."

As Susan Sontag noted in *Illness as Metaphor,* metaphor permits and even encourages giving "disease a meaning—that meaning being invariably a moral one."[11] The metaphor of sin says that those who are infected have the virus *because* they were engaged in specific activities of which many people do not approve. They are, thus, "responsible" for their disease: they "deserve" it. The disease is *their* problem, not the problem of those who do not take part in the disapproved behavior (be it drug use, homosexual acts, or "promiscuous sex," whatever that may mean to the disapproving individual). In addition, the AIDS story created by Death as Punishment for Sin means not only that those who have the virus deserve their fate but also that those who have not engaged in the disapproved behavior are safe from the disease. Death does not visit the righteous. Hence this narrative achieves a double purpose for those who are not infected: they may safely abjure responsibility or concern for those who are infected (because it is their own fault) and they need not worry about their own health.

AIDS as crime is presented in two ways: first, the disease itself is a crime that must be solved. This aspect of the metaphor concentrates on researchers as detectives looking for clues to solve the mystery of AIDS. The AIDS story in this metaphor takes the standard form of the detective story in which the good guys track down the bad guys to stop the continuing crime. The reality of HIV infection doesn't fit this metaphor well and leads to a confusion between whether the "bad guy" is the AIDS virus or the person who carries the virus. The infected individual becomes not only justly punished for his behavior but justly hunted down by others because of his infected status.

The second aspect of the metaphor of AIDS as crime is the disease as supercriminal, a serial murderer who embarks on intercontinental killing sprees. This kind of criminal is so threatening that only the most extreme methods can be used to defeat it. If this disease is a crime, only something bigger, more aggressive, and more powerful than it can be expected to defeat it. Finally, it means fighting crime with crime. Although not referring to AIDS, the advertising campaign for Sylvester Stallone's 1986 movie, *Cobra,* captures the heart of this metaphor/story: "Crime is a disease and Cobra [that is to say, more crime] is the cure." When AIDS is seen as a major crime, it is easy to accept that only a bigger criminal and greater violence can defeat it. Thus, punitive and hostile actions appear to be justified and even necessary in "tracking down" and "defeating" the disease (and its carriers).

The metaphor of medicine as war is so common that we can scarcely imagine any other way of talking about how health care providers deal with diseases and patients. It is commonly said that medicine's job is to fight disease (as opposed to preventing illness). When the practice of medicine becomes war (and the phrase "the war against AIDS" is perhaps the most common metaphor used in the popular press), then the patient becomes the battlefield. When transmission of disease involves an infected carrier, especially an infected asymptomatic carrier, then the metaphor-become-analogue/model of AIDS as war makes the carrier a spy and a traitor. Traitors and spies are internal enemies for whom capital punishment is justified. The enemies are now clearly identified: the virus is the external (foreign) enemy, the carrier the internal (traitorous) enemy. Defeating or capturing one enemy also involves defeating or capturing the other one. Ordinarly we don't worry much about the civil rights of foreigners or enemies and, in time of war, there is certainly no room for such concerns.

The final AIDS metaphor, the metaphor of otherness, is perhaps less an independent metaphor than the result of the previous four: those who are dead, those who are sinners, those who are criminals, and those who are enemy-harboring traitors. These are "the others," outside the general population, as so many speakers and writers have commented.[12] The sense of otherness is demonstrated in the way in which people talk about what "we should do about them" (i.e., those who are infected by HIV). The constant use of the terms leper and leprosy in referring to HIV infection and people with AIDS continually reinforces this sense of otherness, for the leper is perhaps the most persistent and widespread instance we have of human exile. The leper is traditionally outside the human community, both physically and spiritually. He/she is truly seen as something different and "other" than us, for the life of isolation with the sole prospect of slow death has deprived the leper of relationship—that which defines the human community. By enclosing people with HIV infection firmly in the story of otherness and of leprosy, we can treat them less generously, less compassionately, and less fairly. In the same way that foreigners—a different kind of "other"—are seen as ineligible for the constitutional protections guaranteed to American citizens, those with HIV infection can be denied more basic rights derived not from law but from the requirements of human decency.

Metaphors and their encompassing analogue narratives do not merely play themselves out in journalism and dinner table conversation; they play themselves out in real life, in actions that affect other people. The stories on AIDS and HIV infection that hold our attention can influence our thinking and our actions. All five of these metaphors encourage a denial of respect for persons, the single most important principle upon which our ethical analyses are based. Whether the issue is caring for patients with AIDS and ARC, supporting seropositives who are asymptomatic, or providing HIV testing, metaphors that characterize an individual as apart, guilty, and as good as dead will encourage unethical responses; the person is not, in reality, different, guilty, or dead.

THE METAPHORS IN PRACTICE

Care of Patients with AIDS and ARC

The vast number of health care providers who work with AIDS patients have undoubtedly given the best possible care to their patients, which was especially commendable during that period when it was not clear whether the health care worker was at substantial risk of contracting the disease from the patients. Nevertheless, beginning around 1983, there have been numerous stories of failure to provide appropriate care for patients with AIDS because of their perceived difference. Hospitals have refused admission to people with AIDS or shipped them unceremoniously to other hospitals; anesthesiologists have been unwilling to administer anesthesia to them; surgeons have refused to perform lung biopsies; nursing and dietary aides have refused to enter patients' rooms; patients have been unnecessarily isolated within hospitals; nurses have refused to care for them; pathologists have refused to perform autopsies; hospital staff members have insisted upon wearing extraordinary amounts of protective equipment; internists have refused to perform endoscopies; unwritten hospital policies have denied ICU care; AIDS patients have borne the burden of cost constraints by being denied expensive care since they are expected to die anyway; dialysis has been denied for patients with both acute renal failure and chronic end stage renal disease; information about AIDS patients has been bandied about the hospital and beyond its confines as choice gossip; and, most recently, medical students have begun to shy away from internships and residencies at hospitals where there is a substantial AIDS patient census. These responses are all encouraged and even made sensible by the divisive metaphors of AIDS.

Repeated studies have demonstrated the minimal risk that patients with AIDS pose to health care workers if the providers take appropriate protective steps.[13] AIDS and ARC patients are, of course, entitled to all the care and services necessary for their illness and one can hope that as information about the minimal risk permeates the health care professions instances of inappropriate denial of treatment or provision of uncaring treatment will disappear. Staff education, however, tends to be provided at a technical level and is unlikely to alter the intense emotional holding power of the metaphor/narratives that the media have furthered. Most hospitals have had little experience with AIDS patients and thus there is no great impetus for providing any education. Furthermore, many hospitals report that when AIDS education programs are given, few attend.

Hospital ethics committees are increasingly concerned about how to deal with ethical questions surrounding treatment of patients with AIDS, ARC, or positive antibody results. It is not clear what role committees can play in addressing the issues when there are so many conflicting messages being sent.

What, for example, is the ethics committee to say about the commitment to confidentiality when every employee is insisting upon knowing which patients are HIV positive and which are not? Should hospital employees be expected always to use appropriate protective measures when exposed to patient secretions and body fluids? Or must the patients submit to the release of antibody status information, regardless of how stigmatizing it may be, so that the health care workers need only use protective measures when they know they may be at risk? The metaphors that reduce the patient's entitlement to rights leave ample room for insisting that the patient take the risk of stigmatization while the health care provider accepts the benefits of increased convenience and reduced personal anxiety.

Beyond the question of risk to health care providers, however, there are a number of difficult ethical issues that education alone cannot solve. The question of how much treatment the AIDS patient should receive is not limited to medical/technical analysis. Policies—personal or institutional, written or unwritten—that deny ICU care to all AIDS patients are ethically questionable. The metaphor of AIDS as death encourages this view since, the unspoken argument goes, a patient who is as good as dead need not be treated. The President of the Society for the Right to Die, Mrs. A. J. Levinson, was recently quoted in *The New York Times* as saying that "The only good thing to come out of the AIDS epidemic is that many more doctors are thinking twice before doing everything they can to, for instance, cure pneumonia in an AIDS patients. Do these patients want to be cured of pneumonia now so that they can certainly die of AIDS next year?"[14] It would certainly seem more than possible that *even* AIDS patients might like another year of life, especially when that year will probably be spent, for the most part, outside the hospital. There is still a real possibility for what is increasingly being called "quality life." Levinson, however, appears to regard those with AIDS as already dead; the metaphors sustain her attitude.

In a similar vein, R. M. Wachter, a resident at San Francisco General Hospital, reported that AIDS patients were increasingly refusing intensive care and respirator care.[15] He believed that they were being encouraged to do so by physicians who had become seriously depressed by the prospect of so many young patients dying. As a result, housestaff were, perhaps, endorsing patients' refusal of life-prolonging treatment in order to "get it over with quickly."[16] But Wachter, unlike Levinson, sensed that there was something wrong with this, that it was not a celebration of the right to die.

In another San Francisco-based study, clinician-researchers Steinbrook, Lo, Tirpack, and associates, found that people with AIDS significantly overestimated the effectiveness of ICU care in saving the lives of patients with Pneumocystis carinii pneumonia.[17] Yet, they too claimed that more and more patients were refusing life-sustaining care. This apparent contradiction may have a reasonable explanation—for example, those with AIDS may believe that ICU care will prolong their lives but don't want their lives extended because they believe the quality of their lives is too poor. It is also possible, however, that patients are being implicitly or explicitly discouraged from requesting or consenting to life-prolonging treatment (including treatment available in the ICU) by someone else's judgment that their quality of life is not worth maintaining or that the financial cost to the hospital is too high. Since they are as good as dead, since we owe them nothing, there is no need to prolong their lives, suggest the metaphors.

Fortunately, in California, the legislature has provided a solid mechanism by which the patient can control his medical care even when he is no longer competent. Because AIDS involves a considerable risk of central nervous system involvement and thus possible dementia and incompetence, the Durable Power of Attorney for Health Care is an important tool for the patient. In addition, because so many of the AIDS patients are gay men living in nontraditional family arrangements, it is particularly important for them to name the person whom they wish to make decisions for them. Nevertheless, Steinbrook, Lo, Moulton, and associates, found in a second study, that many physicians are not discussing this issue with their patients, even though the patients would like to discuss it.[18] Many patients have not signed durable power statements, perhaps because they do not know about them. Initiating discussion of this issue is extremely difficult, of course, and it appears that such discussion may be avoided unless conscious steps are taken. San Francisco General Hospital has a policy that requires discussing the durable power of attorney with all AIDS patients within 48 hours of their initial admission.[19] Other hospitals, however, are not as aggressive in pursuing this problem. Physicians are frequently reluctant to discuss the use of advance directives such as living wills, natural death acts, or durable powers of attorney with any patient, but this reluctance is so overwhelming with AIDS patients that there must be some deeply seated emotional pull that keeps them from doing so.

Providing or forgoing life-sustaining treatment for AIDS patients has all the ordinary difficulties involved in making such a decision with the added problems of the patient's mental competence to make decisions, and potential conflicts between the patient's family and lover or friends about what the patient would have wanted. The metaphors make it easier for families and caregivers to reject treatment. Although that may be what the patient too, would have chosen, without clear evidence we will only be guessing or imposing our own preferences. To circumvent these problems, hospitals may have to provide special training for certain employees, to ensure that advance directives are discussed with AIDS patients.

Advice to Individuals Who Are Seropositive and Asymptomatic

Asymptomatic seropositive individuals are currently presumed to be infectious (although they may not be) and this presumed infectiousness is thought to be a permanent condition. Issues of particular concern to health care workers with respect to asymptomatic seropositives include: what advice should be given to seropositive pregnant women, to seropositive women who may wish to become pregnant, and to seropositive individuals in general; what responsibilities does the physician have for protecting sexual partners of those who are seropositive; and should some kind of restrictions be applied to seropositive health care providers?

The problem of pregnant seropositive women is not entirely new as there are substantial parallels in genetically transmitted diseases. The infant of a pregnant seropositive woman will not inevitably have AIDS. Assuming that abortion is an ethically acceptable choice, standard ethical analysis would not maintain that abortion was obligatory or even necessarily appropriate since there is some possibility that the abortion will be performed on a fetus that does not and will not have the virus or ensuing disease.[20] Nevertheless, many public heath officers and physicians have suggested that seropositive women should not become pregnant, implying that *they* perceive the risk of the child's contracting AIDS too great to be taken.[21] It would logically follow, then, that abortion would be the appropriate response to pregnancy in these circumstances, and a San Francisco Health Commission Task Force (chaired by pediatrician Moses Grossman) recommended "encouraging abortion for newly pregnant women infected by the AIDS virus."[22] Influenced as we all are by the images the metaphors encourage, it may be difficult to be neutral. We may agree that no one should risk giving birth to a child with AIDS, for it would be like giving birth to a nonhuman. Health care providers may make recommendations against pregnancy and for abortion and sterilization rather than provide information that would allow women to weigh the risks and benefits and to make their own, informed choices.

The physician's responsibility for protecting third parties—especially sexual partners of seropositive individuals—is a very thorny issue. The legal parallel is the *Tarasoff* duty to take appropriate steps to protect known, threatened third parties from dangerous patients in psychotherapy. If a physician knows that a seropositive patient is not informing his/her sexual contacts of the risk, does the physician have a duty to inform that person(s)? Several writers maintain that there is such a duty but suggest that the duty may be met by informing public health authorities.[23] However, if it is generally known that the public health authorities are not conducting contact-tracing, does that end the physician's duty? This issue is going to become increasingly troublesome, but the AIDS metaphors will advise always acting to protect others—the third parties. That is because, within the metaphors, the patient with HIV does not merit consideration, his/her responses, needs, and concerns are not relevant, given the underlying fault/guilt and the need to stop the disease/crime.

The Public Health Service has issued recommendations for counseling individuals who are asymptomatic but seropositive.[24] They include informing past and future sexual partners of seropositive status, informing medical and dental workers of seropositivity, refraining from donating blood, and using "safe sex" practices.[25] There is relatively little disagreement about these recommendations but it may be unrealistic to expect people who are already deeply distressed by their seropositive status to respond affirmatively to these guidelines. Paul Volberding, one of the most experienced clinicians in the country with respect to AIDS, has said that informing a patient that he or she is seropositive is as anxiety-provoking as telling him/her that he/she has AIDS.[26] Given the enormous impact of this information, how will the individual respond to the advice that is given? Telling others of seropositive status—whether professionals, acquaintances, friends, family members, or lovers—risks extraordinary ostracization. Furthermore, the news will almost inevitably be circulated to yet a broader group of people. One may expect confidentiality to be honored within the medical field (even if practice does not meet expectations), but no such expectation exists in the social environment. Very little is known about how to provide these recommendations in a way that will encourage and support compliance. Not much attention has been paid to the inevitable psychological denial that will accompany the receipt of such devastating news. There is, somehow, the assumption that "they" will behave as "we" want them to, even though "we" do not think too much about what sacrifices and burdens that behavior entails.

Seropositive health care workers are not usually seen to pose a particular threat to patients because the primary modes of transmission are sexual intercourse and blood exchange. However, some writers have argued that seropositive health care providers should not be permitted to conduct invasive procedures if there is *any* risk of blood contamination. Health care providers' desire to know about patients' positive antibody status is mirrored by the less-discussed issue of whether patients have a right to know about the positive antibody status of their physician, nurse, or technician. As to the former, there are several pieces of legislation that have recently been introduced in California that would allow all those directly involved in the patient's care to have access to antibody status information. As to the latter, patients will probably not be able legally to have access to information about their health care providers. Nevertheless, the ethical dimension of this question remains and one could surely speculate about whether the metaphors of AIDS, focused as they now are around IV drug users and gay men, will spill over to health care workers who are seropositive, even if they are not members of high risk groups. Recent reports of an unusual delay by the CDC in issuing guidelines about health care providers who are antibody positive and their obligations to their patients suggests that this may already be happening.[27]

Providing HIV Testing

When the HIV antibody test was introduced in March 1985, there were widespread announcements that the function of the test was to screen blood, not persons. However, the test is being increasingly used or recommended for screening people. Currently, the following groups of people are being screened: all members of the military, all military applicants, U.S. military academy students, all blood and plasma donors, all organ and tissue donors, all sperm donors, and, in Nevada, Colorado, Iowa, and Missouri, prisoners.[28] In addition, the following is but a partial list of groups who have been suggested as appropriate for either mandatory screening or routinely recommended voluntary screening: health care workers, health care workers who perform invasive procedures, dialysis patients, pregnant women, patients in hospitals, applicants for marriage licenses, children placed for adoption or foster care whose mothers may be in high risk groups, college students, all members of high risk groups and their sexual partners, hemophiliacs and their sexual partners, candidates for organ transplant, prisoners, prostitutes, patients in chemical dependency hospital units, attendees at sexually transmitted disease clinics, applicants to drug diversion programs, transfusion recipients (prior to March 1985), all women with more than one sexual partner, and health and life insurance applicants.

The public policy issue of testing revolves around weighing the benefits gained by individuals' knowing their antibody status and the risks of that information being used against them. So far little is known about what happens to individuals who are asymptomatic and antibody positive: that is, what benefits accrue to others if the seropositive person chooses "alternative behaviors" to prevent spread of infection, and what social and psychological disadvantages accrue to the individual from knowing their status. As previously noted some physicians have reported that telling a person that he/she is antibody positive is even more psychologically distressing than telling a patient that he/she has AIDS.[29] The general failure in the United States to provide adequate counseling and strong guarantees of confidentiality for those who are found to be seropositive will surely contribute further to this distress. The public fear of anyone who is "tainted" with AIDS may also lead to measures that are extremely harmful to the person who is antibody positive. The benefits from this testing are naturally assumed to be for others, who will then be able to avoid exposure to the virus.

The debate on this issue—which is extremely intense—focuses on whether the burden of preventing the spread of infection should be placed on those who are seropositive or on those who are not. Should those who are presumed to have the virus protect others by changing their sexual behaviors and informing their prospective sexual partners of their antibody status, or should those who are presumed not to have the virus protect themselves by changing *their* sexual behaviors and not engaging in practices that will put themselves at risk? Do you have a duty to find out whether you are seropositive and, if you are, to then take on the burden of protecting others? Or do you have a duty to take on the burden of protecting yourself from risking infection, from becoming seropositive? The divisive metaphors of AIDS make it easy to place the burden of knowledge, stigmatization, and significantly altered behavior exclusively on the "others," on those who are separate and different and who have, in the language of the metaphor, placed "us" at risk because of their sinful and criminal activities. Thus, many health care providers are much more interested in finding out patients' antibody status than in insisting that everyone practice appropriate infection control procedures.

RESOLVING THE METAPHORS

If we are to think about what is just and what is fair in dealing with the complex public and personal issues that the human immunodeficiency virus brings to us, it is necessary first to clear our minds and our language of the metaphors that so easily lead to punitive actions at the individual, the professional, and the government level. Justice and fairness require that if there are to be burdens and benefits, they should be distributed evenly—not all the burdens for those who are seropositive and all the benefits for those who are seronegative.

The metaphors tell a different story, of course. Because they are inherently divisive, they suggest that burdens should be placed on to the guilty, while benefits should go to the innocent. The metaphors emphasize protection of the public health at the expense of the public good. It must be remembered that we are all—sick and well, infected and uninfected—members of that public. The metaphors deny that we live in a human community in which all need to be protected and care for. A culturally accepted story that says one group of people embodies death, sin, crime, war, and otherness is powerful information that suggests that we are not all in this together. Despite the widespread acceptance of these metaphors, they are not necessarily true. Those who are carriers of the HIV virus need to care about and to protect those who are not; those who have not been exposed need to care for and to protect those who have been. It is not that some of "us" need protection and some of "them" need to sacrifice their rights; that some belong to death while others embrace life; that some are righteous and others are sinners; that some are criminals and others their victims; that some are enemies and others loyal and deserving citizens; that some may be cast out, while others are kept securely within. We are all in this together; we are all innocent. Surely those who have been exposed to AIDS have enough to suffer without being victimized by metaphorical myths.

Disease, especially disease that may lead to death, always takes on a dramatic quality. Drama encourages elevated language. A brief stroll through the *Reader's Guide* listings under AIDS will demonstrate the drama that AIDS has provided for readers in the past few years: "Now No One Is Safe," "Battling AIDS," "The Plague Years," "AIDS Panic," "Public Enemy #1," "Death After Sex," "Homosexual Plague Strikes New Victims." The moral meanings of these headlines (and hundreds more) and the metaphors they enclose are shaping public response to this disease. It is giving this disease, as Sontag warned, a moral meaning, but that morality is in our minds not in the disease. If ethical judgments about caring for patients, about restricting viral carriers, and about providing HIV testing are to be based on positive, humane attitudes, it is time to confront the inner meanings our language betrays and then to rid not only our speaking and writing but also our thinking of these metaphors. We cannot begin to consider ethically appropriate responses until we firmly fix in our minds that the over 40,000 Americans with AIDS, the unknown numbers with ARC and lesser illnesses, and the over 1 million currently asymptomatic seropositive individuals are not someone unknown, different, foreign, or alien. They are our friends, our brothers, our sisters, and our children. They are a part of us and, as members of our human community, they *are* us.

NOTES

1. The first articles to deal with ethical issues in a substantial way include *The Hastings Center Report*'s Special Supplement, AIDS: The emerging ethical dilemmas, August 1985; and June Osborn's The AIDS epidemic: Multidisciplinary trouble. *New England Journal of Medicine* 1986:314(12):779–782.

2. HIV (human immunodeficiency virus) is the name chosen by the International Committee on Taxonomy of Viruses to replace the previously used and increasingly confusing names of HTLV-III, LAV, and ARV. See Coffin, J., et al. Human immunodeficiency viruses. *Science* 1986:232:697.

3. Originally published in *The New York Times* and reprinted in the *Los Angeles Daily Journal*, 3/21/86, p. 4.

4. See, for example, the *Los Angeles Times* poll, 12/19/85, §1, pp. 1, 30. Other polls (*Newsweek*, *Time*) have shown similar results.

5. The slowness of perceiving the disease in Africa may, in part, be attributed to the greater prevalence of untreatable disease there, making AIDS just another difficult disease among an abundance of disease.

6. For a discussion of the way in which narratives structure our ethical choices, see Hauerwas, Stanley. *Truthfulness and Tragedy*, University of Notre Dame Press, 1977, especially Chapter 1, "From system to story: an alternative pattern for rationality in ethics."

7. Lakoff, George, and Johnson, Mark, *Metaphors We Live By*, University of Chicago Press, 1980, p. 3.

8. For a fuller discussion of the AIDS metaphors and their sources, see Ross, J. W., Ethics and the language of AIDS, in *AIDS: Ethics and Public Policy*, edited by Pierce and vanDeVeer, Wadsworth, in press.

9. Sontag, S. *Illness as Metaphor*. NY: Vintage Books, 1979.

10. Figures on survival after diagnosis vary somewhat depending upon category patient group, and date selections. For example, San Francisco General Hospital reports a survival time of 21 months from time of diagnosis for those with Kaposi's sarcoma (*Medical Tribune* 1985 July:26(19)3, whereas Landesman et al., report a figure of 224 days from the date of first hospitalization with opportunistic infection (Landesman, S. H.; Ginzburg, H. M.; Weiss, S. H. The AIDS epidemic. *New England Journal of Medicine* 1985:312(8):521–524).

11. Sontag, S. *Illness as Metaphor*.

12. Margaret Heckler was the first to receive wide publicity for using this aspect of the meta-phor when she said that "we must conquer [AIDS] as well before it threatens the health of our general population." As quoted in *Journal of the American Medical Association* (*AMA*) 1985:253(23):3377. Subsequently, it has been commonly used by many speakers and writers.

13. For a discussion of risk to health care providers, see McCray, E. Occupational risk of the acquired immunodeficiency syndrome among health care workers. *New England Journal of Medicine* 1986 April 24:314(17):1127–1132.

14. The *New York Times*, 3/17/86, pp. 1, 13.

15. Wachter, R. M. The impact of the acquired immunodeficiency syndrome on medical residency training. *New England Journal of Medicine* 1985:314(3):177–179.

16. Wachter is not the only one to express this concern. Susan Light, M.D., discussing her feelings about forgoing treatment (for patients other than those with AIDS) as a house staff physician, comments that "I wanted it [i.e., their death] to be over so I would not have to be faced daily with our 'failure' and the visible grief of the family." Letters, *Journal of the AMA*. 1986:255(22):3113.

17. Steinbrook, R.; Lo, B.; Tirpack, J., et al. Ethical dilemmas in caring for patients with the acquired immunodeficiency syndrome. *Annals of Internal Medicine* 1985:103(5):787–790.

18. Steinbrook, R.; Lo, B.; Moulton, J., et al. Preferences of homosexual men with AIDS for life-sustaining treatment. *New England Journal of Medicine* 1985;314(7):457–460.

19. Wachter, R. M. The impact of the acquired immunodeficiency syndrome on medical residency training.

20. Risk figures are reported from 0% to 65%. Recommendations for assisting in the prevention of perinatal transmission of HTLV-III/LAC and AIDS. *Morbidity and Mortality Weekly Report* 6 Dec 1985:34(48):722.

21. The Centers for Disease Control states that "infected women should be advised to consider delaying pregnancy. . ." Ibid., 725.

22. *Los Angeles Times*, 1/6/86, §1, p. 2.

23. See, for example, Mills, M.; Wofsy, C. B., Mills, J. Infection control and public health law. *New England Journal of Medicine* 1986:314(14):931–936.

24. *Morbidity and Mortality Weekly Report* 1985:34:1–5.

25. Centers for Disease Control. Additional recommendations to reduce sexual and drug abuse-related transmission of human T-lymphotropic virus Type III/lymphadenopathy-associated virus. *Morbidity and Mortality Weekly Report* 1986:35(10):152–155.

26. Norbert Rapoza, reporting Volberding's comments, *Journal of the AMA* 1985:253(23): 3463–3465.

27. Newsline. *Physician's Management*. May 1986:26(5):15.

28. Glasbrenner, K. Prisons confront dilemmas of inmates with AIDS. *Journal of the AMA* 1986:255(18):2399–2400, 2404.

29. See, for example, the *Los Angeles Times*, AIDS testing dilemmas: To know or not to know, 4/1/86, pp. 1, 10.

CHAPTER 8

AIDS Overview

PAUL A. VOLBERDING

INTRODUCTION

Since first observed in 1981, the acquired immune deficiency syndrome (AIDS), has become an enormous medical, social, and political problem that requires major commitments of human and financial resources to resolve. As a new disease that primarily affects young adults and that has very high mortality, AIDS has generated intense public and medical interest. Under pressure to act as quickly as possible to find a cure or vaccine for AIDS, medical researchers have sometimes been overly optimistic about the implications of their findings. As a consequence, the public and people with AIDS have sometimes been misdirected toward false hopes or confused by revised interpretations based on new data. Although a cure or a vaccine has not yet been found, much has been learned about the epidemiology, routes of transmission, natural history, and clinical manifestations of AIDS. We now know that the life-threatening diseases associated with AIDS are end-stage manifestations of infection with the human immunodeficiency virus (HIV). As we learn more about the life cycle of HIV, it is becoming possible to develop and test antiviral drugs and immune system modulators to halt progression of the retroviral infection and correct the immune deficiency.

DEFINITION OF AIDS

The Centers for Disease Control (CDC) defined AIDS for surveillance purposes as a syndrome characterized by unusual opportunistic infections and rare malignancies in otherwise healthy individuals with no other reason for immune system compromise.[1] Although somewhat restrictive, this definition enabled public health officials to monitor the rapidly expanding AIDS epidemic even before its cause was known.

In 1983–84 the retrovirus that causes the underlying immunodeficiency

97

was independently identified by researchers in France and the United States. Variously called LAV by Luc Montagnier of the Pasteur Institute,[2] HTLV-III by Robert Gallo of the National Institutes of Health,[3] and ARV by Jay Levy of the University of California, San Francisco,[4] the retrovirus was renamed in 1986 by an international committee on nomenclature[5] and is now known as HIV. Once the virus was cultured and sensitive viral antibody tests were developed, it became possible to understand much more fully the nature, transmission, and epidemiology of AIDS and related clinical syndromes.

HIV infection produces a spectrum of clinical manifestations ranging from no symptoms in some infected individuals to rapid disease progression in others, with death from opportunistic infections or rare malignancies. Within this clinical spectrum, several syndromes have been defined, including the persistent generalized lymphadenopathy syndrome (PGL),[6-8] the AIDS-related complex (ARC),[9,10] and the acquired immune deficiency syndrome (AIDS).[11-13] At first thought to represent discrete manifestations of response to the virus, these syndromes are now understood to be clinical stages of progressive retroviral damage to the immune system.

The CDC recently proposed a new classification system for HIV infection, in which the clinical manifestations of AIDS are categorized as Stage IVC (secondary infectious diseases) and Stage IVD (secondary malignancies).[14] The CDC surveillance definition of AIDS may soon be extended to include severe wasting (Stage IVA, constitutional disease) and dementia (Stage IVB, neurological disease).

MAGNITUDE OF THE EPIDEMIC IN THE UNITED STATES

In the United States more than 35,000 AIDS cases and more than 20,000 AIDS deaths have been recorded.[15] By the end of 1991, these numbers are expected to increase to 270,000 cases and 179,000 deaths.[16] Because the AIDS-related complex (ARC) is not currently a reportable condition in this country, the actual number of people with symptoms of acquired immune deficiency not included in the surveillance definition for AIDS is unknown. However, it is estimated that 10 times the number of people with AIDS may have ARC.

When AIDS was first described in 1981, 95% of cases were among homosexual or bisexual males; today, that percentage has fallen to about 73% of all AIDS cases. Intravenous drug users (IVDUs) account for approximately 17% of cases. Recently, the CDC has begun to differentiate in its reporting between homosexual and bisexual men who are not intravenous drug users (66%) and those who are (8%). Combining homosexual and heterosexual AIDS patients who have a history of intravenous drug use, 25% of AIDS patients may be classified in this group. With evidence of rapid spread of HIV among IVDUs in certain cities,[17–21] the proportion of AIDS cases in this risk group may be expected to increase in future years.

Although white males are disproportionately represented among AIDS cases overall, more than two-thirds of heterosexual IVDUs with AIDS and three-quarters of the children with AIDS are black or Hispanic.[22] The majority of pediatric AIDS cases result from perinatal transmission from infected mothers who are themselves IVDUs or the sexual partners of IVDUs. In the United States, 8% of AIDS cases are women and 92% are men, but in Central Africa, where AIDS has been transmitted primarily among heterosexuals, the ratio of male to female cases is 1.1 male to 1.0 female. To date, only 4% of AIDS cases in the United States have resulted from heterosexual contact, but this percentage is expected to increase by 1991.

The case fatality rate for AIDS is 50%, which means that at any given time approximately half the people diagnosed with AIDS have died. Among patients with the opportunistic infections and rare cancers included in the CDC surveillance definition of AIDS, the two-year mortality approaches 90% and the ultimate mortality is close to 100%.[23] In patients with ARC the two-year mortality is still low, but as many of these patients progress to AIDS, the ultimate mortality may be quite high.

The magnitude of the epidemic is most apparent when measured on a local scale. In San Francisco, a city of 700,000 people, 3,300 AIDS cases have already been reported and 18,000 cumulative cases are expected by the early 1990s. In the cities and hospitals where the majority of AIDS cases are diagnosed and treated, health care resources and systems are already overburdened by the complex medical, psychological, and social needs of AIDS patients. Estimates of the average lifetime costs of care per AIDS patient range from $50,000 to $150,000.[24–26] Costs are lower at San Francisco General Hospital, where a comprehensive system of AIDS patient care was developed. The San Francisco General Hospital model emphasizes coordination among multidisciplinary medical, psychosocial, and nursing staff in an outpatient care setting, integration of inpatient and outpatient care, and close cooperation with voluntary, community agencies in providing psychosocial support, home care, and educational services.[27,28] Lifetime hospital charges at this hospital are about $30,000,[29] but when out-of-hospital costs are included, the cost of care is probably $50,000 to $70,000.

Evidence is accumulating that a majority of people with HIV infection will eventually manifest some symptoms of disease[30,31] and more than half may progress to ARC or AIDS (G. Rutherford, personal communication, 1987). Since 1 to 2 million people in the United States may currently be infected with HIV, and millions more in Africa and other nations, the full impact of AIDS in terms of morbidity, mortality, and socioeconomic costs has only begun to be felt.

TRANSMISSION OF HIV

HIV is transmitted by blood and by direct contact of genital or rectal mucosa with infected semen or vaginal secretions. Although HIV may be found in virtually any body fluid, only blood, semen, and vaginal and cervical secretions are thought to be important in viral transmission. HIV has been detected in saliva and tears, but there is no evidence that the virus is transmitted through these fluids.

Sexual transmission of the virus can occur through vaginal, anal, and possibly oral intercourse. Infected males can transmit the virus to male or female sexual partners, and infected females can transmit the virus sexually to males and perinatally to their unborn infants. Although it is theoretically possible for females to transmit the virus to female sexual partners, lesbians who are not bisexual and do not use intravenous drugs are considered to be at low risk for HIV infection.

In the United States, viral transmission through blood transfusion is less problematic now that blood is being tested for HIV antibodies. However, among intravenous drug users, blood-borne transmission takes place through sharing hypodermic syringes contaminated with infected blood. Because infected intravenous drug users also can transmit the virus sexually, this group may constitute a bridge for viral transmission into the wider heterosexual population.

Health care workers have been concerned about the risks of occupational infection with HIV. Recently, three cases of occupational transmission of HIV following mucocutaneous exposure to infected blood were reported to the CDC. In general, however, studies show that the risks of transmission of the virus to health care workers are very low.[32-34] At San Francisco General Hospital, for example, 300 health care workers agreed to be tested for HIV antibodies. Of the 253 health care workers without other risk factors (i.e., heterosexual, non-IV drug users), not one was found to be infected with HIV despite five years of working with hundreds of AIDS patients. Of 84 health care workers who stuck themselves with needles contaminated by HIV-infected blood, none showed evidence of viral infection. Clearly, if health care workers do not become infected with HIV following years of intense, close contact with AIDS patients, the risk to the general public from casual contact with infected individuals is virtually nonexistent. Studies of household contacts of AIDS patients also demonstrate that casual transmission of the virus does not occur.[35-37]

The risk of HIV transmission varies considerably among different populations. Homosexual men and intravenous drug users who share needles are at very high risk for HIV infection. Heterosexuals who have had long-term monogamous sexual relationships and who do not use intravenous drugs or share needles still have a very low risk of HIV infection in most parts of the world. The determinants of an individual's infectiousness or susceptibility to

HIV infection are unknown at this time. The role of possible cofactors, such as concurrent viral infections or venereal diseases, nutrition, and recreational drug use, in facilitating viral transmission or infection also is unclear.

When introduced into a susceptible population, HIV can be spread very rapidly. In San Francisco, serum samples collected in 1978 from a large group of homosexual men with histories of venereal disease were tested retrospectively for HIV antibodies. This cohort has now been followed for several years by the San Francisco Health Department. Although in 1978 only 4% of serum samples had been infected with HIV, by 1984, 50% of this cohort tested seropositive to the virus, and by 1986, 75% were infected.[38] The epidemiology of AIDS in Central African countries and possibly in other parts of the world suggests that heterosexual populations may be as susceptible to rapid infection with HIV as the homosexual population in San Francisco.[39-43] Retrospective studies document rapid spread of HIV among intravenous drug users, as well. In New Jersey, seroprevalence rates among IVDUs rose from 11% in 1977, to 27% in 1979, to 58% in 1984.[44] Similar rates of increase among IVDUs have been reported in European cities[45,46] and in San Francisco.[47]

PATHOGENESIS AND NATURAL HISTORY OF AIDS

Retroviral infection occurs when HIV attaches to the T4 antigen on the surface of a cell. Many cells appear to carry the antigen, including T-helper lymphocytes, macrophages, and possibly glial cells in the central nervous system. It is not yet known whether infection requires exposure to the naked virus or to cells infected with the virus. After penetrating the nucleus of the cell, the retrovirus integrates its genetic material into that of the cell through the action of a unique enzyme, reverse transcriptase, and can begin to replicate itself.

At various lengths of time following infection, HIV begins to destroy the T-helper cell population, possibly by lysing (disintegrating) these cells following viral replication, or by disrupting hormones responsible for normal cell functioning, or by infecting and destroying the stem cells needed to replenish the T-cell population. Although we do not have good measures of immune competence, the absolute number of T-helper cells is often used as a shorthand for measuring the degree of immune damage caused by this virus. As the immune system is destroyed, patients gradually begin to manifest the variety of symptoms collectively referred to as AIDS-related complex, or ARC. With further immune deficiency, opportunistic infections or Kaposi's sarcoma appear as the overt clinical manifestations of AIDS.

HIV may penetrate the central nervous system very early in the disease process. Evidence for this comes from clinical observations of aseptic meningitis in patients who experience the acute retroviral syndrome within a few weeks following infection.[48] The presence of HIV in the central nervous system has been confirmed by viral culture of cerebral spinal fluid.[49] It is not known whether the dementias and neurologic syndromes associated with AIDS are caused directly by viral infection of brain cells or indirectly through the action of lymphokines or other secreted factors in the brain.

Within eight weeks following infection with HIV, 50% of infected people show a positive result on the ELISA antibody test.[50] Almost all individuals seroconvert within six months following infection. First developed to screen donated blood, the HIV antibody test has also been used to detect the presence of the virus in populations and to monitor the rate of viral transmission in large cohorts of people at risk for infection. The ELISA test, with Western Blot confirmation, is most commonly used, although sensitive and accurate immunofluorescence assays also are available.[51] Regardless of the technique, when properly used in populations with high prevalence of the virus, the antibody test is highly accurate. In populations with low prevalence of the virus, however, the ELISA test produces some false positives.[52] Recombinant antigens are currently being developed to decrease some of the problems associated with HIV antibody testing.

Antibodies to HIV do not appear to function in the same way as antibodies to many other viruses. The hepatitis virus antibody, for example, appears as the antigen disappears, and the presence of the antibody implies immunity to the virus. By contrast, the HIV antibody and antigen appear almost simultaneously, and the presence of antibody implies ongoing viral infection rather than immunity. Thus, a positive HIV antibody test implies that an individual is actively infected, presumably for life, and represents a continuous contagious risk to others through sexual, parenteral, or perinatal routes of transmission.[53-55]

In the past, it was estimated that perhaps 5–10% of people infected with HIV would develop AIDS,[56] but recent evidence suggests that those estimates were much too low. In one study of patients with diffuse lymphadenopathy (mild ARC), 50% of patients developed AIDS within 5 years following HIV infection.[57] It now seems very likely that the majority of infected people will go on to experience some degree of immune deficiency and perhaps overt AIDS. Based on the estimated numbers of people presently infected with the virus, it is anticipated that we will be dealing with an AIDS epidemic for the next 5 to 10 years, regardless of any preventive measures now taken to stop viral spread.

CLINICAL MANIFESTATIONS OF AIDS

Following infection with HIV, many people remain asymptomatic and healthy, often unaware that they are infected, yet capable of transmitting the virus to others. Why some people rapidly develop AIDS following infection and others live in apparent homeostasis with the virus for many years is still unknown. In certain people, various chronic symptoms may be present for some time before an opportunistic infection or cancer appears, but many patients initially manifest Kaposi's sarcoma or an opportunistic infection.

Some infected people experience an acute flulike illness within a few weeks following infection. This acute retroviral syndrome lasts for a mean of eight days and is characterized by fevers, sweats, malaise, lethargy, swollen glands, and other nonspecific symptoms.[58] A transitory erythematous macular rash (reddish patches) is seen in about 50% of these patients. As the immune system becomes progressively impaired, other clinical manifestations may appear, including persistent generalized lymphadenopathy (PGL), oral candidiasis, and oral hairy leukoplakia. In people with PGL, the onset of oral candidiasis or hairy leukoplakia signals an increased risk of rapid progression to AIDS.[59]

The clinical forms of AIDS vary among risk groups; AIDS does not give rise to the same diseases in homosexual men as in heterosexuals. For example, Kaposi's sarcoma is seen at diagnosis in gay men in 30–50% of cases.[60] By contrast, only 2% of hemophiliacs with AIDS have Kaposi's sarcoma. Similarly, *Pneumocystis carinii* pneumonia (PCP), which accounts for more than 50% of all initial AIDS diagnosis in this country, is relatively more common in heterosexuals infected through blood transfusions than among gay men. Lymphocytic interstitial pneumonitis is very rarely seen in adults with AIDS, but it is a common diagnosis in children with AIDS. These differences have not yet been explained. Regional differences also occur in the clinical manifestations of AIDS.[61] In the United States, PCP is the most common opportunistic infection, seen more frequently than esophageal candidiasis and cryptococcal meningitis. In Africa and Haiti, however, PCP is less common than other infections. *Candida* infection and cryptococcal meningitis are the most common AIDS-related infections in Africa and *Candida* and tuberculosis are seen more frequently in Haiti. To some degree, the types of infections manifested in different parts of the world reflect the microorganisms most frequently found in those regions. It is not yet known whether there are genetic influences on the manifestations of AIDS or regional differences in the AIDS virus itself that might cause different reactions to different tissues and, thus, different clinical manifestations of disease.

As the epidemic evolves, changes are taking place in its clinical manifestations. In the United States, the incidence of Kaposi's sarcoma, which accounted for 48% of AIDS cases in 1981, accounted for only 18% of cases in 1986. To understand these changes, we will need ongoing epidemiologic surveillance.

Opportunistic Infections

Opportunistic infections are the most common presenting clinical manifestations that establish a diagnosis of AIDS. These infections are characterized by an aggressive clinical course, resistance to therapy, and a high rate of relapse. Among the infections associated with AIDS are parasitic infections (e.g., PCP, cryptosporidiosis, toxoplasmosis), bacterial infections (e.g., *Mycobacterium avium intracellulare*), viral infections (e.g., invasive cytomegalovirus, invasive herpes simplex virus), and fungal infections (e.g., cryptococcal disease, histoplasmosis).

PCP is the most common opportunistic infection, seen in 55–60% of AIDS patients, and is by far the most common initial presenting diagnosis in AIDS. PCP usually presents with a diffuse pneumonitis. Symptoms include shortness of breath, nonproductive cough, dyspnea (labored breathing) on exertion, chest tightness, and often high fever. At the time of diagnosis, chest x-rays usually are abnormal, showing some increase in bronchovascular/interstitial markings in more than 95% of cases. Although a diagnosis of PCP once required doing a bronchoscopy, it is now diagnosed at many hospitals on the basis of careful microscopic observation of induced sputum. This technique decreases the need for expensive and invasive testing of patients and allows more rapid outpatient diagnosis of this infection.

The standard drugs used to treat PCP are trimethoprim/sulfamethoxazole and pentamidine administered intravenously, orally, or by inhalation. Unfortunately, most patients become allergic to or intolerant of these medications and they must be discontinued. Dapsone, a drug now being tested for use in treating PCP, appears to have substantial activity especially when combined with trimethoprim/sulfamethoxazole.

Malignancies

Several cancers are associated with HIV infection, including Kaposi's sarcoma and various lymphomas. Kaposi's sarcoma, central nervous system lymphomas, and high grade peripheral B-cell lymphomas are believed to result directly from the immune deficiency caused by HIV infection. Other cancers, such as Hodgkin's lymphoma, may not be directly attributable to HIV infection, but their clinical course is definitely altered by it. Hodgkin's lymphoma is seen with increased incidence in homosexual men and follows an aggressive clinical course.

Kaposi's sarcoma (KS), the second most common clinical manifestation of AIDS, is a multicentric disease process that produces reddish or violaceous lesions in various regions of the body simultaneously. Often the lesions are distributed in a striking linear pattern, following the paths of lymphatic drainage. Although the cell of origin is uncertain, tumors appear to arise from the lymphatic endothelium. The earliest KS lesions resemble many other types of lesions commonly seen on the body. At more advanced stages of disease, however, the appearance of the lesions is so striking and typical that biopsy often is not necessary to make the diagnosis. Visceral KS is common, but often clinically silent. In contrast, pulmonary KS is less common, but more aggressive. Generally, patients with pulmonary KS have an extremely poor prognosis.

Unlike many other manifestations of AIDS, KS can be quite disfiguring. In addition to visible lesions, lymphedema of the face of the lower extremities, caused by lymphatic obstruction by the tumor, frequently occurs. AIDS patients with KS are usually the most stigmatized and isolated, often rejected by employers, friends, and family members. Although patients with KS usually die of opportunistic infections rather than the cancer itself, much of the morbidity associated with AIDS is caused by this visible tumor.

Chemotherapeutic agents have some activity against KS, but because they may further impair cellular immunity and increase the risk of infection, their use is controversial. Radiation therapy is used primarily for palliation, to reduce painful lesions of the feet, erosive oral lesions, and areas of extensive lymphedema.

Despite the development of efficacious treatments to control the opportunistic infections and cancers that result from AIDS, their impact on AIDS-related mortality will be minimal until the underlying immune deficiency can be corrected.

ANTIVIRAL THERAPY AND IMMUNE SYSTEM STIMULATION

General Considerations

Several experimental therapies are being developed to correct the underlying immune dysfunction and to interrupt and neutralize the retroviral infection process. The goals of antiviral drug development are both preventive and therapeutic. These drugs might be used to prevent viral transmission by reducing the infectiousness of people already carrying the virus or by reducing the susceptibility of people not yet exposed to it. An important goal is to prevent further progression of disease in infected people. In people with AIDS or ARC, it may be possible to reverse established disease and restore immune function. Much more needs to be learned, however, about the mechanisms of HIV transmission, its natural history, and the pathogenesis of immune deficiency before truly effective antiviral drugs can be developed. Moreover, many practical and economic issues must be resolved before an antiviral drug can be distributed to the millions of people at risk or already infected. For these reasons, efficacious antiviral agents are not expected to be available for many years.

To reduce infectiousness, an antiviral drug would have to markedly decrease viral replication and concentration in semen, blood, and vaginal secretions. To reduce susceptibility to infection, the drug would have to block attachment of the virus to the T4 antigen on cells or neutralize the effects of possible cofactors. To prevent disease progression or to reverse established disease, an antiviral drug must block viral replication without compromising the restoration of normal immune function. The drug also must be capable of crossing the blood-brain barrier to treat infected cells in the central nervous system.

Ideally, to prevent retroviral damage to the immune system, treatment should start almost immediately following infection. However, widespread use of an HIV antigen or antibody test to identify individuals as soon as possible following infection raises several concerns, including potential risks to civil rights and the needless trauma that many people who test false positive will undergo. This last concern is especially relevant if the tests are used in populations with low viral prevalence.

Those issues aside, antiviral drug treatment of infected people poses many other difficulties. Treatment may need to continue for 10 or more years and possibly for life. Experience with other chronic illnesses, such as hypertension, suggests that long-term compliance with drug treatment is extremely difficult to maintain. An antiviral drug for HIV, therefore, must be convenient to take, orally administered, have minimal toxicity and no subjective side effects, and must be inexpensive so that large numbers of people can afford to take it continuously for many years. Thus far, no experimental agent to treat HIV that has been clinically tested meets all of these requirements.

For ethical reasons, the first anti-HIV experimental drugs were tested in patients with advanced disease. Even if a drug is active against HIV, this may be difficult to demonstrate in patients whose immune systems are already severely compromised. Although there is still concern about testing experimental drugs in infected people who are relatively healthy, researchers today are designing clinical trials of drugs in healthier patients to see if a drug such as zidovudine (formerly AZT) might prevent progression of disease.

Immune System Modulators

Attempts to restore immune function through immune system modulators have thus far been unsuccessful. Interferon, an antiviral drug with anti-cancer properties, also stimulates the immune system. In our tests, however, interferon showed no evidence of activity against cytomegalovirus or other viruses, modest activity against Kaposi's sarcoma, and no evidence of boosting the immune system.[62] The most potent immune stimulator that we have tested is recombinant interleuken-2, the lymphokine of the immune system. Even at very high doses, however, this drug showed no benefit.

Several factors may explain why immune stimulators have been unsuccessful in correcting the immune deficiency in AIDS. First, by the time a person has AIDS, the immune deficiency may be so severe that correction is impossible. Second, newly produced T-lymphocytes may themselves become infected with HIV. Third, the worst possibility, immune stimulation may actually exacerbate the immune deficiency by causing cells infected with HIV to proliferate and produce more virus.

Antiviral Agents

Most experimental drug treatments for AIDS focus on decreasing replication of the virus once infection has occurred. Because HIV requires reverse transcriptase to replicate itself within cells, several antiviral drugs are being designed to target this and other enzymes. Drugs like interferon may act to prevent, delay, or slow down the assembly of intact viruses following transcription within the cell.

Suramin was the first antiviral agent against HIV tested in the United States.[63–67] Unfortunately, suramin proved to have no efficacy and considerable toxicity; it led to the death of a number of patients who had not yet developed AIDS. Two of our patients became adrenal insufficient during the trial and still have no detectable adrenal function. Although HIV was no longer detectable in viral cultures of five patients treated with suramin, the disease continued to progress in four of these patients. Tests of HPA 23, the French drug that drew Rock Hudson and many other Americans to Paris when it was first used there, had similar disappointing results in clinical trials. HPA 23 had no effect on clinical outcome even when the virus appeared to be inhibited.

Zidovudine (formerly called azidothymidine or AZT) is the first drug that has showed clear benefits in slowing down, but not preventing, the progression of AIDS. Under the brand name Retrovir (Burroughs Wellcome), zidovudine recently received FDA approval for prescription to AIDS patients who meet certain eligibility requirements. A simple analogue of thymidine, zidovudine is difficult to synthesize and expensive to produce.

Initially developed as a potential antineoplastic (tumor) agent, zidovudine was later found to be very active against HIV in vitro. In a double-blind placebo clinical trial in patients with AIDS and ARC, patients receiving the drug had significantly reduced mortality during the trial compared with those who received the placebo.[68] The trial was terminated at the end of six months, after 16 deaths had occurred among patients receiving the placebo and only 1 death among patients receiving zidovudine. In comparing patients receiving placebo or zidovudine in terms of serious events experienced during the course of the trial (e.g., development of opportunistic infections or Kaposi's sarcoma, or death), researchers found that after the first six weeks of the study, drug recipients appeared to experience fewer serious events than placebo recipients. These indirect indications of zidovudine's effectiveness against HIV are supported by the observation of slightly increased levels of

T-helper cells during the study in patients receiving the drug compared with those on placebo.

Zidovudine has considerable toxicity. Hemoglobin levels often drop dramatically in patients receiving this drug. By the end of the clinical trial, 25% of AIDS patients taking zidovudine required regular blood transfusions to maintain hemoglobin. With the problem of an already limited blood supply in this country, the prospect of thousands of people taking zidovudine on a continuous basis and becoming transfusion-dependent is worrisome but may be reduced when the drug is used in less advanced HIV infections.

The cost for one year's supply of zidovudine has been estimated to be about $10,000. The high cost alone makes this a less than ideal drug for life-long use by thousands of infected people in the United States and may preclude its use altogether in Third World countries with few health care resources. Our experience with zidovudine has helped us to appreciate that even if a drug is active against HIV in vivo, we may have other problems when we try to use it on a large scale.

Research for effective treatments is very important and must go forward, but education remains our most potent weapon to halt the spread of AIDS. Both homosexuals and heterosexuals must be encouraged to follow safer sex guidelines, which include decreasing the number of sexual partners, getting to know partners well before having sexual contact, and using condoms. Among our most pressing tasks is the development of adequate means of communicating information about AIDS to intravenous drug users, members of minority groups, adolescents, and others at risk for HIV infection. In addition to preventing further viral spread, widespread education about AIDS can help to reduce the stigma, discrimination, and psychosocial distress that have so often accompanied an AIDS diagnosis.

REFERENCES

1. *The Case Definition of AIDS Used by the CDC for National Reporting (CDC-Reportable AIDS)*. 1985. (Document No. 0312S). Atlanta, GA: Centers for Disease Control.
2. Barre-Sinoussi, F.; Chermann, J. C.; Rey, F.; Nugeyre, M. T.; Chamaret, S.; Gruest, J.; Daugier, C.; Axler-Blin, C.; Vezinet-Brun, F.; Rouzioux, C.; Rosenbaum, W.; Montagnier, L. 1983. Isolation of a T-lymphotropic retrovirus from a patient at risk for acquired immune deficiency syndrome (AIDS). *Science* 220: 868–871.
3. Gallo, R. C.; Salahuddin, S. Z.; Popovic, M.; Shearer, G. M.; Kaplan, M.; Haynes, B. F.; Palker, T. J.; Redfield, R.; Oleske, J.; Safai, B.; White, G.; Foster, P.; Markham, P. 1984. Frequent detection and isolation of cytopathic retroviruses (HTLV-III) from patients with AIDS and at risk for AIDS. *Science* 224: 500–503.
4. Levy, J. A.; Hoffman, A. D.; Kramer, S. M.; Landis, J. A.; Shimabukuro, J. M.; Oshiro, L. S. 1984. Isolation of lymphocytopathic retroviruses from San Francisco patients with AIDS. *Science* 225: 840–842.
5. Coffin, J.; Haase, A.; Levy, J. A.; Montagnier, L.; Oroszian, S.; Teich, N.; Temin, H.; Toyoshima, K.; Varmus, H.; Vogt, P.; Weiss, R. 1986. Human immunodeficiency viruses. *Science* 232: 697.

6. Pinn-Wiggins, V. W. 1985. Follow-up at 4½ years on homosexual men with generalized lymphadenopathy. *New England Journal of Medicine* 313: 1542.
7. Sirianni, M. C.; Rossi, P.; Scarpati, B.; Ragona, G.; Seminara, R.; Bonomo, G.; Aiuti, F. 1985. Immunological and virological investigation in patients with lymphadenopathy syndrome in a population at risk for acquired immunodeficiency syndrome (AIDS); with particular focus on the detection of antibodies to human T-lymphotropic retroviruses (HTLV-III). *Journal of Clinical Immunology* 5: 261–268.
8. Abrams, D. I.; Mess, T.; Volberding, P. A. 1985. Lymphadenopathy: Endpoint or prodrome? Update of a 36-month prospective study. *Advances in Experimental Medicine and Biology* 187: 73–84.
9. Morris, L.; Distenfeld, A.; Amorosi, E.; Karpatkin, S. 1982. Autoimmune thrombocytopenic purpura in homosexual men. *Annals of Internal Medicine* 96: 714–717.
10. Abrams, D. I.; Kiprov, D. D.; Goedert, J. J.; Sarngadharan, M. G.; Gallo, R. C.; Volberding, P. A. 1986. Antibodies to human T-lymphotropic virus type III and development of the acquired immunodeficiency syndrome in homosexual men presenting with immune thrombocytopenia. *Annals of Internal Medicine* 104: 47–50.
11. Gottlieb, G. J.; Ragaz, A.; Vogel, J. V.; Friedman-Kien, A.; Rywkin, A. M.; Weiner, E. A.; Ackerman, A. B. 1981. A preliminary communication on extensively disseminated Kaposi's sarcoma in young homosexual men. *American Journal of Dermatopathology* 3: 111–114.
12. Rivin, B. E.; Monroe, J. M.; Hubschman, B. P.; Thomas, P. A. 1984. AIDS outcome: A first follow-up. *New England Journal of Medicine* 311: 857.
13. Jaffe, H. W.; Bregman, D. J.; Selik, R. M. 1984. Acquired immunodeficiency syndrome in the United States: First 1,000 cases. *Journal of Infectious Diseases* 148: 339–345.
14. Centers for Disease Control. 1986. Classification system for human T-lymphotropic virus type III/lymphadenopathy-associated virus infections. *Morbidity and Mortality Weekly Report* 20: 334–340.
15. Centers for Disease Control. 11 May 1987. *AIDS Weekly Surveillance Report—United States.*
16. National Academy of Sciences. 1986. *Confronting AIDS.* Washington, DC: National Academy Press, p. 8.
17. Weiss, S. H.; Ginzberg, H. M.; Goedert, J. J., et al. 1985. Risk of HTLV-III exposure and AIDS among parenteral drug abusers in New Jersey [Abstract]. *The International Conference on the Acquired Immunodeficiency Syndrome.* Philadelphia, PA: American College of Physicians.
18. Robertson, J. R.; Bucknall, A. B. V.; Welsby, P. D.; Roberts, J. J. K.; Inglis, J. M.; Peutherer, J. F.; Brettle, R. P. 1986. Epidemic of AIDS-related virus (HTLV-III/LAV) infection among intravenous drug users. *British Medical Journal* 292: 527–529.
19. Angarano, G.; Pastore, G.; Monno, L.; Santantono, J.; Luchese, N.; Schiraldi, O. 1985. Rapid spread of HTLV-III infection among drug addicts in Italy. *Lancet* 2: 1302.
20. Rodrigo, J. M.; Serra, M. A.; Aguilar, E.; Del Olmo, J. A.; Gimeno, V.; Aparisi, L. 1985. HTLV-III antibodies in drug addicts in Spain. *Lancet* 2: 156–157.
21. Chaisson, R. E.; Moss, A. R.; Onishi, R.; Osmond, D.; Carlson, J. R. 1987. Human immunodeficiency virus infection in heterosexual intravenous drug users in San Francisco. *American Journal of Public Health* 77: 169–172.
22. Centers for Disease Control. 11 May 1987. *AIDS Weekly Surveillance Report—United States.*
23. Moss, A. R.; McCallum, G.; Volberding, P. A.; Bacchetti, P.; Dritz, S. 1984. Mortality associated with mode of presentation in the acquired immune deficiency syndrome. *Journal of the National Cancer Institute* 73: 1281–1284.
24. Hardy, A.; Rauch, K.; Echenberg, D. F.; Morgan, W. M.; Curran, J. W. 1986. The economic impact of the first 10,000 cases of AIDS in the United States. *Journal of the American Medical Association* 225: 209–211.
25. Kizer, K. W.; Rodriguez, J.; McHolland, G. F.; Weller, W. 1986. *A Qualitative Analysis of AIDS in California.* Sacramento, CA: California Department of Health Services.

26. Scitovsky, A. A.; Rice, D. P.; Showstack, J.; Lee, P. R. 1986. *Estimating the Direct and Indirect Economic Costs of the Acquired Immune Deficiency Syndrome, 1985, 1986, and 1990.* (Task order 282-85-0061.) Atlanta, GA: Centers for Disease Control.

27. Volberding, P. A. 1985. The clinical spectrum of the acquired immunodeficiency syndrome: Implications for comprehensive patient care. *Annals of Internal Medicine* 103: 729–733.

28. Abrams, D. I.; Dilley, J. W.; Maxey, L. M.; Volberding, P. A. 1986. Routine care and psychosocial support of the patient with acquired immunodeficiency syndrome. *Medical Clinics of North America* 70: 707–720.

29. Scitovsky, A. A.; Cline, M.; Lee, P. R. 1986. Medical care costs of patients with AIDS in San Francisco. *Journal of the American Medical Association* 256: 3103–3106.

30. Abrams, D. I., et al. Lymphadenopathy: Endpoint or prodome?

31. Abrams, D. I., et al. Antibodies to human T-lymphotropic virus type III.

32. McCray, E. 1986. Occupational risk of the acquired immunodeficiency syndrome among health care workers. *New England Journal of Medicine* 314: 1127–1132.

33. Henderson, D. K.; Saah, A. J.; Zak, B. J.; Kaslow, R. A.; Lane, H. C.; Folks, T.; Blackwelder, W. C.; Schmitt, J.; LeCamera, D. J.; Masur, H.; Fauci, A. S. 1986. Risk of nosocomial infection with human T-cell lymphotropic virus type III/lymphadenopathy-associated virus in a large cohort of intensively exposed health care workers. *Annals of Internal Medicine* 104: 644–647.

34. Moss, A.; Osmond, D.; Bacchetti, P.; Gerberding, J.; Sande, M.; Volberding, P.; Levy, J. A.; Carlson, J.; Casavant, C.; Conant, M. 1986. Risk of seroconversion for the acquired immune deficiency syndrome (AIDS) in San Francisco health workers. *Journal of Occupational Medicine* 28: 821–824.

35. Friedland, G. H.; Saltzman, B. R.; Rogers, M. F.; Kahl, P. A.; Lesser, M. L.; Mayers, M. M.; Klein, R. S. 1986. Lack of transmission of HTLV-III/LAV infection to household contacts of patients with AIDS or AIDS-related complex with oral candidiasis. *New England Journal of Medicine* 314: 344–349.

36. Mann, J. M.; Quinn, T. C.; Francis, H.; Nzilambi, N.; Bosenge, N.; Bila, K.; McCormick, J. B.; Ruti, K.; Asila, P. K.; Curran, J. W. 1986. Prevalence of HTLV-III/LAV in household contacts of patients with confirmed AIDS and controls in Kinshasa, Zaire. *Journal of the American Medical Association* 256: 721–724.

37. Fischl, M. A.; Dickinson, G. M.; Scott, G. B.; Klimas, N.; Fletcher, M. A.; Parks, W. 1987. Evaluation of heterosexual partners, children, and household contacts of adults with AIDS. *Journal of the American Medical Association* 256: 640–644.

38. Rutherford, G. W.; Echenberg, D. F.; O'Malley, P. M.; Darrow, W. W.; Wilson, T. E.; Jaffe, H. W. 1986. The natural history of LAV/HTLV-III infection and viraemia in homosexual and bisexual men: A 6-year follow up study [Abstract P99]. *Abstracts of the Second International Conference on AIDS*. Paris.

39. Mann, J. M.; Francis, H.; Quinn, T. C. 1986. Surveillance for AIDS in a central American city: Kinshasa, Zaire. *Journal of the American Medical Association* 255: 3255–3259.

40. Piot, P. T.; Quinn, T. C.; Taelman, H.; Feinsod, F. M.; Minlangu, K. B.; Wobin, O.; Mbendi, N.; Mazebo, P.; Ndangi, K.; Stevens, W.; Kalambayi, K.; Mitchell, S.; Bridts, C.; McCormick, J. B. 1984. Acquired immunodeficiency syndrome in a heterosexual population in Zaire. *Lancet* 2: 65–69.

41. Clumeck, N.; Van de Perre, P.; Carael, M.; Rouvroy, D.; Nzaramba, D. 1985. Heterosexual promiscuity among African patients with AIDS. *Lancet* 2: 182.

42. Van de Perre, P.; Rouvroy, D.; Lepage, P.; Bogaerts, J.; Kestelyn, P.; Kayihigi, J.; Hekker, A. C.; Butzler, J. P.; Clumeck, N. 1984. Acquired immunodeficiency syndrome in Rwanda. *Lancet* 2: 62–65.

43. Kreiss, J. K.; Koech, D.; Plummer, F. A.; Holmes, K. K.; Lightfoote, M.; Piot, P.; Ronald, A. R.; Ndinya-Achola, J. O.; D'Costa, L. J.; Roberts, P.; Ngugi, E. N.; Quinn, T. C. 1986.

AIDS virus infection in Nairobi prostitutes: Spread of the epidemic to east Africa. *New England Journal of Medicine* 314: 414–418.

44. Weiss, S. H., et al. Risk of HTLV-III exposure and AIDS among parenteral drug abusers in New Jersey.

45. Angarano, G., et al. Rapid spread of HTLV-III infection among drug addicts in Italy.

46. Rodrigo, J. M. HTLV-III antibodies in drug addicts in Spain.

47. Chaisson, R. E. Human immunodeficiency virus infection in heterosexual intravenous drug users in San Francisco.

48. Cooper, D. A.; Gold, J.; Maclean, P.; Donovan, B.; Finlayson, R.; Barnes, T. G.; Michelmore, H. M.; Brooke, P.; Penny, R. 1985. Acute AIDS retrovirus infection: Definition of a clinical illness associated with seroconversion. *Lancet* 1: 537–540.

49. Ho, D. D.; Rota, T. R.; Schooley, R. T.; Kaplan, J. C.; Allan, J. D.; Groopman, J. E.; Resnick, L.; Felsenstein, D.; Andrews, C. A.; Hirsch, M. C. 1985. Isolation of HTLV-III from cerebrospinal fluid and neural tissues of patients with neurological syndromes related to the acquired immunodeficiency syndrome. *New England Journal of Medicine* 313: 1493–1497.

50. Melbye, M. 1986. The natural history of human T-lymphotropic virus III infection: The cause of AIDS. *British Medical Journal* 292: 5–12.

51. American Medical Association Council on Scientific Affairs. 1985. Status report on the acquired immunodeficiency syndrome: Human T-cell lymphotropic virus type III testing. *Journal of the Americal Medical Association* 254: 1342–1345.

52. National Institutes of Health. 7–9 July 1986. *The Impact of Routine HTLV-III Antibody Testing of Blood and Plasma on Public Health.* Draft report on a consensus conference, Bethesda, MD.

53. Markham, P. D.; Salahuddin, S. Z.; Popovic, M.; Patel, A.; Veren, K.; Fladager, A.; Orndorff, S.; Gallo, R. C. 1985. Advances in the isolation of HTLV-III from patients with AIDS and AIDS-related complex and from donors at risk. *Cancer Research* 45 (Suppl): 4588s.

54. Groopman, J. E. 1985. Clinical spectrum of HTLV-III in humans. *Cancer Research* 45 (Suppl): 4649–4651s.

55. Centers for Disease Control. 1986. Recommendations for assisting in the prevention of perinatal transmission of human T-lymphotropic virus type III/lymphadenopathy-associated virus and the acquired immunodeficiency syndrome. *Morbidity and Mortality Weekly Report* 34: 721–726;731–732.

56. Sivak, S. L., and Wormser, G. P. 1985. How common is HTLV-III infection in the United States? *New England Journal of Medicine* 313: 1352.

57. Abrams, D. I., et al. Lymphadenopathy: Endpoint or prodome?

58. Cooper, D. A., et al. Acute AIDS retrovirus infection.

59. Metroka, C. E.; Cunningham-Rundles, S.; Krim, M., et al. 1984. Generalized lymphadenopathy in homosexual men: An update of the New York experience. *Annals of the New York Academy of Science* 407: 400–411.

60. Des Jarlais, D. C.; Marmor, M.; Thomas, P.; Chamberland, M.; Zolla-Pazner, S.; Sencer, D. J. 1984. Kaposi's sarcoma among four different AIDS groups. *New England Journal of Medicine* 310: 1119.

61. Volberding, P. 1986. AIDS—Variations on a theme of cellular immune deficiency. In J. C. Gluckman and E. Vilmer (eds.). *Acquired Immunodeficiency Syndrome.* Paris: Elsevier, pp. 191–198. (International Conference on AIDS, Paris, June 23–25).

62. Groopman, J. E.; Gottlieb, M. S.; Goodman, J.; Mitsuya, R. T.; Conant, M. A.; Prince, H.; Fahey, J. L.; Derezin, M.; Weinstein, W.; Casavant, C.; Rothman, J.; Rudnick, S. A.; Volberding, P. A. 1984. Recombinant alpha 2 interferon therapy of Kaposi's sarcoma associated with acquired immunodeficiency syndrome. *Annals of Internal Medicine* 100: 671–676.

63. Broder, S.; Yarchoan, R.; Collins, J. M.; Lance, H. C.; Markham, P. P.; Klecker, R. W.; Redfield, R. R.; Mitsuya, H.; Hoth, D. F.; Gellman, E.; Groopman, J. E.; Resnick, L.; Gallo, R. C.; Myers, C. E.; Fauci, A. S. 1985. Effects of suramin on HTLV-III/LAV infection presenting Kaposi's sarcoma or AIDS-related complex: Clinical pharmacology and suppression of virus *in vivo*. *Lancet* 2: 627–630.

64. Levine, A. M.; Gill, P. S.; Cohen, J.; Hawkins, J. G.; Formenti, S. C.; Aguilar, S.; Meyer, P. R.; Krailo, M.; Parker, J.; Rasheed, S. 1985. Suramin antiviral therapy in the acquired immunodeficiency syndrome. Clinical, immunologic, and virologic results. *Annals of Internal Medicine* 105: 32–37.

65. Rouvroy, D.; Bogaerts, J.; Habyarimana, J. B.; Nzaramba, O.; Van de Perre, P. 1985. Short-term results with suramin for AIDS-related conditions. *Lancet* 1: 878–879.

66. Stein, C. A.; Saville, W.; Yarchoan, R.; Broder, S.; Gellman, E. P. 1986. Suramin and function of the adrenal cortex. *Annals of Internal Medicine* 104: 286–287.

67. Kaplan, L. D.; Wolfe, P. R.; Volberding, P. A.; Feorino, P.; Levy, J. A.; Abrams, D. I.; Kiprov, D.; Wong, R.; Kaufman, L.; Gottlieb, M. S. 1987. Lack of response to suramin in patients with AIDS and AIDS-related complex. *American Journal of Medicine* 82: 615–619.

68. Fischl, M. A.; Richmond, D. D.; Grieco, M. H.; Gottlieb, M. S.; Volberding, P. A.; Laskin, O. L.; Leedom, J. M.; Groopman, J. E.; Mildvan, D.; Schooley, R. T.; Jackson, G. G.; Durack, D. T.; King, D., the AZT Collaborative Working Group. In press. The efficacy of 3'-azido-3'-deoxythymidine (azidothymidine) in the treatment of patients with AIDS and AIDS-related complex: A double-blind placebo-control trial. *New England Journal of Medicine*.

CHAPTER 9

Treatment Issues in AIDS

ELLEN C. COOPER

BACKGROUND

Acquired immune deficiency syndrome (AIDS) presents one of the most complex therapeutic challenges of any disease ever described. While fundamentally a systemic viral infection, its hallmark is a profound immunodeficiency that leaves the human host susceptible to many opportunistic infections (OIs) which eventually lead to death in most patients. The most common AIDS-defining OI in the United States is pneumonia due to *Pneumocystis carinii,* an ubiquitous parasite that causes life-threatening pulmonary infection in the immunocompromised host. Other organisms causing OIs in patients with AIDS include cytomegalovirus (CMV), *Mycobacterium avium intracellulare* (MAI), *Toxoplasma gondii, Cryptococcccus neoformans, Candida albicans,* and *Cryptosporidium.* In addition, individuals infected with the human immunodeficiency virus (HIV)* are at increased risk for developing malignancies, the most common by far being Kaposi's sarcoma (KS). It is not understood why some HIV-infected individuals develop KS, often months or even years before developing their first major opportunistic infection, while others are spared this manifestation of the disease. Epidemiologic evidence suggests the role of a cofactor, which may be particularly prevalent in the male homosexual population.[1]

Once an infected individual develops an AIDS-defining opportunistic infection, median life expectancy is reported as a year or less, while individuals with cutaneous KS as their only AIDS-defining condition have a somewhat longer survival.[2] Individuals infected with HIV may also die of their infection before they develop classic AIDS, for instance, from a progressive wasting syndrome resulting in death without the diagnosis of an OI, or from complications of HIV infection of the brain, causing a debilitating neu-

---

* The primary etiologic agent of AIDS. The virus is also referred to as HTLV-III (human T-lymphotropic virus). LAV (lymphadenopathy associated virus) and ARV (AIDS-related virus).

rologic syndrome called AIDS-dementia complex, not technically an AIDS-defining condition at this time.

Thus it is apparent that the treatment of persons with AIDS requires a multifaceted approach. First and foremost, in a destructive disease process thought to be dependent on continued viral replication, the retroviral infection must be controlled in order for any additional treatment to have lasting benefit. An ideal antiviral therapy would be capable of eliminating the virus from the body, but no such agent is available today even in an experimental stage. HIV appears to integrate into the host DNA of some cells it infects[3] where it presumably remains and is inaccessible to existing compounds which act on actively replicating viruses. This so-called pro-virus may remain latent for long periods of time in some cells, while in others it produces copies of itself and viral proteins in enormous quantities. The result is a lytic (destructive) infection which kills the cell and releases many virions into the extracellular environment which are then able to infect other susceptible host cells. It is also believed that the virus may move from cell to cell directly, without an extracellular phase. An effective antiviral agent could presumably act at one or both phases, by inhibiting the process of viral replication itself or by interfering with viral penetration into uninfected cells. Because there is little optimism that an agent which can selectively destroy integrated viral DNA will be developed in the foreseeable future, it is presumed that antiviral treatment will need to be chronic, probably lifelong. Therefore it is important that it be relatively nontoxic and available in a convenient formulation for outpatient administration (e.g., oral). It should also cross the blood-brain barrier in sufficient quantity to inhibit viral replication in the central nervous system.

The second aspect of AIDS that may require treatment is the immunodeficiency which develops some time after initial infection with HIV, but is always present to a significant extent once an AIDS-defining opportunistic infection develops. The immunodeficiency is primarily cellular, although humoral (contained in serum) immunity is also affected.[4] It may be that in earlier stages of HIV infection, effective treatment of the retroviral infection alone will halt progression of the disease and specific immunotherapy will not be required, but no such agent has yet been demonstrated to accomplish this goal.

For persons with more advanced disease, effective control of the virus may not permit sufficient recovery of immune cells such that specific immunotherapy is not needed. However, some researchers believe that if an effective, nontoxic antiretroviral agent is developed, even the most advanced patients may be able to recover without additional immunotherapy, as long as a minimum critical number of uninfected thymic and stem cells remain.

There are at least three approaches that may be taken in attempting to restore immune function in patients with AIDS. One is passive administration of immune elements (such as immune globulins or white blood cells) with the hope that these substances will provide protection from infection with the multitude of organisms to which the AIDS patient is susceptible. The second approach is to attempt active immunostimulation with an agent having the ability to activate mature lymphocytes and/or induce growth and differentiation of uninfected lymphocyte precursors or stem cells. No such agent has yet been shown to be clinically effective in this manner, although several lymphokines, including interleukin-2 and gamma-interferon, have been studied in small numbers of patients.[5,6] One concern with this general approach has been that lymphocyte stimulation, in the absence of effective antiviral therapy, may accelerate the disease process by making the newly activated lymphocytes more susceptible to infection with HIV, as has been observed in vitro.[7]

A third approach is to replace the major elements of the destroyed immune system by transplanting uninfected stem cells from a healthy person into the infected person (e.g., bone-marrow transplant and/or thymic transplant). While this approach has a number of appealing aspects, transplantation has two important limitations: (1) the need for an HLA compatible donor (i.e., one with similar histocompatibility locus antigens, also known as "tissue transplant" antigens), and (2) the need to control the retroviral infection in the recipient before and after transplantation without causing unacceptable toxicity to the transplanted cells, resulting in a failure of engraftment (some antiretroviral agents currently under study are quite toxic to blood cells). Bone-marrow transplantation (BMT) is also an expensive procedure, with certain risks to the donor (primarily general anesthesia) and to the patient (if the donor is not an identical twin there is the possibility of graft vs. host disease). Progress has been made in the past few years in reducing the potential for this complication in recipients of allogeneic (genetically different) marrow by depleting the donor marrow of mature T-cells, but some studies indicate that this approach may increase the likelihood of graft failure and/or an increased incidence of opportunistic infections.[8,9]

Another facet of treating AIDS patients is the need for effective specific therapies to treat the opportunistic infections. The infections which are AIDS-defining are frequently disseminated and life-threatening and some of them, such as cytomegalovirus (CMV), may exacerbate the immunologic defects in these patients.[10] These infections are caused most commonly by environmental parasites, fungi, mycobacteria, and viruses which generally require a functional cellular immune response in the host for resistance, rather than by the more usual pathogenic bacteria, although serious bacterial infections can also occur in patients with AIDS.[11] As there are many relatively nontoxic antibiotics available, and AIDS patients respond reasonably well to specific antibiotic therapy for bacterial infections, these are not usually fatal. However, there are fewer antiparasitic, antifungal, antimycobacterial, and antiviral agents available, and they are generally more toxic. In addition, since most of the opportunistic infections tend to be both severe and recurrent, intensive initial therapy is required, and prolonged "suppressive" regimens appear necessary following infection with certain organisms.[12]

An additional complication of treating OIs in AIDS patients is the much higher incidence of adverse effects after administration of certain approved medications, in particular, sulfa-containing agents, such as trimethoprim/sulfamethoxazole for Pneumocystis carinii pneumonia (PCP).[13] Medications with hematologic toxicity are also likely to be less well tolerated in AIDS patients because of their already compromised hematologic status secondary to the HIV infection itself.[14]

Comprehensive medical management of AIDS patients requires the use of drugs and other therapies for the treatment of Kaposi's sarcoma and the other malignancies that afflict them. Indolent, cutaneous KS does not usually require treatment unless it poses a cosmetic problem and in that case localized radiation therapy is often temporarily effective.[15] If symptomatic visceral KS develops, more aggressive systemic chemotherapy can be used, although it is not always efficacious. Alpha-interferon is also under investigation for the treatment of KS in AIDS, and has been shown to have preliminary evidence of efficacy, particularly in patients without a prior history of an OI.[16] B-cell lymphomas, especially of the central nervous system, are the second most common AIDS-associated malignancy. This condition is usually fatal within one year despite intensive chemotherapy, which is particularly difficult to administer to already immunocompromised individuals.[17]

An additional aspect of the medical treatment of HIV-infected individuals is the frequent need for symptomatic therapy: (1) for debilitating manifestations of the underlying infection(s) (e.g., fever, headache, diarrhea); (2) for global reactions to the disease process, both organic and reactive (e.g., depression, anxiety, insomnia); and (3) for treatment of side effects (e.g., nausea, vomiting, rashes) of the potent medications often required to treat the primary and secondary manifestations of the disease.

Finally, a special aspect of the treatment of patients with HIV infection is the management of babies and young children with AIDS. While many of the treatment issues in AIDS apply to pediatrics as well, there are several potentially important differences in the pathogenesis and manifestations of the two disease processes which may require refocusing the issues somewhat. Briefly, these differences include the following:[18]

1. an immunologically immature host infected with HIV at a very early stage of development,
2. a generally more rapid progression to death of infected children compared with adults,
3. more frequent and more severe bacterial infections, and
4. an unusual lung disease called lymphoid interstitial pneumonitis as a common disease manifestation.

THE ISSUES

One very important issue which will arise in the management of HIV-infected persons as effective antiviral therapies are developed is the decision as to when in the course of the disease to initiate treatment. The answer is not simple for at least two important reasons, and will probably vary with the particular agent under consideration. First of all, the natural history of HIV infection in terms of the risk of developing AIDS is not well established at this time. While some infected persons clearly develop AIDS rather rapidly (within a couple of years), in natural history studies reported to date,[19,20] the majority of asymptomatic patients have not progressed to AIDS after four to five years, and varying proportions have developed symptomatic disease. It may be that the immune systems of some individuals can effectively contain the virus early during infection and AIDS will not develop. On the other hand, another five years of follow-up may indicate that most, if not all, infected persons will experience progressive deterioration.

At this time, however, the existence of a latent but relatively benign life-long infection with HIV remains a possibility in some individuals, and certainly has precedent in other human viral infections caused by herpes simplex virus, Epstein-Barr virus, hepatitis B virus, and so on. Persons who are naturally able to control the virus, even if only temporarily, may be better off without specific antiviral therapy which carries the risk that treatment may interfere with the ongoing natural host immune response. Such early intervention may thereby actually do harm by permitting the disease to progress more rapidly should the infected individual become unable to continue antiretroviral therapy for some reason (e.g., toxicity, resistance to the drug, drug interactions).

A second reason why it is unclear at what stage of infection initiation of specific antiretroviral therapy will be beneficial is that many of the antiretroviral drugs tested in people have significant toxicities. Zidovudine (approved generic name for azidothymidine or AZT), for instance, has been demonstrated to have benefit in prolonging life in certain patients with AIDS or advanced ARC when given for six months or less. However, it has significant bone-marrow toxicity which could limit its efficacy when it is taken for longer periods of time; for example, the dose may have to be reduced to subtherapeutic levels or discontinued frequently due to severe anemia or granulocytopenia (depressed white blood cell count), or the recovery of lymphocyte number and function may eventually be inhibited by the toxicity of the drug itself. On the other hand, less advanced patients may experience less hematologic toxicity from zidovudine, and therefore be able to tolerate it for longer periods, deriving a net benefit.

The argument for initiation of antiretroviral therapy in asymptomatic patients rests primarily on the twin assumptions that if the spread of the viral infection is halted early, destruction of the immune system will not occur and AIDS will not develop, and that antiretroviral drugs may have a better chance of working in patients with more intact immune systems. At this time there is no way of clearly identifying those asymptomatic infected individuals who will progress to AIDS and therefore are more likely to benefit from early antiviral therapy than those infected individuals who are unlikely to progress, at least in the near-term, and for whom the toxicities of prolonged antiviral therapy may outweigh the benefits. It has been reported that asymptomatic persons who are viremic (that is, have virus in the blood) are at higher risk of progression,[21,22] but this logical risk factor has not been thoroughly evaluated, and in any event, will be difficult to study rigorously until a reliable, interpretable method for culturing patients or assessing "viral load" is established. Several new antigen capture assays which are being developed hold some hope in this regard.[23,24]

Various laboratory immune parameters, such as elevated plasma levels of acid-labile alpha interferon,[25,26] decreased gamma-interferon production by lymphocytes in vitro after stimulation with antigen,[27] declining plasma levels of erythrocyte complement 3B receptors together with triple positive Coombs test,[28] and high serum levels of antilymphocyte antibodies,[29] have been reported by different investigators to be associated with risk of progression, but they have not been studied prospectively in large numbers of individuals. A lower absolute T-helper/inducer (CD4 or T4) cell count in the peripheral blood is generally acknowledged to be correlated with risk of progression, but this association has not yet been studied closely in asymptomatic individuals over the entire spectrum of CD4 counts. In any event it is unlikely that this parameter alone will be a good early discriminator for antiviral intervention in the individual patient because destruction of T-helper/inducer cells is a consequence of HIV infection, and the aim of identifying patients early as candidates for antiretroviral therapy is to prevent this destruction.

A second issue in the treatment of HIV-infected persons involves the concept of immunorestoration: whether it is useful, and if so, at what stage of the disease it may be necessary and what might be the best approach.

Once HIV infection has progressed to the point where clinical immunosuppression exists (manifested as an OI or neoplasm), it will likely be more difficult for antiviral treatment alone to restore health than at earlier stages of disease. As previously discussed, if HIV exists in an integrated but latent state to any significant extent in infected humans, the current and foreseeable types of antiretroviral agents will not eradicate the virus from the body. In most infections, and particularly in viral infections, the aim of anti-infective therapy is to reduce the replication of organisms and associated tissue destruction while the host immune response is developing. Organisms not destroyed by the anti-infective agent are then eliminated or held in check by the body's own newly developed immunity, cellular immune responses being of primary importance in most viral infections.[30] HIV impairs the ability of the body to develop effective cellular immunity by destroying the T-helper/inducer cells which are critical for this function.

There is presently no known immunomodulator capable of restoring lost T-helper/inducer cell function. Bone-marrow transplantation has theoretical promise[31] but has practical problems which will probably restrict widespread application even if it proves efficacious in individual patients. While pharmacologic doses of lymphokines such as interferon and interleukin-2 can be administered to humans, it is unlikely that such a monolithic approach will be of long-term benefit in restoring as complex and intricate a biological mechanism as the immune system (although certainly something would be learned in the attempt). It would seem that an effective immunorestorative agent needs to stimulate the differentiation, production, and maturation of cellular immune elements which are destroyed by HIV, and thereby restore the patient's own ability to resist opportunistic infections.

Because there is no proven or even promising therapy which will completely restore immunocompetence in patients with AIDS, passive immunoprophylaxis has been attempted in the form of immunoglobulin injections. This form of therapy has not been demonstrated to be particularly helpful in adults, probably because they have normal or elevated levels of immunoglobulins, which generally contain antibodies against multiple pathogens acquired earlier in life. In the pediatric population, where there has not been prior exposure to multiple antigens, gamma globulin may be of some benefit in preventing serious bacterial infections.[32] Whether a type of hyperimmune globulin made up of neutralizing or other antibodies to HIV will be of greater benefit remains to be seen.

A second form of passive immunotherapy, aimed at restoring cellular immunity, consists of the repeated transfusion of peripheral blood lymphocytes from a compatible donor.[33] This approach has been further refined to involve the transfer of CD4 cell enriched populations of lymphocytes cultured in vitro to very high numbers under special conditions before transfusion to the HIV-infected recipient. While this procedure is technically less risky to the donor than bone-marrow transplantation and therefore can be performed more frequently, it has not been shown to be of proven benefit and has a disadvantage similar to BMT in requiring an HLA compatible donor. Some investigators feel that intensive lymphocyte therapy may transfer a sufficient quantity of stem cells to essentially substitute for bone-marrow transplantation, but this possibility remains unproven in humans at this time. For any cellular therapy to be effective, it is generally felt that inhibition of HIV replication must be achieved, or infection and destruction of the transferred lymphocytes will occur. Here again, the question of optimal dosage of an antiviral agent is critical, particularly for an agent such as zidovudine whose primary toxicity is hematologic.

A third major issue in treating HIV-infected patients involves therapies for opportunistic infections. Once an OI is diagnosed, initial treatment is usually reasonably straightforward for those infections for which there exists effective and relatively safe drug(s). Special problems in AIDS patients include the generally increased severity of such infections, their high likelihood of recurrence even after successful acute treatment, and the increased incidence of adverse reactions to standard medications.

The treatment of opportunistic infections is further complicated by the fact that for a number of OIs, no approved, effective therapy exists, in part because many of these infections were relatively rare prior to the AIDS epidemic. Examples include infection with *Mycobacterium avium intracellulare* and *Cryptosporidium*. When these infections were recognized as pathogenic in the context of AIDS several years ago, many physicians felt justified in administering experimental therapies based on in vitro susceptibility data or the sparsest of anecdotal reports of apparent efficacy. Thus a number of unproven experimental agents have become available for the "treatment" of certain OIs through a mechanism previously referred to as "Compassionate INDs (Investigational New Drug Applications)," under which unapproved drugs were made available on a case-by-case basis to patients with a particular disease. One problem with this approach, particularly in the context of the AIDS "epidemic," is that after several years it is still not clear whether some of these experimental agents are truly efficacious or in fact harmful, and it becomes increasingly difficult to carry out well-controlled clinical trials because either it is generally deemed "unethical" to withhold active drug from some patients in a placebo-controlled trial because of presumed but not proven or well-characterized efficacy, or interest in the drug is lost, even for conducting controlled trials, because of apparent but not established lack of effectiveness. On balance, it is probably a greater disservice to patients now and in the future to permit the use of unproven drugs on a "compassionate basis" in lieu of adequately controlled, appropriately designed clinical trials in which safety and efficacy can be determined over a relatively limited period of time. The likely consequences of widespread use of unproven drugs in as complex a disease as AIDS include delayed development and approval (if ultimately demonstrated to be efficacious), excessive polypharmacy (administering several drugs concurrently), and the real risk of additional toxicity which is not justified by any benefit to the patient.

For many opportunistic infections, chronic "prophylaxis" or suppressive therapy is another important issue in the treatment of patients with HIV infection. For certain infections, such as cerebral toxoplasmosis, cryptococcosis, and CMV retinitis, chronic low dose therapy following acute treatment is generally accepted as necessary because of the very high relapse rate when therapy is discontinued. For other infections, notably PCP, the value of either primary or secondary prophylaxis is less clear for several reasons. After an initial episode of PCP, the relapse or recurrence rate is under 50% (although the proportion of patients who develop a second episode may increase in patients on zidovudine if life expectancy is increased significantly); acute treatment of a second episode (particularly if detected early) is usually successful although less likely to respond than the first episode; there is concern that resistant organisms may develop with prolonged use of subtherapeutic doses; and the available drugs most appropriate for prophylaxis, such as trimethoprim sulfamethoxazole and pyrimethamine sulfamethionine, contain sulfa components, which are poorly tolerated in many patients with AIDS. In addition, while a number of investigators feel strongly that prophylaxis against Pneumocystis successfully reduces the recurrence rate,[34] this has not been demonstrated in a controlled trial; nor is it known whether successful prophylaxis will in fact prolong survival.

As alluded to previously, another concern in the treatment of patients with AIDS is polypharmacy, or the concurrent administration of a number of drugs, particularly on a chronic basis. When chronic antiretroviral therapy becomes commonplace, the problem of drug interactions from concomitant therapy will become more prominent. Many of the drugs used to treat OIs have significant toxicity at the doses required, and administration of two or more drugs at the same time can be expected to result in additive or even synergistic toxicity, and also possibly to result in diminished efficacy for one or the other agent because of competition for similar metabolic or excretory pathways in the body.

On the other hand, in vitro testing of agents against HIV shows that some combinations of drugs may result in synergistic (more than additive) efficacy.[35,36] Several such combinations of agents are being considered for human trials and at least two have already begun. In these situations, the administration of the second drug is based on a sound scientific rationale under which it is hoped that either efficacy will be improved or toxicity will be reduced or both. Appropriate combinations of proven antiretroviral agents may also be tested, when available, to see if lower and therefore less toxic doses of each drug are effective when administered concurrently, and also to determine whether potential resistance to the drugs by the virus can be prevented or reduced by combining agents with different mechanisms of action. This latter approach has proven utility in the treatment of certain other infections (e.g., tuberculosis),[37] but remains to be established for viral infections, including HIV. A third rationale for combined therapy is the use of an antiretroviral with an immunomodulator in patients with various degrees of immunodeficiency. Again, the aim is to achieve efficacy that cannot be obtained by either therapy alone.

Other important aspects of AIDS, such as prevention of transmission of the virus, are very important but have not generated treatment issues per se until very recently. As clinically efficacious antiretroviral agents become available, questions regarding their usefulness in reducing the chance that an infected individual will transmit the virus to others and their potential role as "prophylactics" if taken immediately before or after exposure to a potential source of infection will surely be raised.

SPECIFIC ANTIRETROVIRAL AGENTS

The antiretroviral drug zidovudine (which is marketed under the trade name Retrovir and manufactured by Burroughs Wellcome Company) is a nucleoside analog which has been demonstrated to delay death and increase the time to development of OIs in certain patients with advanced AIDS-related complex (ARC) or "early" AIDS/OI. In early 1985 it was shown to markedly reduce evidence of HIV replication at low concentrations in laboratory assays,[38] and it appeared reasonably nontoxic in early short-term animal studies. Zidovudine was administered to human beings for the first time in July 1985 at the National Cancer Institute (NCI) in a small pilot study designed to obtain pharmacokinetic data and to study tolerance (toxic effects), first at low doses, and then at higher doses as indicated, in patients with AIDS or advanced ARC.[39] Although this Phase I study, performed largely under the direction of Drs. Samuel Broder and Robert Yarchoan at the NCI, was not designed primarily to study the possible efficacy of the drug, some preliminary but encouraging signs of a beneficial effect were noted, such as increases in the number of helper T-cells in the peripheral blood, weight gains, an improved sense of well-being, improved neurologic function in patients with deficits at entry, and clearing of minor fungal infections in two patients without specific antifungal therapy.

These results encouraged Burroughs Wellcome, in collaboration with university and government scientists, to plan and sponsor a larger multi-center placebo-controlled trial in similar types of patients, that is, certain patients with AIDS or advanced ARC. The goal was to determine if the drug was truly efficacious, or whether the apparent benefits which had been seen in the uncontrolled Phase I trial were either part of the natural waxing and waning of the disease or due to a "placebo-effect" (merely the fact or receiving a potentially helpful drug may cause a patient to feel better, not due to any specific action of the drug itself). Although significant toxicities from zidovudine, primarily hematologic in nature, were seen in the Phase I trial, they were felt to be manageable by blood transfusions and/or temporary reduction or discontinuation of therapy.

Enrollment in the planned six month, 12-center, placebo-controlled trial began in February of 1986 and was complete by the end of June. Two hundred eighty-one patients were enrolled and randomized to receive either zidovudine or a matching but inert placebo. To be eligible, patients with AIDS were required to have recovered from a first episode of PCP within the previous three months, and patients with "advanced" ARC were required to have documented oral thrush and/or recent significant unexplained weight loss, plus one other ARC symptom, such as persistent unexplained fever or diarrhea. All patients were also required to have an absolute T-helper cell count less than $500/mm^3$ and cutaneous anergy (lack of responsiveness) to four specific antigens.

An independent Data Safety Monitoring Board composed of approximately eight individuals (physicians, scientists, ethicists, and statisticians) had the responsibility of reviewing significant toxicity and efficacy data from the trial (such as deaths, incidence of opportunistic infections, and hematologic data) on a bimonthly basis to decide whether or not the trial should be terminated early because of unacceptable toxicity or overwhelming efficacy. On September 10, 1986, the Board convened for a special meeting at the company's request, to review the mortality data which had accumulated over the past month showing an apparent marked imbalance in the number of deaths in the two treatment groups, occurring predominantly in AIDS patients. Eight days later, after a more thorough review of additional data supplied by the company, both the Board and the FDA were convinced that the results were real and apparently due to the drug. At this time, 17 patients receiving placebo and 1 on zidovudine had died, and the Board recommended to Burroughs Wellcome that the placebo be discontinued. It was deemed unethical to continue administering an inactive substance to patients in the face of such strong evidence of efficacy.

The following week a protocol was written which would allow persons with AIDS who had recovered from a histologically confirmed episode of PCP and met certain laboratory criteria to receive zidovudine under a company-sponsored "Treatment IND." This protocol was submitted to the FDA on September 26, 1986 and was approved within two working days.

The National Institutes of Health provided administrative support for this project, and as of this writing (March 1987), over 4000 patients have received zidovudine free of charge from Burroughs Wellcome under the Treatment IND. During the last quarter of 1986, the company further collected, compiled, and analyzed the data from the placebo-controlled trial in order to submit an NDA (new drug application) to the Food and Drug Administration requesting permission to market the drug based on the efficacy demonstrated in the trial. Zidovudine was approved by the FDA on March 19, 1987 "for the management of certain adult patients with symptomatic HIV infection (AIDS and advanced ARC) who have a history of cytologically confirmed Pneumocystis carinii pneumonia or an absolute CD4 (T4-helper/inducer) lymphocyte count of less than 200/mm^3 in the peripheral blood before therapy is begun."

Because so many important unanswered questions remain regarding zidovudine and its use in HIV-infected patients, a number of other clinical trials have been initiated since the company's placebo-controlled trial in AIDS/post-PCP and advanced ARC patients ended in September 1986. In addition, those patients still receiving zidovudine in an uncontrolled extension of this study continue to be monitored closely. Under the 19 recently awarded NIH-sponsored AIDS Treatment and Evaluation Unit (ATEU) contracts, a planned two year placebo-controlled trial in asymptomatic patients with Kaposi's sarcoma was begun in December 1986 along with a large one year dose-comparison study in AIDS/post-PCP patients (zidovudine at 250 mg every four hours compared with a lower dose that is hoped will provide the same benefit with less toxicity). A number of other studies are also planned by NIH, Burroughs Wellcome, and others, including trials in HIV-infected patients with primarily neurologic manifestations (AIDS-dementia complex), in asymptomatic HIV-infected individuals, and in earlier ARC patients with minimal symptoms and higher CD4 cell counts.

At the present time it is desirable to plan placebo-controlled trials in some of these groups of patients, particularly those with a good short-term prognosis, as the risk to benefit ratio of zidovudine has yet to be determined in less ill patients. As discussed previously in this chapter, the toxicity of the drug when given on a chronic basis over many months may reduce the potential benefit the drug appears to have in halting the replication of the virus. The most efficient study design to determine whether or not a drug will be of more benefit than harm is to compare a group of treated patients with a similar group of untreated (or control) patients in a double-blind, randomized trial. It is ethical to do this when the drug is of unknown value in a particular group of patients. Data Safety and Monitoring Boards will review the data from the trials on a periodic basis much as they did for Burroughs Wellcome's placebo-controlled trial.

Another antiviral drug that inhibits HIV replication in some laboratory assays is ribavirin,[40] also a nucleoside analog, which also has in vitro activity against a broad range of other viruses, including respiratory syncytial virus (RSV), influenza A, and herpes simplex virus. It has been tested in humans in various formulations for a number of years, and is approved for use in aerosol form in hospitalized infants and young children with serious RSV pulmonary infection.

Placebo-controlled studies of the oral formulation of ribavirin were begun early in 1986 in asymptomatic HIV-infected patients with chronic lymphadenopathy, and in more advanced patients with at least one ARC symptom (fever, malaise, diarrhea, night sweats, weight loss). Because the manufacturer, ICN Pharmaceuticals, decided to study the drug at earlier stages of disease than did Burroughs Wellcome for zidovudine, it seems unlikely that the dramatic differences in mortality that resulted in the premature termination of the zidovudine trial will be seen in the ribavirin trials. However, if the results are encouraging, controlled trials of ribavirin versus zidovudine in later stages of HIV infection may be undertaken.

No other antiretroviral agents have been tested in placebo-controlled efficacy trials. Suramin, a complex antitrypanosomal agent in human use for years but not approved in the United States, was identified early by NCI scientists as having activity against HIV in the laboratory.[41] Extensive Phase I testing in AIDS and ARC patients over one and a half years identified a maximum tolerated dose, but some patients developed serious side effects, such as adrenal insufficiency, and no clinical efficacy was seen.[42] A placebo-controlled trial was never begun, so it is unclear to what extent adverse events were disease-related rather than caused by the drug. The NIH has recommended that suramin no longer be studied alone for its antiretroviral effects in this disease.[42]

HPA 23, a complex heteropolyanion (compound) developed at the Pasteur Institute in Paris, was discovered to have antiretroviral activity against HIV in vitro and was given to HIV-infected individuals in France beginning in 1983. Early reports of clinical improvement in a few patients generated much interest in the drug,[43] and a Phase I trial was conducted in this country in the fall/winter of 1985–1986. Very little further information has been reported, except for some results from small studies in France.[44]

Foscarnet (sodium phosphonoformate) is an antiviral drug manufactured in Sweden that was initially studied in topical formulation against herpes simplex virus. It also has activity in vitro against CMV and HIV[45] and is currently undergoing studies in Europe in a parenteral formulation. Other antiretroviral drugs, including other nucleoside analogs, are in earlier stages of testing. No clinical benefits have been reported to date.

The approval of zidovudine for the treatment of certain patients with advanced HIV infection raises major issues regarding the testing of other experimental antiretroviral therapies. The design of trials for determining the efficacy and safety of new drugs will be guided by both regulatory and ethical concerns in addition to scientific imperatives. It will be important to compare new agents with zidovudine in those patients for whom the approved drug is indicated (been shown to be of benefit). For other groups of HIV-infected patients for whom there is no approved therapy, placebo-controlled trials will continue to be ethical, and in fact, highly desirable, but may be difficult to implement and complete if many patients at earlier stages of infection choose to risk taking zidovudine even though benefit has not been established.

The specific agents discussed above are believed to act primarily by inhibiting reverse transcriptase, an enzyme critical for retroviral replication. Other approaches to controlling the spread of infection within the host include the use of agents which interfere with the ability of HIV to attach to and penetrate uninfected target cells. It appears that the virus enters the cell after binding to the CD4 molecule,[46] so considerable research has focused on exploring inhibitors of CD4 receptor binding including monoclonal antibodies. AL721, an investigational agent which has been reported to inhibit HIV in cell culture,[47] is said to act by changing the "fluidity" of the cell (or virus) membrane and thus altering critical receptor configuration. A new chemically synthesized peptide is also said to act by interfering with viral attachment. Another approach to antiretroviral therapy which is being actively pursued in the laboratory at this time is the use of synthetic oligonucleotides complementary to viral RNA or proviral DNA, aimed at inhibiting viral replication by interfering with gene transcription and/or translation.[48]

CONCLUSION

At the present time, the medical management of patients with AIDS and related conditions is indeed complex. It consists for the most part of palliative therapies which may improve the quality of life but only temporarily delay the seemingly inevitable outcome—death. Looking to the future, it would appear that the only way to rid society of this disease is by preventing further spread of the virus to currently uninfected individuals, by means of education as to its modes of transmission and eventually by universal vaccination of the susceptible population. The prospects for actual cure of infected persons are dim, in my view. However, with patience, expanded research efforts in "drug discovery" programs, additional well-designed clinical investigations, and a lot of hard work, it may be possible to identify relatively safe antiretroviral agents which, when used alone or in some combination with immunorestorative therapy, will arrest the destructive disease process and improve the infected individual's ability to resist AIDS-related opportunistic infections and malignancies. If such a therapeutic regimen that can be tolerated on a long-term basis is devised, HIV-infected individuals may be able to anticipate a relatively normal life. The demonstration that an antiretroviral agent can delay death and the development of OIs in certain groups of ill patients is certainly an important step in the right direction. Partly because of this achievement, I believe that we can look forward to a rapid increase in the number of new therapies under investigation in HIV-infected individuals, as well as to the development of novel approaches to all aspects of the treatment of this disease and its associated conditions.

I would like to express my gratitude to Dr. Robert Yarchoan of the Clinical Oncology Program, National Cancer Institute, National Institutes of Health, Bethesda, Maryland, and to Dr. H. Clifford Lane of the Laboratory of Immunoregulation, National Institute of Allergy and Infectious Diseases, National Institutes of Health, Bethesda, Maryland, for their helpful comments and critical review of the manuscript. I would also like to thank Ms. Betty McRoy for her technical assistance.

REFERENCES

1. De Jarlais, D. C., et al. "Kaposi's Sarcoma Among Four Different AIDS Risk Groups." *New England Journal of Medicine* 310:1119 (1984).
2. Rivin, B., et al. "AIDS Outcome. A First Follow-up." *New England Journal of Medicine* 311:857 (1984).
3. Shaw, G. M., et al. "Molecular Characterization of Human T-Cell Leukemia (Lymphotropic) Virus Type III in the Acquired Immune Deficiency Syndrome." *Science* 226:1165–71 (1984).
4. Lane, H. C., and A. S. Fanci. "Immunologic Abnormalities in the Acquired Immunodeficiency Syndrome." In *Annual Review of Immunology* Vol. 3, edited by William E. Rapul et al, 477–500 (1985).
5. Lane, H. C., et al. "The Use of Interleukin-2 in Patients with the Acquired Immune Deficiency Syndrome (AIDS)." *Journal of Biological Response Modifiers* 3:512–516 (1984).
6. Lane, H. C., et al. "A Phase I Trial of Recombinant Immune (gamma) Interferon in Patients with AIDS." *Clinical Research* 33:408 A (1985).
7. Barr-Sinoussi, F., et al. "Isolation of Lymphadenopathy-Associated Virus (LAV) and Detection of LAV Antibodies from U.S. Patients with AIDS." *JAMA* 253:1737–1739 (1985).
8. Mitsuyasu, R., et al. "Treatment of Donor Bone Marrow with Monoclonal Anti-T-Cell Antibody and Complement for the Prevention of Graft-Versus-Host Disease." *Annals of Internal Medicine* 105:20–26 (1986).

9. Martin, P. J. "Effects of In Vitro Depletion of T-Cells in HLA-Identical Allogeneic Marrow Grafts. *Blood* 66:664–672 (1985).

10. Rouse, B. T., and D. W. Horohov. "Immunosuppression in Viral Infections." *Reviews of Infectious Diseases* 8:850–873 (1986).

11. Whimbey, E., et al. "Bacteremia and Fungemia in Patients with the Acquired Immunodeficiency Syndrome." *Annals of Internal Medicine* 104:511–514 (1986).

12. Fischl, M., and G. Dickinson. "Acquired Immunodeficiency Syndrome." In *Conn's Current Therapy 1986*, edited by Robert E. Rakel, 25–32. Philadelphia, PA: W. B. Saunders Co., 1986.

13. Gordin, F., et al. "Adverse Reactions to Trimethoprim-Sulfamethoxazole in Patients with Acquired Immunodeficiency Syndrome." *Annals of Internal Medicine* 100:495–499 (1984).

14. Castella, A., et al. "The Bone Marrow in AIDS: A Histologic, Hematologic, and Microbiologic Study." *American Journal of Clinical Pathology* 84:425–432 (1985).

15. Gelmann, E. P., and S. Broder. "Kaposi's Sarcoma in the Setting of the AIDS Pandemic." In *AIDS: Modern Concepts and Therapeutic Challenges*, edited by Samuel Broder, 227–229. New York: Marcel Dekker, Inc., 1987.

16. Krown, S., et al. "Kaposi's Sarcoma and the Acquired Immune Deficiency Syndrome: Treatment with Recombinant Interferon Alpha and Analysis of Prognostic Factors." *Cancer* 57:1662–1665 (1986).

17. Levine, A. M., et al. "AIDS-Related Malignant B-Cell Lymphomas." In *AIDS: Modern Concepts and Therapeutic Challenges*, edited by Broder, 240–241.

18. Parks, W. P., and G. B. Scott. "An Overview of Pediatric AIDS: Approaches to Diagnosis and Outcome Assessment." In *AIDS: Modern Concepts and Therapeutic Challenges*, edited by Broder, 245–262.

19. Polk, B. F., et al. "Predictors of the Acquired Immunodeficiency Syndrome Developing in a Cohort of Seropositive Homosexual Men." *New England Journal of Medicine* 316:61–66 (1987).

20. Francis, D. P., et al. "The Natural History of Infection with the Lymphadenopathy-Associated Virus Human T-Lymphotropic Virus Type III." *Annals of Internal Medicine* 103:719–722 (1985).

21. Rutherford, G., et al. "The Natural History of LAV/HTLV-III Infection and Viraemia in Homosexual and Bisexual Men: A 6-year Follow-up Study (Abstract)." In *Proceedings of International Conference on AIDS*, Paris, 23–25 June, 1986, 99.

22. Kaplan, et al. "HTLV-III Viremia in Homosexual Men with Generalized Lymphadenopathy." *New England Journal of Medicine* 312:1572–1573 (1985).

23. Chaisson, R. E., et al. "Significant Changes in HIV Antigen Level in the Serum of Patients Treated with Azidothymidine (Letter)." *New England Journal of Medicine* 315:1610–1611 (1986).

24. Goudsmit, J., et al. "Expression of Human Immunodeficiency Virus Antigen (HIV-AG) in Serum and Cerebrospinal Fluid during Acute and Chronic Infection." *Lancet* 2:177–180 (1986).

25. Eysler, M. E., et al. "Acid-Labile Alpha Interferon: A Possible Preclinical Marker for the Acquired Immunodeficiency Syndrome in Hemophilia." *New England Journal of Medicine* 309:583–586 (1983).

26. Metroka, C., et al. "Acid-Labile Interferon Alpha in Homosexual Men: A Preclinical Marker for Opportunistic Infections (Abstract)." In *Proceedings of International Conference on AIDS*, Paris, 23–25 June 1986, 80.

27. Murray, H. W., et al. "Impaired Production of Lymphokinecs and Immune Interferon in the Acquired Immunodeficiency Syndromes." *New England Journal of Medicine* 310:883–889 (1984).

28. Lange, et al. "Prospective Study on a Homosexual Cohort: Significance of Persistant Acid Labile Alpha Interferon and Decreasing Erythrocyte Complement 3B Receptors (Abstract)." In *Proceedings of International Conference on AIDS*, Paris, 23–25 June 1986, 73.

29. Cronin, W., et al. "Prognostic Significance of Antilymphocyte Antibodies in Serum of Patients with AIDS and ARC. (Abstract)" In *Proceedings of International Conference on AIDS*, Paris, 23–25 June 1986, 80.

30. Sissons, J. G., and M. B. A. Oldstone, "Host Responses to Viral Infections." In *Virology*, edited by B. N. Fields et al. 266. New York: Raven Press (1985).

31. Lane, H. C., and A. S. Fanci. "Immunologic Reconstitution in the Acquired Immunodeficiency Syndrome." *Annals of Internal Medicine* 103:714–718 (1985).

32. Rubinstein, A., et al. "Treatment of AIDS with Intravenous Gammaglobulin (Abstract)." *Pediatric Research* 17:263A (1984).

33. Lane, H. D., et al. "Partial Immune Reconstitution in a Patient with the Acquired Immunodeficiency Syndrome." *New England Journal of Medicine* 311:1099 (1984).

34. Fischl, M. A., and G. M. Dickinson. "Trimethoprim-sulfamethoxazole Prophylaxis of P. Carinii Pneumonia in AIDS (Abstract no. 436)." In *Program and Abstracts of the 25th Intersciencce Conference on Antimicrobial Agents and Chemotherapy*, 1985.

35. Harshom, et al. "Synergistic Inhibition of Human T-Cell Lymphotropic Virus Type III Replication In Vitro by Phosphonoformate and Recombinant Alpha-A Interferon." *Antimicrobial Agents and Chemotherapy* 30:189–191 (1986).

36. Harshom, et al. "Effects of Combination Antiviral Therapy on LAV/HTLV-III Replication In Vitro (Abstract)." In *Proceedings of International Conference on AIDS*, Paris, 23–25 June 1986, 69.

37. Lester, W. "Tuberculosis." In *Medical Microbiology and Infectious Disease*, edited by Abraham Brande, et al., 977–978. Philadelphia, PA: W. B. Saunders & Co., 1981.

38. Mitsuya, H., et al. "3'-Azido-3'-deoxythymidine (BWA509U): An Antiviral Agent That Inhibits the Infectivity and Cytopathic Effect of Human T-Lymphotropic Virus Type III/Lymphadenopathy-Associated Virus In Vitro. *Proceedings of National Academy of Sciences USA*, 821:7096–7100 (1985).

39. Yarchoan, R., et al. "Administration of 3'-azido-3'-deoxythymidine, An Inhibitor of HTLV-III Replication, To Patients with AIDS and AIDS-Related-Complex." *Lancet* 1:575–580 (1986).

40. McCormick, J. B., et al. "Ribavirin Suppresses Replication of Lymphadenopathy-Associated Virus in Cultures of Human Adult T Lymphocytes." *Lancet* 2:1367–1369 (1984).

41. Mitsuya, H., et al. "Suramin Protection of T Cells In Vitro Against Infectivity and Cytopathic Effect of HTLV-III." *Science* 226:172–174 (1984).

42. Cheson, B. D., et al. "Suramin Therapy in AIDS and Related Diseases. Initial Report of the U.S. Suramin Working Group (Abstract)." In *Proceedings of International Conference on AIDS*, Paris, 23–25 June 1986, 35.

43. Rozenbaum, W., et al. "Antimoniotungstate (HPA 23) treatment of Three Patients with AIDS and One with Prodrome (Letter)." *Lancet* 1:450–451 (1985).

44. Dormont, E., et al. "Virologic and Immunologic Follow-up of 15 Patients with AIDS or AIDS Related Complex, and 4 LAV/HTLV-III Seropositive Patients Treated with Daily IV Doses of HPA 23 During 4 to 15 Months (Abstract)." In *Proceedings of International Conference on AIDS*, Paris, 23–25 June 1986, 34.

45. Sandstrom, et al. "Inhibition of Human T-Cell Lymphotropic Virus Type III In Vitro by Phosphonoformate." *Lancet* 1:1480–1482 (1985).

46. Maddon, P. J., et al. "The T_4 Gene Encodes the AIDS Virus Receptor and Is Expressed in the Immune System and the Brain. *Cell* 47:333–348 (1986).

47. Sarin, et al. "Effect of a Novel Compound (AL 721) on HTLV-III Infectivity In Vitro." *New England Journal of Medicine* 313:1289–1290 (1985).

48. Zamecnik, P. C., et al. "Inhibition of Replication and Expression of Human T-cell Lymphotropic Virus Type III in Cultured Cells by Exogenous Synthetic Oligonucleotides Complementary to Viral RNA." *Proceedings of the National Academy of Sciences* 83:4143–4146 (1986).

CHAPTER 10

Choosing Therapies

CHUCK FRUTCHEY

MEDICAL TREATMENTS

The decisions involved in choosing treatments are difficult for people with AIDS and ARC. For many, the decisions require both information and analytical skills that they may not have.

A physician should be consulted before pursuing any treatment plan; however, all decision-making authority should not be surrendered. The decisions ultimately remain the patient's and preparation is necessary to make them intelligently. A person with AIDS should use doctors, friends, and other people with AIDS/ARC as resources, but should retain and exercise the right to make choices about his or her own health.

Unlike many alternative therapies, where the effectiveness of the treatment is not certain, with medically supervised therapies there is usually a great deal known about the treatment process—its benefits and possible negative side effects. The patient should find out all pertinent information, investigating even those therapies not likely to be chosen, to understand why they may or may not be appropriate. The clinician should encourage the patient to ask lots of questions, and to keep asking if something is explained and is still not understood. Many patients will probably have to learn new things about how the human body functions in order to increase their knowledge to make appropriate decisions. Health care providers should be prepared to refer the patient to other resources for information they cannot provide.

The patient should also be made aware that in some cases no therapy at all may be an option. Some people, such as those with early and nonaggressive Kaposi's sarcoma, do not always need treatment. For other people, there may only be one type of medication to treat a particular infection which requires immediate attention. After the infection has been eliminated, however, patients may be able to "safely" stop treatment, or take some time to consider which treatment is best.

Since the treatment of most opportunistic infections in AIDS is fairly straightforward, the most difficult decisions will involve investigational drugs. In order to make an intelligent choice about a drug program, it is first necessary to understand how these programs are run and what are the possible side effects of the drugs.

Every drug trial involving humans is divided into four phases after first testing the drug in animal studies. During Phase 1, the drug is monitored for toxicity (harmfulness) and tested to see how the body processes or metabolizes it. In Phase 2, the test moves on to find out how effective the drug is in controlling the disease or its symptoms. Phase 3 introduces many of the elements we normally think of for "controlled" studies. In this stage, the study participants are randomly divided into two or more groups. One group receives the investigational drug at a dosage that is based on Phase 2 results. The other group will get a harmless, inactive compound, usually a sugar pill or equivalent, known as a placebo. Neither the researchers nor the participants know who is getting the drug and who is getting the placebo. This is called a "double-blind" study. Phase 4 studies are ongoing studies of the drug's effects and usefulness in clinical practice.

Double-blind studies are extremely important in proving whether or not a new drug is worthwhile. It is important for the participants not to know what they are receiving because it is very common for people taking placebos to show some improvement, simply because they *think* they are taking an effective medicine. At the same time, it is important for the researchers not to know which patients are receiving the placebo so that they are not prejudiced when evaluating the participants.

There has been a lot of criticism lately about the "immorality" of giving people placebos when they are very sick. But without placebo-controlled studies, it would be impossible to know if any observed benefits were the result of the drug or merely the participants' desire to get well. The mind can be a very powerful tool in healing and designing experiments that take this into account is necessary to evaluate the real cause behind a drug's apparent success. Even with the drug AZT, which has become more widely available though all of the effects are not fully understood, the initial evidence that it was useful came from double-blind, placebo-controlled studies. Only when the results are dramatically successful or unsuccessful can a solid determination of efficacy without placebo controls be made. (As we progress in our study of drugs to treat AIDS, it will become possible to replace the placebo with a drug whose effectiveness is known and measure the new drug's effectiveness against it. This is a variation of placebo-controlled studies and satisfies the same requirements.)

In the long run, the method of controlled trials benefits more people than uncontrolled drug testing ever would. But it is important for the patient participating in one of these studies to understand that it may or may not be beneficial. Investigational drug protocols are not the same as a proven, effective treatment or cure. The drug may be a failure or cause adverse side effects which could make the condition of the participant worse.

When considering whether to be a participant in a study, the patient should discuss the pros and cons of the experimental drug with a doctor. Important questions for the patient to ask him- or herself and the doctor include: How sick am I? Will this new drug interrupt another treatment that I am already receiving that is effective? How do I feel about entering the study? What are the existing statistics on the efficacy of the drug?

If the patient is not fully committed to participating, he or she should not do so. If the patient is not very sick, he or she may not want to participate in a study which may have serious side effects that worsen the current status of the disease. On the other hand, the patient may decide that intervention at an early stage—while he or she still feels well and strong—is the most promising course to take.

AZT provides a good illustration of this situation. AZT is now available to certain people with AIDS (those who have had *Pneumocystis carinii* pneumonia or who have a helper T-cell count less than 200). It is being tested on other AIDS and ARC patients, as well as on some asymptomatic seropositive individuals. Some people in the latter group may want to take a conservative approach and not take the drug. Since the drug does have several adverse side effects, most notably a depression of bone marrow function, a healthy asymptomatic seropositive person may choose to wait and see if the benefits outweigh the risks. Others, who may be more anxious about their future, may decide that enrolling in an experimental program with AZT is a reasonable bet, hoping that an early intervention might prevent the disease from progressing. At present, there is no scientific basis on which to make this decision. Personal feelings are the best guidelines.

The patient who decides to participate in a drug study must be reminded that he or she has the right to withdraw at any time. If the patient feels, for whatever reason, that the study is harmful, he or she can drop out of the investigational program. Whether the individual has AIDS, ARC, or is asymptomatic seropositive, the decision to enter an experimental drug program should be made with great care and consideration.

ALTERNATIVE THERAPIES

The term "alternative therapies" is defined here as all types of intervention against disease that are not part of the Western medical tradition. This covers a wide range of treatments—everything from acupuncture, yoga, and other non-Western traditional practices, to visualization, mega-vitamins, light therapy, and swallowing crushed gem stones. Many alternative therapies have much documented success and some have theoretical frameworks to explain how they work. Others are newer and although they seem to have some benefit, it is difficult to identify what is actually causing the effect—the patients' expectations, the therapy, or mere chance. There are also alternative treatments that are suspect or have clearly been discredited. If a person is considering using one of these therapies, it is helpful to be able to distinguish those that may work from those that probably won't.

A major problem in evaluating alternative therapies for AIDS/ARC is the lack of hard data. While many of these therapies seem promising, very few have been rigorously tested in controlled experiments. Without such testing, as mentioned previously, it is impossible to be sure how much healing is due to the therapy, how much is due to the placebo effect, and how much is due to chance. A group of people must be carefully followed through a particular therapy and its impact measured in order to determine what percent of people have benefited from utilizing the therapy. Some therapies, such as acupuncture, have a proven effect in one area (painkilling), but not in others (immune boosting).* Other therapies, such as visualization, seem to work well in some situations but have yet to be studied to understand their applications and their limitations.

There are many alternative therapies that deserve more careful study, but at this time very few are being examined. This is due not only to a preference for traditional Western medicine on the part of the doctors and financial sponsors, but also to the suspicion or fear of being tested on the part of many alternative practitioners. Many alternative therapists feel it is unfair to give some patients a placebo in a controlled study. Yet, little concern is expressed for the much larger number of people who must, therefore, choose a therapy without knowing whether it is helpful or useless.

It's nearly impossible for an individual to be aware of all of the therapies, what they purport to do, and how effective they are, especially with the rapidly changing AIDS/ARC therapies. A practical solution is to have certain guidelines and questions that can be used for any therapy being considered. The following guidelines were developed mainly for evaluating alternative, nonmedical therapies, but most can be applied to discussions with a medical doctor about drug therapies as well.

The first step for the patient to take is to identify a primary care physician. Even if a patient decides to pursue an alternative therapy, there is no substitute for being followed by a doctor who can monitor vital signs, blood work, and so on. Any alternative practitioner who advises staying away from physicians should not be trusted. Likewise, using a doctor who warns people against considering any alternative therapy is not a wise choice.

It is also important for different caregivers to communicate with one

---

* G. Chen, S. Li, and C. Jiang. Clinical studies on neuropsychological and biochemical bases of acupuncture analgesia. *Journal AM. J. Clin, Medicine* 14(1 and 2):84–95 (1986).

another so they do not say or do things that will contradict each other or the therapy being followed. For example, a doctor and an herbalist may be prescribing medications which can react adversely with each other and endanger the patient. If each practitioner knows what the other is doing, dangerous situations can be avoided. The patient's medical record is usually the most complete description of health and disease history, so it is useful to have traditional as well as alternative treatments recorded there. However, this again points to the necessity of having clear communications among all caregivers.

If a patient decides to pursue an alternative therapy, it is advisable that careful research be done. There are various means for gathering information, such as asking friends or acquaintances for recommendations or asking at health education centers and/or public agencies for referrals. The patient should collect as much information as possible before making a choice of therapy. He or she may decide to pursue more than one therapy but, again, the different practitioners must be advised to talk with each other.

After deciding on a therapy, there are several important considerations in choosing a caregiver. First, who is the caregiver and what is his or her reputation? Are they any colleagues with the same specialty who will provide a reference? Is it possible for the patient to talk with previous patients? If the therapist is not known in the community or can provide no references, look for another one. Also ascertain whether the therapist has done any previous work with persons with AIDS/ARC and how long the therapy has been practiced.

Another consideration is whether the caregiver can explain the therapy in a way that makes sense to the patient. Is the alternative practitioner eager to answer questions? Is he or she willing to talk to a doctor or other caregivers? What is the underlying philosophy from which the therapist operates? Therapists who insist solely on faith and spurn hard data are likely candidates for quackery. If the patient gets explanations that sound more like gibberish than reasoned thought, he or she should think twice about whether to trust this person with his or her health.

The relevance of the therapy to the individual's condition is also a concern. Does the therapy seem to make sense and is it consistent with the patient's own philosophy? Can the patient believe in it or does it seem more like hype than healing? Is it affordable? Some alternative therapists maintain that belief in the effectiveness of the therapy is crucial to its efficacy. If the patient doesn't believe in the therapy, he may be wasting his time and resources.

Other questions that the patient should ask when evaluating the available therapies include: have the number of people who have utilized the therapy, the number who have improved, the extent of improvement, any potential side effects, and possible cross reactions with other drugs or conditions been documented? Has this therapy ever been used to treat AIDS/ARC? Does the therapist take a complete case history before and after therapy? Are adequate records being kept? How is confidentiality maintained?

There are a number of actions the patient should take while receiving therapy. He or she should monitor him- or herself by keeping a log or notes. The therapist should, of course, also be doing this, but it can be useful for the patient to have person records to compare and to be able to provide accurate information to the practitioner. If there is no improvement after what seems like a reasonable amount of time, then further questions should be asked. Above all, the patient should continue to ask questions and be a part of the therapy, not just a passive recipient. The therapy should not be continued if the patient feels it is useless or harmful. The patient should also make sure that financial considerations are taken into account. Rent, food, and other necessities should not be sacrificed for the treatment. Most practitioners are willing to make some financial arrangement that is workable.

These questions and considerations can help the patient carefully explore alternatives. Although the benefits of some alternative therapies cannot be currently explained, neither can they be denied. Having an open mind about treatments is good, but chasing after cures without a critical eye may result in financial losses or, worse, physical harm. The patient should understand at the outset what he or she expects to gain, and how to know when that has been achieved. Perhaps the most vital factor in gaining or maintaining wellness is concentrating on being well, rather than spending enormous amounts of time or energy on sickness. It is possible to get well with AIDS/ARC, and it is important to know this fact. But the old adage still applies: Buyer beware!

The testing of experimental drugs or alternative treatments is a very important part of the ongoing attempt to control AIDS/ARC. People who participate in these studies are performing a valuable service which will help many people. But it is important to evaluate any treatment realistically. A hopeful attitude is essential; blind faith can have disastrous effects.

The best advice to a patient: Be an expert on your condition and know what is being done to and for you.

CHAPTER 11

The New Death among IV Drug Users

DON C. DES JARLAIS
CATHY CASRIEL
SAMUEL FRIEDMAN

INTRODUCTION

Intravenous (IV) drug users are the second largest group of persons to have developed AIDS in the United States and Europe. Of the 33,720 cases of AIDS in the United States, 5565 (17%) are among heterosexual IV drug users and 2550 (8%) are among male homosexual/bisexual IV drug users (reported through 6 April 1987).[1] In Europe, 600 (15%) of the 3898 cases have IV drug use as their primary risk factor, and 98 (3%) have IV drug use and male homosexual activity as risk behavior (reported through 31 Dec. 1987).[2] The metropolitan New York area has by far the greatest concentration of AIDS cases in which IV drug use is the primary risk factor, with 3248 cases in New York and 901 cases in New Jersey. These two states account for 75% of all U.S. cases in which IV drug use is the primary risk behavior.

There is great variation in HIV seroprevalence rates among IV drug users in different areas. High levels of seroprevalence—rates of 50% or greater—have been reported in the New York City area,[3,4] Edinburgh,[5] northern Italy,[6] and Spain.[7] Very low rates (4% or less) have been found in southern New Jersey,[8] London,[9] New Orleans,[10] and Glasgow.[11] At present there is no good explanation for this wide variation, although the date at which HIV was first introduced among IV drug users in a local area is undoubtedly one of the reasons.

Transmission of HIV among IV drug users occurs primarily through the sharing of drug injection equipment, with heterosexual transmission apparently playing a relatively minor role (see [12] for a review). The behavioral factors most frequently associated with HIV seropositivity are the frequency of drug injection[13-15] and the sharing of needles across friendship groups as in the use of "shooting galleries" (places where one can rent equipment which is then returned for other IV drug users to rent and use).[16–18] In cities where formally organized shooting galleries do not exist, the use of "house works" (injection equipment that a drug dealer keeps to lend to customers) may be the functional equivalent.

Once HIV is established among IV drug users in a local area, this group can become the dominant means of transmission to heterosexuals and perinatal transmission. In New York City, 87% of the heterosexual transmission cases have been from IV drug users to regular sexual partners who do not inject drugs, and 80% of the perinatal transmission cases have been in the children of IV drug users.[19]

The AIDS epidemic is having a very complex effect on IV drug users in Western societies. AIDS is leading to many changes in this subculture, some of which have been spontaneous and others of which have been in response to public health prevention efforts. The connection between IV drug users and heterosexual transmission of HIV is forcing many public health and political authorities to reassess previous attitudes regarding the nature and importance of illicit drug injection in society.

The theme of AIDS as a new way of dying for IV drug users will be used to integrate many (though clearly not all) of the effects of AIDS on the injection of illicit drugs. Consideration of death and IV drug use prior to the AIDS epidemic provides a good starting point for the analysis.

DEATH IN THE DRUG USE SUBCULTURE

Death was quite common in the IV drug use subculture prior to AIDS. The death rate for drug users in treatment was about 1.5% per year. Estimates of death rates among IV drug users out of treatment have ranged from 3.5% to 8% per year (see [20] for a review). The major factor accounting for the higher rate of out-of-treatment deaths was narcotic overdoses. In fact, prior to AIDS, an overdose was considered the prototype for the cause of death among active IV drug users.

Overdose deaths primarily come from taking a much stronger than usual dose of heroin, so that whatever tolerance has been developed is not sufficient to prevent a fatal respiratory depression. Heroin that can cause an overdose is thus also able to give a very good "high" (if the user exercises appropriate caution). This association between a strong dose of narcotic and overdose death has led many heroin dealers to name their personal "brands" with variations on the theme of overdosing-death. Black Death, Broken Hearted Killer, Death, Death Row, Death Wish, Killer, Killer 1, Kiss of Death, OD, OD (black star), Strangler, Suicide, and The Killer have all been used in the marketing of heroin in New York City.[21] Without being overly psychoanalytic, one may assume a fundamental ambivalence towards overdose deaths among IV drug users. While an overdose death clearly means facing the terrors of dying, as well as loss of the pleasures of using drugs, approaching this form of death also has a connotation of intense pleasure, and can be seen as a justifiable risk in the search for the peak of drug-induced euphoria.

AIDS VERSUS OVERDOSE DEATH

Death from AIDS is very different than death from an overdose. Table 1 presents some of these differences. The variation in the time duration between an overdose death and an AIDS death is fundamental. Death from a narcotic overdose will often occur within several minutes to an hour after taking the drug. During this time the person will usually be unconscious, so there is a very limited amount of time in which to realize/experience the overdose. In contrast, dying from AIDS is usually quite protracted. There may be many years from initial HIV infection to the development of clinical symptoms, days to years between the development of symptoms and the development of diagnosed AIDS, and then perhaps another year or more until death. Both an overdose or AIDS may lead to an IV drug user's death; it is, however, the relative lack of time between an overdose and death compared to the lengthy time between an AIDS diagnosis and death that leads to many of the differences in the psychology of the two forms of death.

The brief time span of an overdose is generally experienced as a narcotic euphoria (though there is some possibility that the IV drug user may become aware and alarmed about a potential overdose prior to losing consciousness). AIDS typically involves physical weakness and incapacitation, along with extended periods of pain associated with the opportunistic infections that arise as a result of the HIV-induced immunosuppression. The two types of dying may be considered almost complete physical opposites—sensations of intense pleasure versus extended debilitation and protracted pain.

An overdose death is basically asocial, although assistance to combat the overdose usually will be provided if others are present. Thus, to the extent

TABLE 1   Characteristics of Overdose and AIDS Deaths

Characteristics	Overdose death	AIDS death
Time duration	Immediate	Protracted
Physical characteristics	Euphoria	Pain, debilitation
Social reaction	Asocial	Isolation, strained relationships, potential intense guilt
Comparison to stressful life	Release	Worsening, leading to suicidal thoughts
Contingent on drug use	Stopping drug use eliminates risk	Often independent of continued drug use

that social relationships are involved in an overdose situation, they are likely to be supportive. The shortness of time between the taking of the overdose and loss of consciousness, however, does not provide much opportunity for social interaction; therefore, from the perspective of the person who has taken the overdose, the event as it occurs is primarily asocial.

The months from AIDS diagnosis to death permit many opportunities for social interaction between the IV drug user with AIDS and others. Despite the commitment and care of many of the health care providers, social interactions are likely to be extremely difficult for the IV drug user with AIDS. Friends who are also drug users may refuse to visit when the patient is in the hospital, out of (a mistaken) fear of casual contact transmission and a (generally correct) perception that current IV drug users are not welcome visitors in most hospitals. Family members may refuse to see the patient, again out of fear of casual contact transmission and also the emotional stress of an impending death. Friends and family may simultaneously feel guilt for not having done enough to prevent the drug dependency that led to AIDS and a "blame the victim" anger at the IV drug user for having brought the disease upon himself or herself.

If the IV drug user has a sexual partner who does not inject drugs, or has young children, there is the possibility of transmitting the virus to the partner and/or child. In this case the direction of any transmission is evident and there is the potential for extreme anger and guilt in all parties concerned. While an overdose death is essentially asocial, the interpersonal relationships after a diagnosis of AIDS are very complex and may cause as much distress and suffering as the physical symptoms of HIV infection.

These differences between overdose and AIDS deaths for IV drug users can be summarized as follows. An overdose death contains many elements of escape—it can be a quick and euphoric release from a troubled life. Death from AIDS, in contrast, is a prolonged experience in dying, combining physical debilitation, pain, and troubled interpersonal relationships. Many IV drug users, when comparing the two types of death, have expressed a preference for an overdose death, and have even suggested that they might deliberately take an overdose if they believed they had AIDS.

A word needs to be said at this point about the possible effects antiviral drugs such as AZT might have on the comparison between an overdose death and an AIDS death. Clearly, any antiviral drug that arrests the progression of HIV infection and prevents persons from dying from AIDS will change the psychology of HIV-infected individuals. The major difference between AIDS and overdoses, however, is in the time period prior to death. An antiviral drug with significant and unpleasant side effects, that requires frequent medical monitoring, and does not fully protect against transmission to others, and that must be taken frequently enough that others became aware of the person's condition, may actually heighten the differences between AIDS and an overdose. Thus much of the psychology of AIDS would still apply even if an antiviral drug that prevented death were readily available to IV drug users with HIV infection.

ACTUAL RESPONSES TO AIDS DIAGNOSES

Although the potentially traumatic effects of an AIDS diagnosis on the psychological functioning of IV drug users should not be underestimated, such a diagnosis very rarely leads to suicide or psychotic breaks. A more common reaction is the desire to regain health and to enter treatment immediately so that the period between diagnosis and death need not be spent trying to hustle drugs on the street. The stress of an AIDS diagnosis can be positive: it is clearly capable of eliciting great courage and strength among IV drug users and their families and friends. Some IV drug users have responded by joining AIDS prevention efforts aimed at current IV drug users.

RISK REDUCTION

Given that AIDS is a new form of death, one would expect IV drug users to have a significant interest in learning about AIDS and to show substantial behavior changes in order to avoid developing the disease. There is consistent evidence that IV drug users in New York City are relatively well informed about AIDS and that many have altered their behavior to reduce the risk of AIDS. In 1984, we conducted a survey of methadone maintenance patients in Manhattan.[22] Essentially all knew of AIDS, and over 90% knew that sharing drug injection equipment was a means of transmitting the virus. Thirty percent personally knew someone who had developed AIDS; 59% reported that they had changed their behavior to reduce their risk; 54% reported changes in their use of needles and syringes, with an increase in the use of sterile/cleaned equipment and a reduction in the number of persons with whom they would share injection equipment the most frequently mentioned changes.

Selwyn and colleagues[23] from Montefiore Medical Center in New York City conducted a similar study in 1985. It sampled IV drug users from a methadone maintenance program and from a prison detoxification service. The results were almost identical. Almost all subjects knew that AIDS was transmitted through the sharing of drug injection equipment, and over 60% had modified their use of injection equipment in order to protect themselves against AIDS. Again, increased use of sterile injection equipment and fewer numbers of people with whom one would share injection equipment were the two most common methods of risk reduction.

Validation of these self-reported changes in needle use behavior comes from our studies of the marketing of illicit sterile injection equipment in New York City. There has been a notable increase in the demand for and marketing of illicit sterile needles and syringes since 1984,[24,25] which supports the self-reports of greater use of such equipment in our own and the Montefiore studies.

These behavior changes among IV drug users in New York City occurred before the establishment of any large-scale prevention programs aimed at reducing AIDS within this group. This risk reduction should therefore be seen as a result of the general information about AIDS transmitted through the mass media and the oral communication networks of the IV drug use subculture rather than the result of any specific prevention campaigns.

Evidence that IV drug users alter their behavior to avoid AIDS is not limited to the New York area, where the large number of cases of AIDS among this group would serve as a signal of the need to reduce their risk. Ongoing research in Amsterdam and San Francisco shows that methods of risk reduction had begun in those cities *prior* to the development of many AIDS cases among IV drug users. Coutinho[26] reports increasing use of the "free needle exchange" program in Amsterdam in response to concern about AIDS in that city. Biernacki and Feldman[27] report that IV drug users in San Francisco were aware of AIDS by the end of 1985, and that a "significant minority" had changed their behavior to reduce the chances of developing AIDS.

REACTION OF DRUG ABUSE TREATMENT STAFF TO AIDS

AIDS as a new form of death has led to changes not only in the behavior of IV drug users themselves, but also in drug abuse treatment programs. In addition to the differences between an overdose death and an AIDS death summarized in Table 1, there is another that is particularly significant for drug abuse treatment programs. Stopping drug use eliminates the threat of an overdose death. Because of the long latency period between initial HIV infection and the development of clinical HIV disease, however, a person may stop drug use and still die from AIDS. This fact creates problems for drug abuse treatment staff in their attempts to motivate drug users to avoid IV drug use.

The reactions of drug treatment programs and staff in New York City have varied over time. Four stages have been observed in their responses to the AIDS epidemic (see [28] for a full presentation of these stages). These stages are similar to, but not identical with, the stages that Kübler-Ross[29] observed in medical patients who receive diagnoses of fatal conditions. They are also similar to the stages in response to stress that have been described by Selye.[30]

As within the Kübler-Ross schema, the typical first response among treatment staff to the AIDS crisis can be termed denial. Denial among drug abuse treatment staff consists of trying to continue treating IV drug users as if the epidemic was not affecting them. Initially this was done by simply not devoting any organizational resources (including staff time) to AIDS-related issues. Later, other methods, such as trying to screen out persons exposed to HIV from entry into the program, evolved.

It would be a fundamental mistake to see this denial as a simple failure to respond to a pressing issue. There are several psychological reasons for the reluctance of drug abuse treatment staff to address AIDS issues or to want to work with HIV-infected persons. The fear of casual contact transmission is one reason. While there is no evidence that HIV can be transmitted by casual contact, the reluctance of scientists to rule out absolutely any such possibility encourages the fear that it could happen. Drug abuse treatment often involves the collection of urine samples (in methadone programs) and the use of common eating facilities (in residential programs) both of which can serve as foci for fears of casual contact transmission.

Drug treatment staff generally have had very little training or expertise in working with infectious diseases, particularly incurable ones like AIDS. Previous experience with infectious diseases is likely to be confined to acute infections that are referred for medical treatment and are cured. They have had essentially no experience with counseling persons with long-term, fatal illnesses; they are neither professionally nor emotionally prepared for counseling persons who may die regardless of any behavior changes or medical interventions. Drug treatment staff are also not trained to counsel on sexual and/or perinatal risk reduction measures that are essential for effective AIDS prevention efforts among IV drug users.

Drug abuse counseling is already a task that is often emotionally frustrating. But there are certain rewards and feelings of accomplishment when, for instance, one sees reduction or elimination of drug use and improvement in the life situations of the clients. AIDS seems to ask drug abuse counselors to make a career change and become AIDS counselors. This new career involves hypothetical exposure to a deadly virus, confronting one's own sense of mortality, learning new counseling skills, and accepting the possibility that clients may die despite the best efforts of the client, the counselor, and medical personnel. Taking all these factors into account, denial can be considered a perfectly reasonable reaction to the AIDS epidemic; it should not be taken as an indication of lack of commitment on the part of drug abuse treatment staff.

It would be impossible to prevent all HIV-infected drug abusers from entering a specific treatment program. Ethical, legal, and technical reasons prohibit full exclusion. It then becomes a matter of time until someone in (or related to) the program develops an AIDS-related illness. This will provoke a second stage of response—panic. The fears of casual contact transmission become acute. Even for persons who do not have this fear, emotional difficulties in acknowledging their own mortality make for difficult interpersonal interactions with the AIDS client. During this stage, drug abuse treatment personnel have sometimes acted in ways that were actively harmful to the HIV-infected clients. They may have dismissed such people from the treatment program or, if allowed to stay, the persons with HIV infection may be required to attend at odd hours when they will not be seen by other clients in the program. AIDS need not occur in a person currently in treatment to provoke the panic stage among the staff. Panic has also arisen in response to HIV infection in the spouse of a current client, leading to the client being initially expelled from the program.

The third stage in the responses of drug abuse treatment staff to AIDS may best be termed coping. This stage includes full education about AIDS for all staff and active education/prevention efforts for all clients. Fears of transmission by casual contact, if not completely eliminated, are not permitted to interfere with the provision of drug abuse treatment services. Education includes acknowledging the fact that the great majority of persons in drug abuse treatment programs must be considered at risk for HIV infection either because they may continue to inject drugs if they are in outpatient programs or they may not successfully complete residential programs. Education efforts also include describing the dangers of heterosexual and perinatal transmission and explaining preventive measures which can be taken (such as the use of condoms, which may be distributed by the program). Effective liaisons are established to provide medical services to any persons who might develop HIV-related illnesses, while continuing their drug abuse treatment services.

The fourth stage, which has been observed among some drug abuse treatment personnel, may be termed burnout. Even after one has developed the necessary skills and prepared oneself emotionally, involvement with AIDS patients can be highly stressful. New cases of disease develop among previously infected persons. And as more IV drug users are infected, it becomes increasingly difficult to keep the remaining unexposed persons from being infected. Obviously the need for behavioral changes to prevent heterosexual and perinatal transmission also intensifies. Simply keeping current with new developments in the field can consume enormous amounts of time. The need for additional resources always seems to run ahead of the ability to develop new resources.

However, burnout need not be seen as inevitable among drug abuse treatment staff dealing with AIDS. Self-help groups composed of persons working in similar areas but in different organizations can be very useful for providing emotional support as well as practical problem-solving techniques. It must be realized, however, that when the coping stage is reached, all problems associated with adapting to the AIDS epidemic may not be resolved. The possibility of staff burnout still remains.

AIDS PREVENTION PROGRAMS FOR IV DRUG USERS

A wide variety of AIDS prevention programs for IV drug users have been established throughout the United States and Western Europe (see [31] for a review).

For the benefit of analysis, it is useful to categorize these AIDS prevention programs into two phases (an extended version of this analysis is presented in [32]). The first phase is general AIDS education. It focuses on informing people that AIDS is spread through the sharing of drug injection equipment and contains exhortations for IV drug users to stop injecting, or if they do continue, to stop sharing injection equipment. This information can be disseminated through the mass media, distribution of posters and pamphlets, and AIDS education sessions conducted in drug abuse treatment programs. It is then typically further spread through the oral communication networks of the IV drug use subculture.[33] This basic AIDS education does appear to motivate substantial numbers of IV drug users to alter their behavior, with increased utilization of available sterile injection equipment and a reduction in the number of persons with whom they share equipment being the most common changes. Such responses to AIDS information, however, are best described as risk reduction and not risk elimination. There is certainly no evidence that the amount of risk reduction that has occurred thus far has been sufficient to stop the spread of HIV among IV drug users in any geographic area.

The second phase of AIDS prevention among IV drug users is providing face-to-face education in conjunction with additional means to change their behavior. Face-to-face education about AIDS offers several potential advantages over general (mass media, pamphlets, posters) forms of education. Problems with language and the use of technical terms can be addressed because the participants have the opportunity to ask questions if there is something they do not understand. Of perhaps greater importance is the opportunity for nonverbal "emotional" communication in the face-to-face setting. The educator can assess the audience's emotional response to the content of the message and, if need be, modulate his or her presentation so that the seriousness of the AIDS threat can be conveyed without raising anxiety to the point where psychological denial of the problem becomes the dominant response. The AIDS educator can also convey nonjudgmental sincerity, explaining that AIDS really does require behavior changes and is not simply another scare tactic to try to get drug users to give up drugs. Ex-addicts can be used effectively as AIDS educators. They are positive role models—they have been successful in reducing their risk for developing AIDS—and have a greater ability to communicate with drug users who can identify with them.

The face-to-face situation allows the health educator to probe for the aspects of AIDS that are of greatest concern to the individuals in the program. It may be the threat of infecting the drug user's children, the pain and debilitation of AIDS, or the difficulty of hustling drugs when ill. Preliminary data from an ex-addict health educator/outreach program in New York indicate that the ex-addicts have been adopting this strategy of tailoring the prevention message to the concerns of the individual recipient, and that this leads to greater interest in seeking additional counseling and greater expressed intentions of behavior change.[34]

Once IV drug users have been motivated to modify their behavior to avoid AIDS, the means for those changes must be provided. That public officials have shown increased willingness to provide these services is an indication of the effect the AIDS epidemic is having on attitudes towards IV drug use. Supplying IV drug users with sterile drug injection equipment is one way to help IV drug users change behavior that puts them at risk for AIDS. Sterile needles and syringes can be purchased legally in most Western European countries and in the great majority of the states in the United States. Prescriptions for the sale of needles and syringes are required in Sweden and in many of the states here that have large concentrations of IV drug users. The lack of a prescription requirement, however, does not necessarily mean that sterile injection equipment is actually available to IV drug users. Pharmacists in many areas have typically refused to sell needles and syringes to persons suspected of injecting drugs, and there are also laws against the possession of "narcotics paraphernalia" in many jurisdictions. The laws requiring prescriptions have been changed in Switzerland[35] and France[36] specifically as measures to reduce AIDS among IV drug users.

"Needle exchange" systems, in which IV drug users can exchange used injection equipment for new sterile equipment are a way of increasing the means for risk reduction among IV drug users with the advantage of providing for safe disposal of many of the used needles and syringes. Needle exchange systems for the prevention of AIDS have been established in Holland, the United Kingdom, and Australia. (The needle exchanges in Holland were actually established as hepatitis control measures prior to the AIDS epidemic, but have been greatly expanded because of AIDS.)

Needle exchange systems (or changing laws that restrict the legal availability of sterile injection equipment) have not yet been instituted in the United States. They have been considered and rejected in New Jersey and California, and, as of April 1987, an exchange system is under consideration in New York. The American alternative to making sterile injection equipment legally available is teaching IV drug users how to sterilize used injection equipment. Bleach, alcohol, and boiling in water can all be used to sterilize injection equipment. There are programs in San Francisco, New York, New Jersey, Chicago, Baltimore, and Washington, D.C. that instruct IV drug users in sterilization procedures. Most of these programs use trained ex-addicts as the instructors. (The instructors also provide general AIDS education, emphasizing that stopping drug injection altogether is a better way to reduce the risk of AIDS.)

Provision of additional drug abuse treatment is another method of increasing the means for AIDS-related behavior change among IV drug users. To the extent that treatment leads to the cessation of IV drug use, the risk of exposure to HIV through the sharing of injection equipment has been eliminated. Even if treatment does not lead to complete elimination of further drug injection, it might still be successful in terms of AIDS prevention. Following "safe injection" procedures appears to be most difficult when a person is using drugs at the level of physical addiction (where sudden cessation of drugs will be followed by withdrawal symptoms). Withdrawal symptoms are sufficiently unpleasant that almost all IV drug users report that if they are in withdrawal and do have drugs to inject, they will use whatever injection equipment is readily available.[37] Thus, if treatment leads to levels of drug use less than those associated with physical addiction, the likelihood of risk-reduction behavior is greatly increased. More treatment programs for drug abuse have been created in New York, New Jersey, San Francisco, and Sweden as an AIDS prevention measure. The National Institute on Drug Abuse in the United States and several European countries, including the United Kingdom and the Federal Republic of Germany, are planning to expand treatment facilities.

As noted earlier, there is consistent evidence that phase one—basic AIDS education—leads to risk reducing behaviors among IV drug users. Measuring the effectiveness of the phase two prevention programs is clearly a much more difficult task, as the effects of these programs must be separated from the ongoing behavioral changes associated with basic information about AIDS and the effect that ever-increasing numbers of HIV-infected persons has on IV drug users. While it is too early to determine the efficacy of the phase two AIDS prevention programs, there are a number of aspects that are worth noting. The programs appear to be well accepted by IV drug users. Reports of the face-to-face education programs indicate that current IV drug users show considerable interest in learning more about AIDS and that the educators have relatively little difficulty in establishing rapport.[38-40]

Many IV drug users are extremely responsive to the face-to-face education programs. As previously mentioned, many of these programs provide education on how to sterilize drug injection equipment (or, as in Europe, actually provide free sterile equipment). Prior to the establishment of these programs, the objection was made that providing means for "AIDS safe injection" would "encourage drug abuse." Contrary to this expectation, the available data show that the progams have either no effect on the levels of drug injection or actually influence many IV drug users to seek treatment to reduce their levels. There is no evidence that the needle exchanges in Amsterdam[41] and in Liverpool[42] have led to any increases in illicit drug injection in these cities. In Amsterdam, the number of IV drug users entering treatment has increased during the period the needle exchange programs (data is not yet available on entry into treatment for other cities with needle exchanges). Early reports on the face-to-face education programs also indicate that many current IV drug users respond to these programs by seeking treatment to reduce their levels of drug injection.[43-45] Thus, while the data still must be considered preliminary, it appears that AIDS prevention programs that include methods of "AIDS safe injection" do not "encourage drug abuse," and may in fact serve to motivate drug users to enter drug abuse treatment programs.

It is clear that AIDS is provoking behavior changes among IV drug users as no other health threat has ever done before. The AIDS prevention programs, however, have generally presented AIDS as a fatal threat to IV drug users and have not usually focused on the differences between AIDS and other threats to the lives of drug users. More research needs to be done to determine what specific aspects of AIDS are most likely to lead to sustained risk reduction and how to individualize the prevention messages to reach different IV drug users. The face-to-face education programs do present a good mechanism for both obtaining data on the responses of current IV drug users to various aspects of AIDS and for presenting individualized prevention messages.

THE NEW DEATH AND NEW IV DRUG USERS

One particularly important aspect of AIDS as a new form of death is how it affects recruitment into IV drug use. There is a relatively high turnover among IV drug users. Within a "stable population" of IV drug users, an estimated 10–20% leave active IV drug use annually,[46] through death, successful treatment, or simply their own efforts to stop injecting drugs. These people are then replaced by new IV drug users. Because of this high turnover, control of HIV within the IV drug use population will require either that the number of new drug injectors is reduced or that new injectors adopt "AIDS safe injection" practices as they are initiated into IV drug use.

How concerns about AIDS are incorporated into IV drug recruitment is particularly interesting, since initial IV drug use almost invariably involves sharing injection equipment,[47] and "fear arousal" techniques have traditionally been ineffective in preventing youth from drug experimentation.[48] (The failure of the possibility of death to prevent drug use applies to legal drugs such as nicotine and alcohol as well as to illicit drugs.)

A research project in New York City is examining new recruitment into IV drug use through a longitudinal study of persons who are heavy users (but not injectors) of heroin and cocaine.[49] The central experimental component of this project is a training group that prepares heroin and cocaine "sniffers" (persons using the drugs intranasally) to manage situations that might otherwise trigger their initiation into drug injection. The training is based on drug prevention efforts developed from social learning theory. Experimental and control subjects are monitored over time to evaluate the training group's success in preventing drug injection and exposure to HIV.

Data from the first 40 heroin sniffers recruited for the study revealed complex but generally positive attitudes towards heroin use. Twenty-five of the subjects had no prior drug treatment history. While few actively opposed treatment, many felt they could control their use and therefore did not need treatment. Ten were trying to stop using heroin; the rest planned to continue using it.

Although subjects were knowledgeable about AIDS and needle transmission, fear of AIDS was rarely the primary reason for remaining a sniffer. Rather, subjects were averse to needles, considering injection a more advanced stage of addiction. Sniffing was seen as less dangerous, less addicting, and easier.

Subjects had rejected encouragement by IV drug users to inject for the "rush." Yet over half thought they might indeed inject "to get a better high." Eleven said they might inject because of peer pressure and ten to avoid withdrawal. A small, but disturbing number (eight), thought they might inject if clean needles were available. Other reasons cited for injecting were: to appease curiosity, to conquer a phobia, and to minimize drug-induced damage to one's nose. Thus it would appear that AIDS has not yet become a dominant reason for avoiding drug injection, even in New York City, where over 3000 cases of AIDS have occurred among IV drug users.

The first group randomly selected to participate in the training showed a very positive response. Out of ten people contacted by telephone, eight came to the first session and seven of these made a commitment to return. There was a 98% attendance record over the course of the training, and the group collectively decided to extend the number of meetings from four to six to cover additional AIDS/drug use issues. While AIDS was not initially considered a major reason for not injecting drugs, the subjects were quite responsive to the intervention designed to reduce their risk of developing AIDS.

A major concern about the connection between IV drug use and AIDS has not yet emerged in the young people who are at high risk to begin injecting drugs and who live in the city with the largest number of IV drug-related AIDS cases. There does, however, appear to be an underlying receptivity to AIDS/IV drug use prevention efforts. Much more research is needed to determine the best methods for utilizing that receptivity.

"NON-AIDS" DEATHS AMONG INTRAVENOUS DRUG USERS

AIDS-related illnesses and AIDS deaths are already having a profound impact on IV drug users, drug abuse treatment programs, and medical care facilities in the New York City area, Spain, and Italy. Given this impact, it is almost ironic to note that there is probably a major underestimation of the amount of HIV-related mortality among IV drug users.

There has been a dramatic increase in deaths among IV drug users in New York City since HIV was first introduced into this group in the middle to late 1970s. The death rate among the group has increased from 257 in 1978[50] to approximately 2000 in 1986.[51] Half of these deaths can be attributed to diagnosed AIDS or ARC.[52] The others have been caused by various factors, including epidemic increases in tuberculosis, non-pneumocytis pneumonia, and endocarditis. Research is currently underway to examine the relationship between these greater numbers of death and HIV infection. At present, the best estimate is that HIV-related deaths among IV drug users are at least 50% greater than the official AIDS/ARC counts.

CONCLUSION

IV drug users are a critical group in efforts to control HIV infection in the United States and Europe. They form the second largest group of persons who have developed AIDS, and they are the major sources of heterosexual and perinatal transmission. The threat of AIDS has already led to much more risk reduction behavior among IV drug users than would have been expected, considering their behavior with respect to other health threats. When AIDS is thought of as a new way of dying much of the data on IV drug user behavior changes and the reactions of drug abuse treatment staff to the AIDS epidemic can be comprehended. Further exploration is needed to discover how best to incorporate the unique aspects of AIDS into prevention programs—particularly prevention programs for persons who are not yet injecting drugs—and what the full range of effects of HIV infection will have on the health of IV drug users.

REFERENCES

1. Centers for Disease Control, AIDS Surveillance. Personal communication, 1987.
2. Brunet J. B. WHO AIDS European Coordinating Center. Personal communication, 1987.
3. Marmor, M.; Des Jarlais, D. C.; Cohen, H.; Friedman, S. R.; Beatrice, S. T.; Dubin, N.; El-Sadr, W.; Mildvan, D.; Yancovitz, S.; Mathur, U.; Holzman, R. Risk factors for infection with human immunodeficiency virus among intravenous drug users in New York City. AIDS: An International Bimonthly Journal. Forthcoming.
4. Weiss, S. H.; Ginzburg, H. M.; Goedert, J. J., et al. Risk for HTLV-III exposure and AIDS among parenteral drug abusers in New Jersey. Paper presented at the International Conference on the Acquired Immunodeficiency Syndrome (AIDS), Atlanta, 14–17 April 1985.
5. Robertson, J. R.; Bucknall, A. B. V.; Welsby, P. D., et al. Epidemic of AIDS related virus (HTLV-III/LAV) infection among intravenous drug users. *British Medical Journal* 292:527–529 (1986).
6. Angarano, G.; Pastore, G.; Monno, L., et al. Rapid spread of HTLV-III infection among drug addicts in Italy. *Lancet* ii: 8467:1302 (1985).

7. Camprubi, J. SIDA: Prevalencia de la infeccion por la IVH en los ADVP: Situacion actual y posibilidades de la actuacion. *Comunidad y Drogas* 2:9–22 (1986).
8. Weiss, S. H., et al. Risk for HTLV-III exposure and AIDS among parenteral drug abusers in New Jersey.
9. Jesson, W., et al. Prevalence of anti-HTL-III in UK risk groups. *Lancet* I:155 (1986).
10. Ginzburg, H. NIDA. Personal communication, 1986.
11. Follett, E. A. C.; McIntyre, A.; O'Donnell, B. HTL-III antibody in drug abusers in the West of Scotland: The Edinburgh connection. *Lancet* I:8478:446–447 (1986).
12. Des Jarlais, D. C.; Friedman, S. R.; Marmor, M.; Cohen, H.; Mildvan, D.; Yancovitz, S.; Mathur, U.; El-Sadr, W.; Spira, T. J.; Garber, J.; Beatrice, S. T.; Abdul-Quader, A. S.; Sotheran, J. L. Development of AIDS, HIV seroconversion, and co-factors for T4 cell loss in a cohort of intravenous drug users. *AIDS: A Bimonthly Journal.* Forthcoming.
13. Follett, E. A. C., et al. HTLV-III antibody in drug abusers in the West of Scotland.
14. Weiss, S. H., et al. Risk for HTLV-III exposure and AIDS among parenteral drug abusers in New Jersey.
15. Schoenbaum, E. E.; Selwyn, P. A.; Klein, R. S., et al. Prevalence of and risk factors associated with HTLV-III/LAV antibodies among intravenous drug abusers in methadone programs in New York City. Paper presented at the International Conference on AIDS, Paris, 23–25 June 1986.
16. Marmor, M., et al. Risk factors for infection with human immunodeficiency virus among intravenous drug users in New York City.
17. Selwyn, P. A.; Cox, C. P.; Feiner, C., et al. Knowledge about AIDS and high-risk behavior among intravenous drug users in New York City. Paper presented at the International Conference on AIDS, Paris, 23–25 June 1986.
18. Chaisson, R. E., Moss, A. R.; Onishi, R.; Osmond, D.; Carlson, J. R. Human immunodeficiency virus infection in heterosexual intravenous drug users in San Francisco. *American Journal of Public Health* 77:169–172 (1987).
19. New York City Department of Health. Personal communication, 1987.
20. Des Jarlais, D. C. Research design, drug use, and deaths: Cross study comparisons. In *Social and Medical Aspects of Drug Abuse,* edited by G. Serban. New York: Spectrum, 1984.
21. Goldstein, P. J.; Lipson, L.; Preble, E.; Sobel, I.; Miller, T.; Abbott, W.; Paige, W.; Soto, F. The marketing of street heroin in New York City. *Journal of Drug Issues* 14:553–566 (1984).
22. Friedman, S. R.; Des Jarlais, D. C.; Sotheran, J. L., et al. AIDS and self-organization among intravenous drug users. *International Journal of the Addictions.* Forthcoming.
23. Selwyn, P. A.; Cox, C. P.; Feiner, C.; Lipschutz, C.; Cohen, R. Knowledge about AIDS and high-risk behavior among intravenous drug abusers in New York City. Paper presented at the Annual Meeting of the American Public Health Association, Washington, D.C., 18 November 1985.
24. Des Jarlais, D. C.; Friedman, S. R.; Hopkins, W. Risk reduction for the Acquired Immunodeficiency Syndrome among intravenous drug users. *Annals of Internal Medicine* 103:755–759 (1985).
25. Des Jarlais, D. C., and Hopkins, W. Free needles for intravenous drug users at risk for AIDS: Current developments in New York City. *New England Journal of Medicine* 313:23 (1985).
26. Coutinho, R. A. Preliminary results of AIDS studies among IVDA in Amsterdam. Paper presented at Workshop on Epidemiological Surveys on AIDS: Epidemiology of HIV Infections in Europe Spread among Intravenous Drug Users and the Heterosexual Population, Berlin, 12–14 November 1986.
27. Biernacki, P., and Feldman, H. Ethnographic observations of IV drug use practices that put users at risk for AIDS. Paper presented at the XV International Institute on the Pre-

vention and Treatment of Drug Dependence, Amsterdam/Noordwijkerhout, the Netherlands, 6–11 April 1986.

28. Des Jarlais, D. C. Stages in the response of the drug abuse treatment system to the AIDS
    epidemic in New York City. *Journal of Drug Issues.* Forthcoming.

29. Kübler-Ross, E. *Living with Death and Dying.* New York: Simon and Schuster, 1981.

30. Selye, H. *The Stress of Life.* New York: MacMillan, 1978.

31. Friedman, S. R.; Des Jarlais, D. C.; Goldsmith, D. S. An overview of current AIDS preven-
    tion efforts aimed at intravenous drug users. *Journal of Drug Issues.* Forthcoming.

32. Des Jarlais, D. C., and Friedman S. R. AIDS prevention among intravenous drug users:
    Phases one and two. Forthcoming.

33. Des Jarlais, D. C.; Friedman, S. R.; Strug, D. AIDS among intravenous drug users: A
    socio-cultural perspective. In *The Social Dimensions of AIDS: Methods and Theory,* edited by
    D. A. Feldman, and T. A. Johnson. New York: Praeger, 1986.

34. Mauge, C. Personal communication, 1987.

35. Ancelle, R. Personal communication, 1986.

36. Brunet, J. B. WHO AIDS European Coordinating Center.

37. Des Jarlais, D. C., et al. AIDS among intravenous drug users: A socio-cultural perspective.

38. Kleinman, P. H. Personal communication, 1987.

39. Feldman, D. A. Personal communication, 1987.

40. Jackson, J. New Jersey Department of Health. Personal communication, 1987.

41. Buning, E. Amsterdam's drug policy and the prevention of AIDS. Paper presented at the
    Conference on AIDS in the Drug Abuse Community and Heterosexual Transmission,
    Newark, N.J., 31 March–1 April 1986.

42. Parry, A. Needle swop in Mesey. *Druglink, The Journal on Drug Misuse in Britain* 2(1):7
    (1987).

43. Kleinman, P. H. Personal communication.

44. Feldman, D. A. Personal communication.

45. Jackson, J. Personal communication.

46. Frank, B.; Schmeidler, J.; Johnson, B.; Lipton, D. S. Seeking truth in heroin indicators:
    The case of New York City. *Drug and Alcohol Dependence* 3:345–358 (1978).

47. Des Jarlais, D. C., et al. AIDS among intravenous drug users: A socio-cultural perspective.

48. Schaps, E.; DiBartolo, R.; Churgin, S. *Primary Prevention Research: A Review of 127 Program
    Evaluations.* Walnut Creek, CA: Pyramid Project, Pacific Institute for Research and Evalua-
    tion, 1978.

49. Des Jarlais, D. C., Friedman, S. R.; Casriel, C.; Kott, A. AIDS and preventing initiation into
    intravenous (IV) drug use. Unpublished manuscript.

50. Des Jarlais, D. C., et al. Risk reduction for the Acquired Immunodeficiency Syndrome
    among intravenous drug users.

51. New York City Department of Health. Personal communication.

52. Stoneburner, R.; Guigli, P.; Kristal, A. Increasing mortality in intravenous drug users in
    New York City and its relationship to the AIDS epidemic: is there an unrecognized spec-
    trum of HTLV-III/LAV-related disease? Paper presented at the International Conference
    on AIDS, Paris, 23–25 June 1986.

CHAPTER 12

The Patient with AIDS: Care and Concerns

SR. PATRICE MURPHY
GRAHAM BASS
CAROLE DONOVAN
BETSY SELMAN

INTRODUCTION

Where can a person afflicted with acquired immune deficiency syndrome (AIDS) turn for care? There is no easy answer to this question. Terminally ill persons are frequently spurned by traditional medical care, and this is all the more likely to occur when the person has AIDS. Currently 90% of persons with AIDS are homosexual or bisexual men, or intravenous drug users. Homosexuals and drug abusers have often been rejected by their biological families. The tendency toward homophobia in our society, intensified by a fear of death, has caused many social institutions as well to reject homosexuals, particularly those with AIDS. In some cases, lovers, friends, health care practitioners, and clergy abandon persons with AIDS due to the fear of contagion. Indeed, where can a person with AIDS turn for care?

To whom can persons suffering from AIDS turn if not to nurses, social workers, physicians, therapists, clergy, and volunteers who have been educated to confront the innumerable complexities of caring for the terminally ill patient with cancer, renal failure, pulmonary disease, and other dreadful illnesses? As hospice caregivers we have learned that symptoms of these diseases can be managed. So, too, can AIDS! We have seen miracles in our work; we are seeing them with AIDS patients and their families and friends. The work of the Supportive Care Program of St. Vincent's Hospital and Medical Center in New York City illustrates a hospice-related program which helps to care for those with AIDS.

The mission of St. Vincent's Hospital from its earliest days has been to serve the sick and poor of New York City. When St. Vincent's Hospital opened its doors in 1850, it was to provide care for the very poor, and often seriously ill, immigrant populations pouring into New York City. Today the mission remains the same, only the population using its services has changed, reflecting the changing demographics of the area and the needs of the times. Currently the issues of AIDS, the homeless, and the underserved are foremost in the Medical Center's concerns.

Located in the heart of Greenwich Village, St. Vincent's Hospital and Medical Center, with a bed capacity of 813, is the oldest community hospital in lower Manhattan, an area which continues to report the greatest incidence of AIDS in the nation. Although patients come from all five boroughs as well as New Jersey, St. Vincent's is the primary provider of acute medical care to residents of the area that immediately surrounds the hospital, commonly known as Chelsea and Greenwich Village. These two communities alone comprise half of the residental population of lower Manhattan and are home to a significant homosexual population. Almost 30% of the homosexual population are men between the ages of 18 and 44, and nearly half of the households are single persons living alone or together with a non-relative.

St. Vincent's has long been active in providing for the gay community's medical needs. Consequently, the staff are particularly aware of the special health care needs of this population. Since 1981 St. Vincent's Hospital has treated over 700 patients with AIDS. Eighty percent of the individuals live in Manhattan; 50% live within the hospital's immediate geographic area. The number of AIDS admissions has increased from a total of 20 in 1982 to nearly 500 in 1987. In late 1983, staff of the Supportive Care Program with expertise in caring for the terminally ill felt that this Program could provide care to AIDS patients. And so the staff began—slowly but determinedly—to incorporate AIDS patients into the Program. Currently patients with AIDS comprise approximately 70% of the Program's participants. The goal of the Program is to provide coordinated comprehensive services and caring through a multidisciplinary approach which enables patients to return to, and remain in, the familiar surroundings of the home environment and, when desired, to die at home.

The team at St. Vincent's Supportive Care Program includes physicians, nurses, social workers, pastoral counselors, and trained community volunteers. Because of the nature of the work, all are invited to explore the pastoral dimension, no matter what their official professional capacity. "Pastoral" here is defined in a broad sense, as distinct from the professional role of the pastoral counselor which often (but not always) applies to the clergy and religious from many faiths who are specifically trained to help people cope with existential and transcendent issues. In this broad definition, the pastoral dimension is the aspect within each human being which recognizes the intrinsic value of each other being and understands the very real connection existing among all people. This dimension needs to be encouraged in anyone who wishes to be of genuine service to a person with AIDS or to the patient's loved ones. In such a capacity we are constantly confronted by our own limitations. Are our unexamined biases regarding homosexuality or drug abuse obstacles to seeing the patient's inherent worth? Are we willing to accept the real human relationship we have to the addict with AIDS who perhaps is still abusing drugs, or to the young gay man denying his diagnosis (and mortality) who continues to be active sexually? How do we relate to the parents who disown their dying child because of his sexuality or abuse of drugs or to the despairing patient contemplating suicide because he has lost hope? These questions continually challenge our attitudes and judgments.

A nurse in the Program quickly realizes that the physical care which he or she extends to his or her patient, as taxing and complicated as it becomes due to the complex symptomatology of AIDS, is only part of the total picture. The emotional, psychosocial, and spiritual aspects are all intertwined. With the diagnosis of AIDS, the physical and the metaphysical come crashing together. There are the physical agonies of Kaposi's sarcoma (KS) lesions, Pneumocystis carinii pneumonia (PCP), intractable diarrhea, encephalopathy, neurological impairment, fevers and sweats, blindness, and exhaustion. Along with these physical ailments are the agonizing metaphysical questions for the patient and the caregiver: "Why me?" "Am I being punished?" "Did God make a mistake when he created me?" "Am I to blame for my illness?" "What was the meaning and purpose of my life?"

These questions form an important component of the care of AIDS patients. However, the purpose of the following ancedotes is to illustrate primarily the medical aspects of care, in particular the treatment of opportunistic infections which are often fatal to persons with AIDS.

JAMES

James was a 54-year-old gay male whom the Supportive Care nurse visited at his home for five weeks. Although there had been other opportunistic infections, his main problem at that time was a *Cryptosporidium* infection. This is a protozoan gastrointestinal illness which, in those with normally functioning immune systems, produces what is sometimes known as "travelers' diarrhea," a bothersome but usually self-limiting condition which "runs" its course and, perhaps with some symptomatic treatment, departs. In AIDS patients, however, it can become an intractable diarrhea, with continuous watery stools, incurable and often unimprovable, leading to physical exhaustion, dehydration, electrolyte imbalance, and eventually death. The latter is often welcomed as an end to an existence which many patients consider to be not worth living.

Such a patient was James. Fiercely independent during his adult years, he was a renowned collector of fine antiques and furniture, and his refined taste and artistic sensibility extended to all areas of his life. This man was found in bed lying in his stool on the nurse's first visit. Having been cleaned only 15 minutes previously in the ongoing, losing battle to keep dry, clean, and comfortable, he was once again wet, soiled, and most uncomfortable. Lomotil had been tried, but it literally failed to stem the flow, followed, equally unsuccessfully, by Imodium. James felt hopeless about any other possibilities. Both he and the young relative who was helping to care for him were exhausted by his constant diarrhea and the efforts involved in trying to keep him comfortable.

After evaluating the situation, the nurse suggested that a rectal tube might provide some immediate relief, if not from the diarrhea itself then at least from the incessant discomfort. James and his relative expressed interest, and the nurse inserted a large, #20 2-way Foley catheter with a 5-cc balloon, lubricated with KY jelly, with the distal end attached to a 2000-cc bedside drainage bag. The insertion itself was the occasion for some humor on the part of James, who commented acerbically that it was an attempt to relate sexually to him. This was the first glimpse of anything other than hopelessness and depression that had been seen in him on that visit. The balloon was inflated with 5 cc of air; immediately, watery stool proceeded to flow through the tube into the drainage bag. Determining that his caregiver felt able to assume the task of removing and reinserting the tube periodically to give the rectal mucosa a rest, the nurse instructed him in the technique of doing so and found him an apt pupil. The caregiver knew that the nurse would be available by phone or in person as necessary to deal with any problems that might arise. Due to the excellent care he had been receiving, James's skin was still in good condition despite the difficulty in keeping him clean. The nurse reinforced the principles and techniques of good skin care, however, to avoid additional problems.

That night, for the first time in many days, James and his caregiver were able to get uninterrupted sleep. And for the first time in weeks, James could lie on a dry, clean sheet with some degree of comfort.

The next step was to see if there could be any success in actually stemming the tide. The nurse spoke with James's physician, who ordered Paregoric. Although the diarrhea did not cease, it did slow down somewhat, so that the 2000-cc bedside drainage bag needed to be emptied only once every 24 hours rather than every 12 hours or less.

James was receiving home Total Parenteral Nutrition (TPN) at night through a Hickman catheter. TPN is a solution of protein and other nutritional elements to compensate for reduced food intake. His latest blood tests, however, had shown a rising blood urea nitrogen (BUN) and troublesome serum electrolyte changes. His physician ordered certain changes in the TPN formula and extra intravenous replacement fluids to correct the imbalances as much as possible. All of this was done at home, since James was adamant about not wanting to return to the hospital. However, at this point, he became adamant about something else as well—he had had enough. Weak, dependent, unable to pursue his interests, vocational or avocational, that made life worth living, he was ready to die. While his own religious beliefs did not permit suicide, he was not willing to do anything to prolong life. The nurse and James talked about this at length, including his caregiver, who had the most difficulty with the idea of not continuing the fight for life, in the discussions. Eventually the caregiver came to understand and respect James's decision to refuse any further TPN or IV fluids. Over the next week, James became progressively weaker, slipped into a coma, and died peacefully.

THOMAS, STEVE, AND JACKIE

Thomas was an actor and a dancer—one of the best! He had been on Broadway and in major films. At the age of 26 he was one of the few who was always working. His physical grace, skill, and appearance were central to his work and to his sense of self. And he had a large, dark purple lesion right on the tip of his nose.

Steve had similar lesions all over his face and body. His eyes were swollen shut, and large, angry, purple weltlike marks adorned his body.

Jackie had only a few lesions. But they were on his legs and the bottoms of his feet, and caused him excruciating pain when he tried to walk or even stand. He spent almost all of his time in bed.

All three patients had Kaposi's sarcoma, a normally rather innocuous form of cancer appearing as dark patches on the skin and usually affecting elderly men of Mediterranean or Middle Eastern descent. As manifested in AIDS, Kaposi's sarcoma (KS) knows no limitations, neither of age nor ethnic descent or extent of dissemination. Thus far it is not curable. Various chemotherapeutic treatments such as bleomycin or vincristine seem to help for a while. Indeed, the lesions and swelling can change dramatically, with lesions becoming smaller and lighter-colored. But upon completion of the chemotherapeutic regimens, the lesions seem to return within weeks, redoubled, almost as if the chemotherapy itself had provided renewed vigor. This was the case time after time.

KS does not always appear in such virulent fashion. Many patients have only a few rather unobtrusive lesions and remain in that condition for long periods of time. Others, like Steve and Jackie, seem to be completely overwhelmed by KS, internally as well as externally. Although the lesions themselves are not usually painful, they can be agonizing if, as in Jackie's case, they are on a part of the body that must bear weight or pressure.

The nurse noted an ironic phenomenon—many of these young men, often involved in professional theatre, dance, fashion, or some other pursuit that involved their physical appearance professionally or socially, would, like Thomas, get a KS lesion in the worst of all places—right on the tip of their nose, resulting in an often grotesque, clownlike appearance. This phenomenon becomes understandable when one realizes that KS is actually a sarcoma of the capillary lining, and therefore, an area of the body particularly well endowed with capillaries—such as the nose—would be a likely site for the appearance of the lesions. Unfortunately, the only current alternative to chemotherapy—radiation therapy—does not do much to improve their appearance. For Thomas, cosmetics helped. A young makeup artist for a TV soap opera volunteered her expertise to develop a makeup that could be matched to the individual patient's skin tone to cover the most blatant facial lesions. This allowed Thomas and Steve, with lesions on their faces, to go out in public with less self-consciousness.

A combination of narcotics, chemotherapy, and radiation therapy to his feet allowed Jackie to have increased comfort for a few weeks. However, the KS lesions on his feet were so abundant, interfering with his blood circulation, that his feet became gangrenous. Before a decision could be made on this latest development, Jackie went into respiratory failure due to KS lesions in his lung. He was intubated, and, a few days later, despite all efforts, died.

Steve's KS led to such facial swelling that his eyes could not open. For a patient whose main pleasure in life at this terrible time was to watch videos on a VCR that he had bought with his remaining money, until the death that he knew was approaching would overtake him, the loss of his vision was torturous. Maintaining a semi-Fowler's or Fowler's position (the head of the bed elevated from one to two feet) in bed, and using cold packs on his eyes, helped reduce the swelling somewhat. But it was ultimately the use of steroids that proved most successful. These drugs are generally contraindicated for AIDS patients, for they may mask infection, cause immunosuppression, and delay healing. But in Steve's case, they allowed him weeks of life that were meaningful to him. Shortly thereafter, the KS lesions affected his lungs, causing eventual respiratory failure.

Thomas's case of Kaposi's sarcoma never became a life-threatening problem, aside from the extent to which its appearance made him feel that his life was not worth living. Psychological counseling and support, giving him opportunities and the encouragement to express his feelings of loss and anger, were vital. During his last months he was able to come to terms with much that had at first seemed completely and incomprehensively overwhelming. His death a few weeks later was due to a cytomegalovirus (CMV) infection which impaired his pulmonary and gastrointestinal functioning.

RODNEY

Rodney had been diagnosed with AIDS for several months. He had herpes on the whole left side of his face, but it was not the herpes simplex of the cold sore, it was herpes zoster ophthalmicus. The virus had affected the left eye, producing blindness. Torturously painful and itchy, it looked as if some blistering scalding process had attacked the whole left side of his face from jaw to temple. Herpes zoster is caused by the varicella zoster virus—the same virus which causes chickenpox. The first exposure to this virus causes chickenpox and usually the virus is subsequently destroyed. However, it is possible that some viruses lodge in nerve ganglia and remain dormant until reactivation by an unknown mechanism. If the body is unable to fight because its immune system is unable to initiate and maintain the effective response to destroy the varicella zoster viruses, the viruses will continue to multiply, spreading down the sensory nerves to the skin and causing the infection herpes zoster. Rodney's depressed immune system was unable to respond adequately to these viruses. The intense pain of his left eye and surrounding facial area was due to the virus having attacked the ophthalmic branch of the trigeminal nerve.

It is necessary to be on a constant "herpes watch" with AIDS patients, for the herpes simplex virus can strike almost anywhere—face, eyes, mouth, genitals, rectum, or other areas of the body. It can present as an innocuous-appearing sore, or, as in the case of Rodney's herpes zoster ophthalmicus, as an overwhelming catastrophe. Acyclovir is the treatment of choice, used either topically or systematically, and although it does not "cure" the patient of the virus, it can drive the infection into remission. Sight once lost does not return and the scars in cases such as Rodney's remain. But the acute intense discomfort, the severe burning pain, the open weeping sores, can be resolved with treatment. However, chronic, less intense pain may persist.

Rodney suffered bravely and at length; healing was a slow process because of the immunosuppression of AIDS. Suddenly, one evening during the healing period, Rodney became confused and disoriented as to time, person, and place; he was threatening and abusive to nurses, angry at anyone who approached him. Always gentlemanly and thoughtful in the past, this behavior took everyone by surprise, and a number of consults were arranged immediately. The consensus of the professionals called to evaluate Rodney's sudden eruptive behavior and disturbed mental activity was that he was suffering from herpes encephalitis. Encephalitis is a severe inflammation of the brain which can be caused by a virus such as herpes. Intense lymphocytic infiltration of brain tissue and the leptomeninges (soft cerebral and spinal membranes) can cause cerebral edema, degeneration of the brain's ganglion cells, and diffuse nerve cell destruction. Herpes encephalitis also produces symptoms that vary from subclinical to acute and often fulminating disease.

It was at least 72 hours before Rodney became more subdued. Decadron to reduce cerebral edema, sedatives for restlessness, Dilantin to prevent convulsions, and aspirin or Tylenol for headaches and fever were administered; he responded eventually. But Rodney has never been fully himself again. Once eager to share thoughts and feelings, intellectually curious, loving to read, listen to music, watch TV, and just enjoy being with and socializing with others, he is now considerably less energetic, more passive and quiet—even listless. While the headaches associated with the herpes infection are long gone, new physical discomforts have replaced them—paresthesias (pricking sensations) of feet, legs, and sometimes parts of his trunk, and varying degrees of foot pain. Weight loss is also apparent, although Rodney's home health aide prepares meals and in-between snacks which he continues to eat adequately. The greatest loss to Rodney seems to be that of the sight in his left eye. Deprivation of the ability to read has been an influence in his increasing apathy and listlessness. What is saddest for those caring for Rodney over many months is the gradual physical, emotional, and mental deterioration that is so much part of this disease.

BOB AND MIGUEL

Words were Bob's life. His job was tracing certain words back to biblical times to see how usage had changed. It was exacting, painstaking work. How cruel then that Bob's illness caused progressive loss of speech until he was mute, a left-sided paralysis, and a partial loss of vision. Bob seemed like a person who had suffered a stroke. He also had hallucinations and paranoid ideas. A psychiatrist worked with him during the months he was hospitalized, but it was not clear whether Bob had become acutely psychotic or had lost his ability to communicate from some destruction of his brain. Because of his helpless condition, an aide was hired to be with Bob 12 hours each day. Tommy—the aide—arrived, a gift from the gods.

Tommy helped Bob move from bed to chair, played tapes of Bob's favorite music, and encouraged him to eat his meals sitting up in a chair. After weeks of making no sounds, Bob suddenly called out one morning to the floor nurse, "MacGregor, get in here!" From that point on, Bob began to speak again. No one understood what had caused him to stop talking or to start again. Bob could now respond to questions but could not initiate conversation. Finally, he was discharged and Tommy continued to care for him Monday through Friday. Tommy carried out a passive range of motion exercises with him, kept the radio tuned to a classical music station, and read aloud concert reviews as ways of providing various forms of stimulation. Any mispronunciation of a composer's name prompted a correction from Bob. In talking with Bob it was clear that his recent memory was intact and, occasionally, that he could recall past information. Once when Tommy and the Supportive Care nurse were talking about an old Abbott and Costello movie, Bob suddenly interjected "Hey, Abbott!" Costello's frequent cry. At times Bob would become fixated on an idea and pursue it over and over. "Tommy, I won't have to have exercises anymore, will I?" he would ask and then repeat the question again in 15 minutes. Tommy patiently reassured him each time.

Bob's physicians believed that he suffered from progressive multifocal leukoencephalopathy (PML). PML is a demyelinating disease caused by a papovavirus that produces blindness, aphasia, hemiparesis (paralysis of one side of the body), and ataxia (impaired ability to coordinate muscular movement).[1] But any number of other neurological changes can occur in these patients and can be caused by viral as well as nonviral organisms.

Loss of recent memory is often the prelude to further neurological problems. Miguel, for example, would report that he could not remember simple things. He had no other neurological changes at the time and no such changes were being reported in the literature. Miguel became progressively more ill with fevers and diarrhea. Simultaneously, he became more and more noncommunicative and withdrawn until he could no longer speak. He would look at whomever was speaking to him but staff members had the impression that there no longer existed a person who could understand or respond on any level.

Some patients with neurological changes complain of numbness and tingling of their fingers, toes, and balls of their feet. It is not known what causes these sensations nor how to relieve them. Occasionally patients with Kaposi's sarcoma, that may or may not be visible, find walking extremely painful. Thick, rubber-soled shoes or slippers may offer some relief. Pain medication such as MS Contin seems to take the edge off the pain but offers no lasting relief. Some patients are put on Tegretol, others on Dilantin, in an effort to alleviate the neurological discomfort. Again results are disappointing.

What seems to help these patients most is allowing them to talk freely about the changes they are experiencing and then make practical suggestions to help them maintain certain functions. For example, if a patient is having difficulty walking, perhaps a walker or wheelchair is in order. Passive or active ranges of motion exercises may do more for morale than for muscle tone, but may be worth trying. Either heat or cold may reduce the intensity of pain. Often it is reassuring to the patient to know that what he is experiencing is part of the physical manifestations of the disease, not something that is psychological.

MARTIN AND ALAN

Martin had been diagnosed as having AIDS for about eight months. He had a number of medical problems—Kaposi's sarcoma and a cytomegalovirus infection among them. He complained of joint pain in his right wrist—an achiness and difficulty flexing it. There was no sign of inflammation or swelling, but eventually a great red lump developed on the outer aspect of his wrist. Soon similar lumps appeared on his thighs. His right ankle became so painful that he could not bear to have even the weight of a sheet on it. Martin always had an elevated temperature and so it was difficult to determine if his usual rise to 100 degrees or more was a signal for some new infectious process.

Martin was admitted to the hospital, his ankle was opened and cultured.

The report read *Mycobacterium avium intracellulare* (MAI). A regimen of anti-tuberculosis drugs were now added to his growing list of medications. MAI is one of a group of atypical mycobacteria. These organisms are not transmitted person-to-person but, rather, are acquired from the environment—for example, from soil or dust. The organism can cause a variety of reactions—lymphadenitis, pulmonary infections, cutaneous infections.[2] The organs commonly infected are bone marrow, liver, spleen, gastrointestinal tract, and lymph nodes.[3] Thus, anemia and pancytopenia (marked reduction of blood components) can occur; liver function tests can be abnormal; malabsorption and weight loss can result.[4]

Hot soaks to Martin's wrist helped ease his discomfort as did a footboard to lift the covers from his feet. Tylenol and codeine were the drugs of choice for pain because other analgesics upset his stomach. But knowing the cause of an infection and administering the drugs which resolve the illness in others does not necessarily change the course of illness for a person with AIDS. Martin continued on a downhill course and finally wished only to be kept comfortable. He wanted what he perceived to be his non-life to end.

Martin had been a fashion designer. When he knew he could no longer work 16 hours a day, he closed his business. Despite his difficulties, Martin maintained his sense of humor and kept a twinkle in his eyes. During the last days, he spoke often about his wish to die and to be with God. One of the Supportive Care Program's volunteer clergy visited regularly with Martin and reassured him, "We're praying for you." Martin rolled his eyes and said, "I know. That's the problem. It's working and I'm still here."

Alan was the director of an elementary school that he had established. He was an exacting person; he would call the manufacturer of the drug he was receiving to check the protocol he was on and to learn more about the drug's side effects. When he was assessed for acceptance in the Supportive Care Program, Alan expressed his concern about his diminished vision. He said that it seemed as though he had a veil over his left eye. The nurse encouraged him to visit an ophthalmologist who found that a wooly exudate on the retina represented a cytomegalovirus infection of the right eye.

Cytomegalovirus (CMV) is classified as a herpes virus and an infection resulting from it is considered to be a sexually transmitted disease.[5] Alan's visual changes are typical of those in patients who have CMV retinitis. The changes usually progress and are irreversible. Often retinitis signals active systemic CMV infection. CMV can be isolated from a number of body secretions and excretions—saliva, blood, urine, stool, secretions of the uterine cervix, semen, and breast milk[6]—and in the immunosuppressed patients can cause "hepatitis, pneumonitis, arthralgias, retinitis, and signs of disseminated disease."[7] Pneumonitis is generally the most common outcome of CMV infection, after fever and mononucleosis. Patients report fever, nonproductive cough, and dyspnea (shortness of breath), often associated with hypoxia (a deficiency of oxygen). The liver and gastrointestinal tract may also be affected by CMV.[8]

To slow the retinal destruction by the virus, Alan was admitted to the hospital for drug therapy. A Hickman catheter was inserted to begin treatment with an experimental drug, DHPG, which he then continued to receive at home.

During the Supportive Care nurse's visits to Alan, he would often evaluate whether or not his vision was changing by reading book titles from across the room, using only his affected eye. In general he found that the visual distortion made it impossible to engage in constructive activities, which distressed him and was a frequent source of complaint to his nurse.

There are a number of ways to alleviate the distress caused by visual distortion. Wearing a patch over the affected eye may help eliminate the conflicting images. Alan found it helpful to wear dark glasses both indoors and out. Safety must be stressed, however. The patient should be reminded to turn his head to check traffic when crossing streets to compensate for the loss of peripheral vision. Using recorded books may relieve the patient's frustration in attempting to read. Patients usually do eventually accommodate to their diminished vision but they need ample opportunities to express their sorrow and anger over the loss of yet another function that compromises self-image and independence.

TOM AND ROY

On a home visit, Tom's lungs were clear to auscultation (listening with a stethoscope). His respiratory rate was 24, his pulse was 84. Yet Tom reported that walking across the room—a small room at that—made him short of breath. He had no fever, but did have a persistent nonproductive cough. A call to his doctor resulted in Tom being placed on the list of for hospital admission. Various tests were then carried out in the hospital and it appeared that Tom most likely had *Pneumocystis carinii* pneumonia (PCP). Once hospitalized, Tom was placed on intravenous pentamidine because of a previously established allergy to Septra, the medication of choice. His respiratory condition worsened. He was asked if he wished to be placed on a respirator if it became necessary and he replied, "Yes." Within four days of admission, Tom was intubated, placed on a respirator, and transferred to the medical intensive care unit.

PCP is one of the more common infections to occur in patients who have AIDS.[9] Its course is difficult to predict: it can rapidly cause death within days or it can progress slowly and resolve itself. Even a chest x-ray can be difficult to interpret. The typical x-ray of a patient with PCP shows bilateral interstitial and alveolar infiltrates. It can however, also appear normal.[10] Septra is the drug of choice, but for those who develop a sensitivity to it, pentamidine is given. Pentamidine can, however, cause either hypoglycemia or hyperglycemia for which insulin may be required. It can also cause renal dysfunction, requiring dietary restrictions of potassium and protein.

Tom remained in the intensive care unit until he could be weaned from the respirator, which happened about one week following his admission. He was then discharged home one week later. His kidneys had been mildly damaged by the pentamidine therapy. With help from a dietician, Tom worked out a diet that was low in potassium and protein. Six weeks later his renal function studies returned to normal.

Roy's bout with PCP also began insiduously. He ran slight fevers and developed a persistent nonproductive cough. Initially his x-ray demonstrated no abnormalities. He was placed on a course of erythromycin because of his cough and fevers. Within ten days, however, Roy began to complain of shortness of breath. Testing now revealed what seemed to be a PCP infection. Roy was admitted to the hospital and Septra therapy was begun. Four days after admission, he spiked fevers to 105 degrees which were followed by drenching sweats and chills. By the second week, his temperature had dropped to 99 degrees and he was ambulatory. By the third week, Roy was home again.

What is so difficult with the respiratory infections these patients experience is accurately determining what is going on in the patients' chests. Respiratory infections in some patients result in permanent changes in auscultory sounds—wheezes for some, diminished breath sounds for others, depending on what residual damage has occurred in the lung tissue. The type of cough also varies from patient to patient. The dry persistent cough seems to be the most annoying and difficult to control. Robitussin is usually the first line of defense moving to elixir of terpin hydrate with codeine for more disruptive coughs.

What seems to be a consistent finding, however, is the unpredictability of AIDS and its manifestations. A careful history needs to be elicited and recorded each week. Clues need to be pieced together to make some sense out of the many symptoms that result from the alterations of many systems. And, as always, the patient needs to be heard, to be comforted, to be reassured. Clearly he knows that little is really known about this disease and that not much is available to combat it.

Despite the uncertainty, despite the despair that comes from knowing friends who have died from this disease, the patient most often remains clearheaded about what is to come and prepares for his death by having his will drawn up and power of attorney assigned. Some patients are able to work on fragmented relationships with family and friends, repairing them where possible and, if not, at least acknowledging the relationship. The courage of each patient throughout their illness is awesome.

CAREGIVERS AND THE EXISTENTIAL

In their psychic pain—helpless and often hopeless—patients with AIDS pose thought-provoking, sometimes threatening, questions and reflections to their caregivers, particularly to nurses. How do we respond to the questions of a 35-year-old, "Will I be brave enough?", or a 23-year old, "What will it be like—the end I mean?"

There is no single answer to such questions. The responses come from deep within each one of us—unique, as each of us is unique, issuing from levels that are deep and personal and spiritual. Levels where each of us commune with our God.

It is vital—possibly more vital than the medical treatment we administer—that we caregivers really be in touch with our innermost selves, with the essence of our spirit of caring, which is love. The following reflections provide us food for thought.

> *. . . And fear ruled.*
> *At first a lump appeared.*
> *On the body, the size of an egg.*
> *Then did spots cover the body,*
> *Then came the fever*
> *With vomiting,*
> *With coughing,*
> *Then swiftly—death.*
> *And despair ruled.*
> *Mothers abandoned their*
> *Children lest they themselves*
> *Be contaminated*
> *The young in fear*
> *Abandoned the aged, ...*
> *Fathers barred the door to sons*
> *And sons cast out infected fathers,*
> *Priests abandoned the infected*
> *And physicians, the dying.*
> *And the Death spared none:*
> *Neither bishop nor priest,*
> *Neither lad nor lass,*
> *Neither scholar nor student,*
> *Master nor journeyman,*
> *Neither merchant nor sailor*
> *Neither artisan nor smith; . . .*
> *Then did despair reign:*
> *There was no herb, no poultice,*
> *Neither cordial nor gold,*
> *No balm nor drink*
> *Nothing could prevent the Death.*
>
> *Then did anger reign:*
> *There was the howling*

And cursing,
Many shouted blasphemies
And cursed the day their
Mothers bore them,
Then did many curse God,
Then all gave way to silence.

This bleak description is taken from a monologue in a play written about Julian of Norwich, a fourteenth-century writer, mystic, and spiritual guide.[11] Julian survived two epidemics of the Black Plague. The fear, despair, and anger of which she speaks is easily applicable to the contemporary tragedy of AIDS. We twentieth-century humans respond in a similar way to our ancestors from the Middle Ages when dealing with a major catastrophe. The fear (however irrational) of contracting a terrifying illness, the despair of a terminal prognosis, the resulting anger at oneself, someone else, or God, are some of the compelling pastoral issues that confront the person caring for AIDS patients and their loved ones. The pastoral person doesn't presume to answer these questions but, rather, searches with the patient through the maze of pain and confusion. The path through this suffering may sometimes lead to vast unexplored places in the heart, or to stony walls that seem inpenetrable. The key throughout this cooperative journey is trust—trust that must be placed in the healer within the patient and in the covenant between this inner healer and the very heart of God. The pastoral person must be comfortable working within "kairos," God's time, and using a new language that emphasizes the interrogative form more than the declarative.

There are so many times with AIDS patients when their experience and our response transcends words. The power of communicating our care and acceptance nonverbally to our patients cannot be stressed enough. Nurses, volunteers, and pastoral counselors can say so much with a simple touch. One of our Program's pastoral counselors describes her experiences with a patient with AIDS.

> I remember visiting one of our first patients with AIDS in 1983. He was a young, extremely talented, and handsome man at the height of his career as a college professor when he was diagnosed. He was very angry and had alienated several of his caregivers. I listened and I listened to his anger and fear and to my anger and fear. Eventually the trust began to grow between us. During one visit, the frustration and pain spilled out in tears. He cried, "No one has touched me in months." Procedures had been done to him, he had been jostled, poked, and prodded, but the most basic human contact of a warm reassuring touch had been absent. Although my presence was helpful, it was ambiguous. I was contributing to the mixed message, "I really care about you and accept you, but you are an untouchable." "Being with" Joseph had to move from empathic conversation, to a more totally empathic presence, to a more primary physical level. It meant working through my own fears of contagion and intimacy. It meant putting my hands where I said my heart was. After this revelation, with his permission, I began to do body work with him. I used techniques gleaned from massage, polarity, therapeutic touch, visualization, and meditation. Almost every time I visited, he would ask with a shy grin,

"Are you going to do that relaxing spiritual stuff today?" I'd say, "Sure, if that's what you'd like," after which, we would do little or no talking. I could see the tension leave his face and body as he relaxed. Usually he would drop off to sleep, a wonderful result because his anxiety prevented him from getting the rest he so badly needed. These quiet sessions together did so much to deepen the trust between us. Ironically, the traditional pastoral issues and questions emerged as a result of this silent time together. I would urge caretakers to become proficient in some form of body work and meditation. It is an invaluable tool in working with AIDS patients.

As Supportive Care workers, we are truly connected to our patients and to each other. We teach each other and we minister to each other. It is a constant mystery in the healing arts—who is healing whom? What broken part of ourselves is being healed as we extend ourselves to another? Recently, on a particularly gray, muggy August afternoon, I (Betsy Selman) sat in my office, damp and miserable, complaining about life in general. There was suddenly a small commotion in the doorway. I went to see who had arrived. Paulette, our secretary, had gone over to the hospital to help one of our AIDS patients make the block-long trip to our office for the weekly AIDS support group. There sat Charles (a young man whose sweet and gentle disposition was reflected in his face) in his wheelchair. He had been attached to a dialysis machine for several days and there had been moments during this last hospital stay when we thought that we would lose him. He sat in his wheelchair and wept (exhausted, but exhilarated to have made it)—not because of his life-threatening illness, but because it was the first time in a month that he had been outside. His tears of gratitude at simply feeling the hot, humid air stunned me. That part of me that complains and takes so much for granted was stilled for a moment, and was given gentle instruction in gratitude and humility. Understanding that we are the patients, even as we are the caregivers, expands the pastoral dimension and improves the quality of our caring.

CONCLUSION

We know with certainty from experiences in the Supportive Care Program that hospice, palliative care, and supportive care programs are viable options and invaluable resources for patients with AIDS and their families, particularly as alternatives to hospitalization and routine home care.

Hospices have been affirmed and further challenged in their efforts by Elisabeth Kübler-Ross, who in her keynote presentation at the First Annual American Conference on Hospice Care in June 1985, said, "A hospice that doesn't accept AIDS patients should not be called a hospice."[14] She stated that the special mission of hospice practitioners was to care for all dying patients with unconditional love; that is, love under any condition.

For all hospice practitioners facing the complex issues surrounding the AIDS crisis, the policy adopted by the National Hospice Organization in November 1985 provides guidance, inspiration and challenge.[12]

> The National Hospice Organization believes that the care of AIDS patients is as important as the cure of the AIDS disease. NHO affirms the pioneering work of our members in making hospice care accessible to AIDS sufferers and responsive to their needs. Those hospices which have pioneered palliative care for AIDS patients symbolize what hospices ought to do in fulfilling the standards and principles of the National Hospice Organization. NHO encourages all hospices to serve AIDS patients.
>
> NHO understands that fear, stress, confusion, and lack of experience and resources may be obstacles to the care of AIDS patients in hospices just as in the rest of our society. The special needs of the AIDS patient and family should not be understated, but should be understood.
>
> The significant issues posed by AIDS and the access of AIDS patients to hospice care must not result in avoidance, denial, or desertion by those to whom these patients can turn for help. The special needs of the AIDS patient call for the best in us as hospices and as hospice people.

We can only agree with this statement.

REFERENCES

1. Levy, Robert M., et al. Neurological manifestations of the Acquired Immunodeficiency Syndrome (AIDS): Experience at USCF and review of the literature. *Journal of Neurosurgery* 62:482 (April 1985).
2. Reese, Richard E., and Douglas, R. Gordon, Jr. *A Practical Approach to Infectious Diseases.* Boston, Toronto: Little Brown and Company, 1983, p. 405.
3. Holmes, King K., et al. *Sexually Transmitted Diseases.* New York: McGraw-Hill, 1984, p. 699.
4. Ibid., p. 699.
5. Ibid., pp. 474, 477.
6. Ibid., p. 475.
7. Mandell, Gerald L., et al. *Principles and Practice of Infectious Disease.* New York: John Wiley, 1979, p. 1317.
8. Ibid., pp. 1308–1319.
9. Holmes, King K. *Sexually Transmitted Diseases*, p. 695.
10. Ibid., pp. 695–696.
11. Janda, Julian J. *A Play Based On The Life of Julian of Norwich.* New York: The Seabury Press, 1984, p. 40.
12. *News Briefs:* NHO adopts policy on AIDS patients. *American Journal of Hospice Care:* 8–9 (March/April 1986).

CHAPTER 13

Children with AIDS

MOSES GROSSMAN

The enormous worldwide attention and publicity that have attended the AIDS epidemic have essentially bypassed the problem presented by infants and children. There are good reasons for this. The number of cases reported in both children and adolescents in the United States as of January 1 of 1987 is less than 2% of the total number of some 28,000 cases. Much of the political and legislative focus has been on the homosexual and bisexual transmission of the disease, which does not include children. The number of adults and children infected by blood and blood products has been relatively small and will not grow, because of the success in screening and protecting blood and blood products from contamination by the human immunodeficiency virus (HIV). The principal pool of infected children has come from infants born to infected women, most of them intravenous drug users; these cases have been concentrated in a very few communities—New York, Newark, Miami, and Los Angles.[1,2] The country at large so far has had no need to face this difficult problem.

This has not been the case in Central Africa however. There the disease has affected many men and women in almost equal numbers and a very large number of children have become infected by vertical transmission. It has now become clear that heterosexual transmission is not an exclusively African phenomenon and the expectation is that the United States will also see an increase in heterosexual transmission and thus an increasing number of affected children.

EPIDEMIOLOGY

There are four ways in which children can acquire infection with the HIV virus: by vertical transmission from the mother, through infection carried by blood; through blood products or transplanted organs; through child abuse; and, finally, for adolescents, through sexual intercourse—homosexual or heterosexual with an infected partner. By far the most important route of transmission is the perinatal one. Some 75% of the 425 cases reported to date are due to perinatal transmission from infected mothers. This infection is transmitted during pregnancy, labor, and delivery from mothers infected with the virus, who themselves may or may not have symptoms.[3] The risk of infection to a baby born to an HIV-infected mother has not been firmly established. If a mother is HIV positive and has had one baby with AIDS or has the disease herself, the risk of infection of the newborn appears to be 50–65%. In the case of an asymptomatic pregnant woman with an HIV infection, the risk is somewhat lower but has not been quantified. What determines whether the infant will or will not be infected is not known.

Early statistics from the Center for Disease Control showed that 18% of children reported to have AIDS acquired this infection from blood or blood products; many were hemophiliacs receiving factor VIII or IX concentrates; some had open heart surgery and some had transfusions in the newborn nursery. This percentage will go down significantly since no new infections have been occurring as a result of the screening of all blood donors.

There is no published information on HIV infections as a result of child abuse. An unconfirmed report suggests that three children have been infected by this route. A prospective study is currently in progress.[4] As for adolescents getting infected as a result of sexual intercourse, clinically the issues are no different from adult infection; legally and socially, the issues are quite different because the adolescents are minors in the eyes of the law. It is important to emphasize that not a single youngster has been found to be infected as a result of *casual* contact. Several well-controlled studies involving well over a hundred children have confirmed that children living in households with family members who have the disease have not acquired the infection over two or three years of exposure.[5-8]

CLINICAL CONSIDERATIONS

The large majority of reported cases of children who acquire HIV infection from their mothers have appeared normal at birth. A few infants have been reported by Marion et al.[9] from New York who appear to have unusual dysmorphic (improperly developed) features—growth failure, microcephaly (small head), hypertelorism (widely spaced eyes), a prominent forehead, and a flat nasal bridge that might represent an embryopathy (diseased development of the embryo) due to this infection. However, the majority of infants appear normal, have a normal weight gain, and are asymptomatic for the first eight or nine months of their life. During this asymptomatic period the infant is truly "in limbo" as far as the diagnosis is concerned. The HIV antibody test is positive, but during this period it is not clear whether these are solely maternal antibodies or whether the infant is making antibodies as well. After a year of life, maternal antibodies disappear and antibody positivity at this point is tantamount to being infected. The recovery of HIV virus from the infant is diagnostic of an infection but viral cultures can only be done in a relatively few research laboratories at the present time. A test for HIV-IGM antibodies would be enormously helpful diagnostically. Such a test is not available at present; it is possible that this test or a test for the presence of the virus not requiring culture techniques (antigen detection or DNA probe) will become available soon; that would certainly help to clarify the infant's status and help with issues of placement, foster care, and adoption.

Infected infants begin to be symptomatic somewhere between eight and fifteen months of age. Initial signs and symptoms are failure to thrive, chronic diarrhea, and developmental delays. Lymphadenopathy (enlarged lymph nodes), hepatomegaly (enlarged liver), and splenomegaly (enlarged spleen) develop. Unlike adult patients, these children are peculiarly susceptible to common bacterial infections such as otitis media (middle ear infection) and pneumonia. Two findings which are peculiar to children are parotid (salivary gland) swellings and lymphocytic infiltrative pneumonitis.[2] As the disease progresses, opportunistic infections that are the hallmark of this disease appear; these include Pneumocystis carinii pneumonia; infection with *Mycobacteria*, principally of the *Avium intracellulare* group; candidiasis (yeast infection); toxoplasmosis (infection with minute parasite); and many others. The brain is infected with HIV, resulting in many neurologic manifestations. A very common laboratory finding is hypergammaglobinemia. Lymphopenia (decreased number of lymphocytes), an almost constant hallmark of the adult disease, is uncommon in children. The reversal of the ratio of T-suppressor cells (T4) to T-helper cells (T8) is not as reliable a diagnostic sign in children as it is in adults.[10]

The spectrum of infection ranges from asymptomatic individuals through ARC (AIDS-related complex) and AIDS, the most serious form of the infection. The CDC definition of pediatric AIDS is quite restrictive. Essentially, it is the same as in adult patients but does include biopsy-proven lymphoid interstitial pneumonia. There are probably a significant number of children who clearly have the disease but do not fit the present definition. Ammann has proposed a less restrictive classification.[11] His proposal would define children with AIDS as those with (1) a history of a risk factor (2) polyclonal hypergammaglobinemia (increased amount of gamma globulin) and T-cell immunodeficiency, and (3) presence of HIV antibody or viral isolation. Primary immunodeficiency, adenosine deaminase deficiency, and nucleoside phosphorylase deficiency should be excluded.

At the present time there is no standard definition of ARC in children. These are symptomatic children with HIV infections who fail to qualify for the strict definition of AIDS.

The prognosis in children has been as dismal as it has in adults. The majority live less than three years and die with opportunistic infections. A few have survived longer periods of time—as long as six years. Their clinical course is often complicated by very serious social circumstances, including serious illness and often loss of the mother from the same disease.

There is no *specific treatment* for the infection at the present time. Attention to nutrition and prompt treatment of both the common and opportunistic infection is important. The administration of prophylactic sulfa trimothoprim to prevent pneumocystis infection should be attempted. The adverse reaction rate is not as high as it is in adult patients. Some advocate monthly prophylactic intravenous gammaglobulin in an attempt to prevent the occurrence of common infections, an approach which makes sense but has not yet been demonstrated to be effective. Specific anti-HIV viral drugs have not yet been tested in children.

PERINATAL ISSUES

Management of perinatal HIV infections has to begin with education of women in the high risk group. At the present time it is a fairly clearly defined group—intravenous drug users, sexual contacts of infected men or men in a high risk category, and recipients of blood or blood products between the years 1979 and 1985. As heterosexual transmission of HIV infection spreads, such educational efforts will have to involve an ever-enlarging group. The first steps are to have the potential mothers-to-be consider whether they might want to get tested before they contemplate pregnancy and to provide information about the effect of HIV infection on the infant. Women in the high risk group who become pregnant should be strongly counseled to be tested for HIV infection during the first trimester; those who are positive may wish to consider the termination of pregnancy because of the deleterious effect of pregnancy on the immunologic status of the mother herself as well as the serious import for the infant.[3] We recommend repeating the antibody test during the third trimester for those women who were negative earlier. This second test will identify women whose antibodies to HIV develop later in pregnancy. We feel that it is very important to inform the delivery room personnel when delivery of an infected mother is imminent. While HIV infection is not spread by *casual* contact, the massive presence of bodily fluids and placenta, all of them containing virus, requires that infection control precautions be taken to protect delivery room personnel.[12–14]

It is equally as important to inform the pediatrician if the mother is antibody positive. The baby is not infectious once the first bath has been given. The only precautions necessary in the nursery are in the handling of blood and body fluids. However, more important for the infant, if the infant is at risk of having been vertically infected, personnel should be more vigorous in treating minor infections. One would also not wish to give the infant live virus vaccines (in the United States where the risk of disease is low; immunization is recommended in Africa) until the infant's status is clarified.[15]

A special problem arises if the baby requires *shelter or foster care,* a situation which arises commonly in this group because of maternal medical and social problems. In that setting one would urge voluntary disclosure on the part of the mother of the antibody status to a single responsible person with assurance of maximal confidentiality. If the mother is unwilling to do so, court-mandated testing of the baby might be considered. This is a serious decision that requires consideration of the likelihood of the baby being vertically infected, the risk of negatively labeling the baby, and the benefit of the medical caretaker and the foster parent being able to provide better, more enlightened medical care for the infant. The *adoption* of babies from this high risk category presents similar problems. Considering the grave nature and cost of the disease and the high mortality it is only right that the adoptive parents should understand all of the facts, including the infant's antibody status. Detailed guidelines for these considerations have been published.[13,16]

Foster care placement of infants positive for HIV antibodies has been a very difficult issue in several communities. Despite convincing evidence that the infection is not transmitted by casual contact foster parents have been reluctant to accept these infants in their homes. Some communities have been successful in appealing to better educated foster parents, in some cases with a background of health care education to accept these infants. Other communities have had to resort to some form of institutional care for these infants, an alternative which is less likely to meet their development and emotional needs than an individual foster home.

DAY CARE

The guidelines of the Center for Disease Control[16] suggest that children with HIV infections be allowed to lead as normal a life as possible and that the advantage of receiving an education in the regular classroom outweighs the risk of being in school and being exposed to infections. We need not consider the risk to others because the evidence that HIV infection is not transmitted by casual contact is really quite strong.[5,6,8] The CDC guidelines do mention that for preschool children or neurologically disabled children who cannot control their body secretions, a more restrictive setting might be advisable. Perhaps of even greater importance is the fact that children attending day care centers have a greatly increased incidence of infections of all types. Shielding these HIV-infected children from excessive exposure to common infection might have quite an important bearing on how or if their HIV infection progresses to the clinical phase. For all these reasons we feel that as a general practice children with HIV infections should not be in regular day care settings until they are three years old. If child care is needed, individual arrangements for care in the home should be made. After the age of three, each child's medical situation should be reviewed and optimal placement in day care recommended.[17] For the majority of the children, regular day care placement will probably be suitable.

PREVENTION

While research on developing various treatment modalities and the development of a vaccine are important, the only realistic approach to the problem of AIDS at this time is prevention. In the case of pediatric AIDS, it is the prevention of infection of women of child-bearing age and the avoidance of pregnancy in women known to be infected, as well as the consideration of termination of pregnancy when it is diagnosed in HIV-infected individuals. To this end the stress on education is of utmost importance. The education of women in high risk categories as well as general education of young people about HIV infection and its consequences. No group is more important than early teenagers. This is the time of life when sexual experimentation is prevalent, the use of contraceptive devices including condoms is mostly neglected, and "magical" thinking of the teenager suggests that she or he is immune from consequences. We hope that educational efforts with this group will be more successful in preventing the birth of children with AIDS than they have been in preventing teenage pregnancies.

REFERENCES

1. Rogers M. F. AIDS in children: A review of the clinical, epidemiologic and public health aspects. *Pediatric Infectious Diseases* 4:230, 1986.
2. Rubinstein, A. Pediatric AIDS. *Current Problems in Pediatrics* 16:365–409, 1986.
3. Scott, G. B., et al. Mothers of infants with the acquired immunodeficiency syndrome. *The Journal of the American Medical Association* 253:363, 1985.
4. Dattel, B., and Coulter, K. Personal communication.
5. Friedland, G. H., et al. Lack of transmission of HTLV-III/LAV infection of household contacts of patients with AIDS or AIDS related complex with oral candidiasis. *New England Journal of Medicine* 314:344–349, 1986.
6. Kaplan, J. E., et al. Evidence against transmission of human T-lymphotropic virus/lymphadenopathy-asociated virus (HTLV-III/LAV) in families of children with the acquired immunodeficiency syndrome. *Pediatric Infectious Diseases* 4:468–471, 1985.
7. Mann, J. M., et al. Prevalence of HTLV-III/LAV in household contacts of patients with confirmed AIDS and controls in Kinshasa, Zaire. *The Journal of the American Medical Association* 256:721–724, 1986.
8. Sande, M. A. Transmission of AIDS: The case against casual contagion. *New England Journal of Medicine* 314:380–382, 1986.
9. Marion, R. W., et al. Human T-cell lymphotrophic virus type III (HTLV-III) embryopathy: A new dysmorphic syndrome associated with intrauterine HTLV-III infection. *American Journal of Diseases of Children* 140:638–640, 1986.
10. Shannon, K. M., and Ammann, A. J. Acquired immune deficiency syndrome in childhood. *Journal of Pediatrics* 106:332–342, 1985.
11. Ammann, A. J. The acquired immunodeficiency syndrome in infants and children. *Annals of Internal Medicine* 103:734–737, 1985.
12. Centers for Disease Control. Recommendations for assisting in the prevention of perinatal transmission of human T-lymphotrophic virus type III/lymphadenopathy-associated virus and acquired immunodeficiency syndrome. *Morbidity and Mortality Weekly Report* 34:721–732, 1985.

13. City and County of San Francisco Department of Public Health Perinatal and Pediatric AIDS Advisory Committee. Guidelines for control of perinatally transmistted human T-lymphotrophic virus-type III/lymphadenopathy associated virus infection and care of infected mothers, infants, and children. *San Francisco Epidemiological Bulletin* 2(1):1S–16S, 1986.

14. Grossman, M. HIV infections in children: Public health and public policy issues. *Pediatric Infectious Diseases* 6:113, 1987.

15. Halsey, N. A., and Henderson, D. A. HIV infection and immunization against other agents. *New England Journal of Medicine* 316:383, 1987.

16. Centers for Disease Control. Education and foster care of children infected with human T-Lymphotrophic virus type III/lymphadenopathy-associated virus. *Morbidity and Mortality Weekly Report* 34:517–521, 1985.

17. Committee on Infectious Diseases American Academy of Pediatrics. Health guidelines for the attendance in day care and foster care settings of children infected with HIV. *Pediatrics* 79:466, 1987.

CHAPTER 14
Public Schools Confront AIDS

ELIZABETH P. LAMERS

INTRODUCTION

The acquired immune deficiency syndrome (AIDS) was not immediately identified as a separate disease when it first appeared in the United States. Initially, a sharp rise in the incidence of Kaposi's sarcoma, a rare and usually fatal type of cancer, was noticed, especially among homosexuals. This was later associated with a rise in the number of cases of *Pneumocystis carinii* pneumonia in the same population. When the disease now known as AIDS was identified in 1981 it was not thought to be contagious. What had been called the "Gay Epidemic" and the "Haitian Disease" was finally named Acquired immune deficiency syndrome, or AIDS, in 1983.

AIDS initially appeared to be limited to homosexuals and intravenous drug abusers. However when AIDS appeared among hemophiliacs and recipients of blood transfusions, the general population began to feel vulnerable. By March 23, 1987, 33,158 cases of AIDS had been diagnosed and 19,192 deaths (58% of the total number of cases) had already occurred. A plague mentality arose; amid fearfulness, misinformation, and overreaction to the disease, some in society looked for a scapegoat. Even though scientific knowledge and understanding of the virus and resulting pathology developed rapidly, AIDS patients and their families nonetheless became the new untouchables. Legislators in California, Texas, and Ohio introduced bills to segregate persons identified as AIDS-infected from the general population. Some fundamentalist ministers preached that AIDS is divine retribution for living an unnatural (that is, homosexual) lifestyle. In May 1983, Patrick Buchanan, former director of communications at the White House, wrote in a syndicated column in a style reminiscent of a fire and brimstone preacher that "[homosexuals] have declared war on nature, and now nature is exacting an awful retribution."[1] Attributing blame for a new and unexplained disease is not a new phenomenon. Cotton Mather (ca. 1663–1728) stated, "Sickness is in fact the whip of God for the sins of many."[2]

When AIDS first appeared, scientists observed patterns of association of the disease with particular segments of the population, but only subsequently demonstrated the mechanism of transmission of the virus. Journalists used terms such as "sexual contact" and "sharing of bodily fluids" in reporting on AIDS, leaving many people with little idea of how AIDS is spread. Even the literature from the Centers for Disease Control and other health authorities has perpetuated some of the misunderstanding, with polite terms such as "casual contact" and "intimate contact" used to describe the method of transmission of the AIDS virus. A poll conducted by the *New York Times/CBS News* in September 1985, showed that nearly half of those polled thought they could catch AIDS by sharing a glass with an AIDS patient, although it was documented by epidemiologists and other scientists that AIDS could be transmitted only by sexual contact or by exposure to infected blood, including maternal-fetal transmission. The fact that AIDS had been transmitted by blood transfusions led a number of people to mistakenly assume that it was therefore unsafe to give blood.[3]

Both *Newsweek* and the *Washington Journalism Review* criticized media coverage for being less than explicit about the mode of AIDS transmission.[4,5] Some reports actually suggested that casual contact could spread the disease. Others resorted to exaggeration, for example: "Now No One Is Safe From Aids," *Life*, July 1985; "School Cook Dies of AIDS: He Chopped Green Beans & Roast Beef," *New York Post*, September 12, 1985; "Aids Child Bites Classmate, Now Both Are Doomed," *Weekly World News*, November 12, 1985. The fact that the medical community has stated that it considers AIDS a relatively difficult disease to contract for those who are either celibate or monogamous has not been totally reassuring. In fact, *Newsweek* reported that physician attempts at reassurance about AIDS has caused some people to distrust doctors. An example of this distrust was shown by a New York City mother who said she was keeping her child out of school because "We are afraid our children will catch the disease even if those so-called, quote-unquote experts say it is impossible."[6]

HISTORICAL OVERVIEW

The public health aspect of classroom education has an interesting, if brief, history. Children were first educated at home by their parents. Gradually, small informal groups (for example, cousins or neighbors) were educated in a specific home. Eventually these small groups evloved into formal schools, the precursor of our current school systems. As the number of children in a classroom increased, the chances of infectious diseases spreading from child to child also increased.

Even today, during the first year of a child's schooling parents often notice an increase in the frequency of infections in their child. Some parents may wonder if school is really worth the risk of illness. However, the frequency of infections usually decreases after the first year of school as children develop a broader immunity to viral respiratory infections and as they receive the formal and informal instruction in personal hygiene which in and of itself reduces transmission of many microorganisms. Viral diseases are spread not only from child to child; child to parent transmission has also been confirmed. The *New England Journal of Medicine* recently reported that children in day-care centers had transmitted cytomegalovirus (CMV) to their parents.[7] This is especially serious for pregnant women because CMV can be passed to the fetus. It has been demonstrated that CMV infection in pregnant women has resulted in a 10% increase in the rate of birth defects. A significant literature has developed surrounding infectious disease control in school-based settings.[8] The public health implications of viral infections acquired in a classroom setting are more complicated than was formerly thought.

Serious infectious diseases which once were a part of childhood are now largely eradicated due to immunization, antibiotics, and improvements in sanitation. Schools generally require that all entering students provide evidence of having been inoculated against diphtheria, tetanus, pertussis, measles, mumps, rubella, and polio. Some school districts also require testing for exposure to tuberculosis. In California, children whose parents have personal or religious objections to inoculations may enter school without the usual medical certificate of inoculations. The parents of these children must sign an affidavit that they are opposed to inoculations on personal or religious grounds and that they (the parents) understand that in the event of an outbreak of a contagious disease their children will be excluded from school until the outbreak has subsided.

Until the current AIDS crisis, epidemics in Western society were largely a thing of the past. The annual recurrence of influenza is usually described as an "outbreak" rather than as an epidemic. Polio, the last epidemic, when considered retrospectively infected relatively few, but affected many in terms of the fear of death or disability associated with the disease. Between 1915 and the introduction of the Salk vaccine in 1955 over 500,000 persons contracted polio. Fifty-seven thousand (11%) died, and many others were left with residual paralysis.[9] This statistic helps put into perspective the current AIDS epidemic wherein 19,192 (58%) have died as of March 23, 1987.

During the 1940s entire towns were sprayed with DDT in an effort to kill flies, despite a lack of evidence that the polio infection was transmitted by insects. Because most polio cases occurred in late summer, many school openings were delayed. Milwaukee (1944) declared a citywide quarantine, prohibiting children from leaving their own yards during the season of peak polio contagion.[10]

DISEASE AND THE CLASSROOM

Ever since children have been brought together for public education, the classroom has served as an arena for resolving larger issues. The conflict between scientific Darwinism and religious creationism escalated from the classroom to the famous Scopes "monkey trial."[11] The social issue of integration versus segregation was played out in classrooms in the South in the 1950s.[11] The religious issue of prayer in the classroom became a major political issue in the early 1960s.[11] The educational issues surrounding AIDS have already attracted the attention of parents and religious groups who have strong feelings about what subjects may be taught in the classroom.[12]

The basic conflict involved is one of rights and responsibilities. The rights of the individual must be preserved. The rights of society must be protected. The school has the responsibility to educate and must operate in the public interest. The school also makes educational decisions on behalf of the parents (*in loco parentis*).

AIDS is a public health issue. The school as a representative of the public interest has a responsibility to teach the facts necessary to reduce the spread of AIDS. To properly teach these facts the school must present information that some parents find objectionable on moral and religious grounds.

For example, education about AIDS requires that children be taught the basic facts about sex, birth control, and drug abuse. It is apparent that the most effective approach is to present this information *before* the children become involved in sexual activity and drug abuse. It is not enough for schools to support sexual and drug abstinence. Children need to know the facts so that over time they can make decisions based upon sound knowledge. If this were a perfect society, moral persuasion would be sufficient to reduce the spread of AIDS. The teenage pregnancy rate shows, however, that this is not a perfect society. Public health issues demand a broad, reasoned, educational approach to AIDS. The general adult tendency to want to shield children from unpleasant realities must, in this instance, yield to the imperative of providing children with life-saving information. Rabbi Steven Robbins of Temple Emanuel in Beverly Hills, California has stated the problem even more bluntly, "If you have any problems about talking to your child about AIDS, it may come down to a condom or a casket for your child."[13]

For 20 years the classroom has been relatively free from public health concerns. Immunization against polio eliminated the last major epidemic among school-aged children. The development of effective treatment for tuberculosis meant that schoolchildren who formerly were isolated in sanatoriums could now attend school, once they were past the infectious stage of the disease. The availability of safe and effective immunization against diphtheria, pertussis, tetanus, measles, rubella, mumps, and polio has made the classroom a relatively safe gathering place for children.

One major medical development of the past two decades that has affected the classroom environment for many children has been improvements in treating childhood cancer. Because of new therapies, children with cancer who formerly left school, never to return, are now able to experience remission or even complete cure. Children now return to the classroom during the maintenance phases of treatment. As childhood cancer has become treatable, it carries less of a stigma. But some parents still fear their child can "catch" cancer from a schoolmate with the disease. Classroom teachers have learned to cope with the child with cancer returning to the classroom. Courts have frequently upheld the rights of children with disabilities to remain in the classroom and to receive the necessary assistance to obtain an education.

AIDS presents a challenge to schools for several reasons. The classroom has been relatively "safe" for over two decades; the fact that it is presumed not to be "safe" any longer is itself a threat to some parents. The mortality rate for those with AIDS exceeds that associated with polio or cancer. The mechanisms of AIDS transmission raise moral, religious, and sexual connotations that are threatening for many adults. This presents an added dimension to the challenge facing teachers and school boards to design educational programs which provide the information and motivation necessary to eliminate the further spread of the disease. The fear of their children "catching" AIDS from an infected classmate has caused parents to question recognized medical authorities.

It is known that the AIDS virus is not a stable virus like the polio virus. The human immunodeficiency virus (HIV) mutates rapidly. Given our present knowledge and technology, one-time immunization against HIV seems an unlikely method of effective prevention. The current lack of any immunization against or effective treatment for AIDS raises the spectre of an epidemic threat to all segments of the population for years to come.

SCOPE OF THE PROBLEM IN SCHOOLS

Because AIDS is transmissible and thus far incurable, school boards have had a difficult time deciding whether or not to admit a child with AIDS. *The Harvard Medical School Health Letter* points out, "There appears to be no cogent reason for excluding such children (with AIDS) from the classroom, unless they have behavior problems, such as habitual biting, that could lead to transmission of the virus."[14] The same letter recommends the establishment of local task forces to conduct confidential case-by-case reviews. Articles in *The New England Journal of Medicine* state that the AIDS virus is not transmitted by casual contact, even within a family unit in which there is close contact with the infected person (sharing household items or household facilities, washing items used by AIDS patients, or hugging or kissing them).[15,16] In a recent study designed to determine routes of transmission, the AIDS virus was isolated from only 1 of 83 saliva samples, although the virus was detected in 28 of 50 blood samples from the same population.[16]

The American Medical Association (AMA) has suggested that preschoolers with AIDS not be admitted to day-care centers because they might bite or scratch other children and may not yet be completely toilet trained.

The AMA suggests that these factors might contribute to the spread of the virus. However, physicians emphasize that school-age children do not pose a health threat to their classmates and should be allowed to participate in the same activities as healthy youngsters.[17] Although the child with AIDS does not pose a contagious threat in the classroom, the natural progression of the disease leads to a point where immunosuppression in the ill child causes the classroom to become a threat. The immunosuppressed child cannot tolerate viral and bacterial organisms that pose no threat to healthy classmates. At this point the child with AIDS should be removed from the classroom to a setting (for instance, home) where there is limited exposure to pathogenic organisms.

The Education For All Handicapped Children Act of 1975 (Public Law 94-142) was enacted to ensure that all children, whether handicapped or not, receive an education. Therefore the question is not "should the child with AIDS be educated," but "how and where should the child with AIDS be educated." There are various ways of educating handicapped children within the educational system. Some can be educated in classrooms within hospitals, others in segregated classrooms within regular schools or in segregated classrooms in schools for handicapped children. Still others can be educated at home, either by a home teacher, or with a video link to the classroom. While educating a child in a special class or at home may satisfy PL 94-142 and the educational needs of the child, these solutions do not necessarily satisfy the child's social and psychological needs. It has long been recognized by educators that schools impart more than book learning. School boards that have segregated handicapped children have been challenged by parents who claim that the social and psychological dimensions of a regular classroom are as important as the instruction received.

Different school boards have handled the problem of the student with AIDS in different ways.[18-23] Most school boards have not taken any action until faced with a student or teacher with AIDS. Some boards (e.g., Beverly Hills, CA) have set up panels of medical experts to review cases as they arise.[23] In certain situations, the question of admitting a student with AIDS to school could not be resolved by the school board, and has been referred to a local court.[24] A decision by the courts in favor of admitting the child does not necessarily resolve the matter. For example, when a Kokomo, Indiana court determined Ryan White had the right to return to class, parents of his schoolmates raised a $12,000 bond to continue their fight to exclude him.[25] In other school districts, parents have withdrawn their children rather than have them attend classes with a student known to have AIDS. Not only have AIDS patients been barred from attending school, but there have also been instances of children or siblings of AIDS patients being barred from school until proven to be uninfected.[26-28]

The case of "Mark" of Swansea, Massachusetts has unfortunately been the exception rather than the rule.[29] Mark has AIDS and has been allowed to attend public school largely through the efforts of the school superintendent, John McCarthy. McCarthy learned the scientific facts about AIDS and educated the community by arranging for physicians to meet with teachers and parents. McCarthy had more credibility in his community than do many other superintendents. He has been a teacher and administrator in Swansea for three decades, and he has taught or coached several of the town's school board members. Nonetheless, his judicious approach to obtaining the pertinent information and providing the appropriate resources serves as a model of enlightened leadership.

Teachers as well as students can be infected with the AIDS virus. As yet, there is no clear pattern of how school boards handle the problem of a teacher with AIDS. The National Education Association (NEA) opposes mandatory testing of teachers for AIDS and has stated that teachers with AIDS should be permitted to keep their jobs.

School boards also must consider the economic implications of the decisions regarding the education of the child with AIDS. Will a school board's decision result in a costly lawsuit? If it is decided that the child with AIDS should be placed in a special education class, will the cost be borne by the school or district, or can the expense be covered by a state or federally funded program? The majority of the monies a school district receives from the state is determined by the daily attendance of students. By admitting a student with AIDS, a district may risk losing income if other students refuse to attend out of fear or in protest. In many school districts multiple and prolonged withdrawals would constitute a financial hardship.

School districts also must consider the possibility of a future lawsuit if another child becomes seropositive and the infection can be traced to the readmitted student with AIDS. Because at present there is no cure for AIDS, some school boards are reluctant to tell parents that their children are safe in a classroom with a child with AIDS. The long incubation period of the AIDS virus (months to years) compounds the uncertainty. The current epidemic demands that school boards act now, although the consequences of their actions may not be known for years.

At present, school-aged children with AIDS were infected either in utero or by later transfusion with AIDS-contaminated blood or blood products. The number of children infected by contaminated blood is expected to decrease as methods of processing blood extracts improve, as new means of screening donors are utilized, and as methods are refined to test blood for the presence of the AIDS virus. The majority of children infected in utero are the offspring of intravenous drug users. Some of these children, ill at birth, never leave the hospital. Of those that do go home, most do not survive to school age.[30] At present the number of children infected antenatally with AIDS is increasing. An education program for IV drug users could decrease these numbers even though this population is notoriously difficult to change. (See Chapter 11.) Dr. Rubinstein, professor of pediatrics at New York's Albert

Einstein College of Medicine, has stated, "These [the infants known to have AIDS through maternal transmission] are the very sick children. A much larger number are infected but not very sick yet. Nobody knows how to label them. We are talking about maybe 2000 children."[31]

EDUCATION IN THE CLASSROOM

Education regarding behaviors to prevent the spread of the AIDS virus offers the greatest hope of containing this epidemic. Students must be taught the basic facts about the transmission of AIDS. Dr. Edward Gomperts, director of the hemophilia center at Children's Hospital in Los Angeles states the need: "Imagine the scenario of high schools with sexually active kids hooked on drugs and infected with AIDS. We could have a generation of infected kids."[32] Dr. C. Everett Koop, Surgeon General of the United States, has asked for AIDS education to begin in elementary school. This poses a problem to some school districts, since effective education about AIDS requires discussing subjects previously considered "taboo" in elementary classrooms: homosexual practices and birth control. To be effective in combating the spread of AIDS, educational materials must be clear and explicit. Parents who have been reluctant to allow heterosexual sex education in schools may be even more resistant to allowing their children to be exposed to concepts of homosexuality and the use of condoms. To eliminate any discussion of homosexuality and "safe sex" would be to ignore important parts of the problem and solution. The Los Angeles Unified School District has developed a new curriculum on AIDS and sexually transmitted diseases for junior and senior high school students. By the end of the 1986–87 school year this new program will be extended to sixth grade students. A number of other school districts across the country are also developing comparable courses designed to halt the spread of AIDS.

As more persons with AIDS return to school, students need to learn how the AIDS virus can and cannot be transmitted. They need to know that persons with AIDS can be touched and hugged without fear of becoming infected. They must learn that the AIDS virus can not be transmitted to uninfected members of the same household in the course of ordinary day-to-day living. Students also need more than facts, however; they need time to discuss their fears and feelings with teachers who have been properly educated regarding the social, psychological, physical, and public health aspects of this unique disease.

When a student dies of AIDS, his or her classmates will need support in dealing with their feelings of loss and grief. They will have questions about AIDS, death, and grief that require answers. They will need encouragement to verbalize their feelings as well as support to attend funeral services and to convey condolences to the bereaved family.[33,34] Teachers must become familiar with the mechanisms of grief. They need to know that some students may become more aggressive and outspoken while others may cry, withdraw, or even develop (transient) exemplary behavior.[33,34]

Ideally, students, teachers, and parents will work together to meet the challenges presented by AIDS. If the problems are faced openly, creative solutions supportive of social and psychological growth can replace some of the early reflexive adjustments made out of fear and misunderstanding.

AIDS AND THE MEDIA

The projected morbidity and mortality resulting from the AIDS pandemic mandates the development of coordinated educational and social approaches to provide all people with basic, factual information about the disease, its mode of transmission, and methods to reduce the risk of infection.

The media (newspapers, television, magazines, radio, videotapes) has a significant place in the lives of students. It has been estimated that the average elementary/secondary student spends six hours per day watching television and considerable other hours watching videos, reading magazines, or listening to the radio. Sexually oriented advertising is commonly used to market a variety of products, from automobiles to music and clothing. Sexual themes play a central role in the entertainment industry. Popular songs frequently contain references to overt sexual activity. There is evidence to suggest the existence of a strong "copy cat" phenomenon in adolescent behavior.[35] Does the same sort of imitative behavior pertain in sexual matters? And, if so, does it represent a public health threat in terms of the transmission of AIDS?

Media programming supportive of casual sexual involvement would undoubtedly dilute the effectiveness of instructional programs designed to foster abstinence, restraint, and "safe sex." Planning for and implementation of instructional programs to reduce the transmission of AIDS should include a review of media impact on the behavior of those for whom the courses are designed. Current evidence of government concern for monitoring the content of radio programming has recently appeared.[36]

Since release of the Surgeon General's report on AIDS, sex education and the use of condoms has gained wide exposure in the media. Discussion in the media regarding the use of condoms has suddenly weakened the taboo against advertising birth control devices on television and in newspapers. The major networks, once reluctant to offend a substantial segment of their audience, have used concern about AIDS as a means of justifying the acceptance of condom advertising. The same networks also continue to offer many hours each week of sexually provocative programming with no more than a disclaimer that "the material in the following show may be offensive to some."

Newspapers, like television, have appeared to operate under a double standard: while refusing to accept advertising for birth control devices, they have continued to allow the use of sexually provocative material to market a wide variety of products. The AIDS crisis appears to have allowed both television and newspapers to accept advertising for condoms on the basis that their use will reduce the transmission of AIDS. But it is doubtful if the media will spontaneously reexamine its attitude toward accepting and programming sexually provocative material. It is unlikely, also, that newspapers and television will make the quantum leap from mentioning the term "safe sex" to accurately describing safe sex practices.

CONCLUSION

AIDS presents a complicated social, psychological, and public health challenge to educators and school boards. Resolution of the problems will depend upon learning the medical facts about AIDS, developing effective strategies for educating students with AIDS and their classmates, and developing educational programs designed to reduce the transmission of the AIDS virus.

In the absence of any effective treatment for AIDS and with no immediate prospect of the development of a vaccine, education offers the only hope of limiting the spread of this dangerous disease. It has been predicted that tens of millions of people will die of AIDS (worldwide) during the next 10 years. The number of people of any age who contract the virus can be influenced by the development and implementation of effective educational programs. Content aimed at understanding and preventing this devastating disease though the assumption of appropriate preventive behaviors on the part of the individual and the community is essential to the well-being of all. Public schools play a significant role in preserving the health of all members of society and in assuring the vitality of future generations.

REFERENCES

1. Alter, J. Sins of omission. *Newsweek*, Sept. 23, 1985, 25.
2. Morrow, L. The start of a plague mentality. *Time*, Sept. 23, 1985, 37.
3. Adler, J.; Greenberg, N. F.; Hager, M.; McKillop, P.; Namuth, T. The AIDS conflict. *Newsweek*, Sept. 23, 1985, 18–24.
4. Diamond, E., and Bellitto, C. M. The great verbal coverup. *Washington Journalism Review*, March 1986, 38–42.
5. Alter, J. Sins of omission.
6. Adler, J., et al. The AIDS conflict.
7. Pass, R. F.; Hutto, C.; Ricks, R.; Cloud, C. A. Increased rate of cytomegalovirus infection among parents of children attending day-care centers. *New England Journal of Medicine* 314(22):1414–1423 (May 29, 1986).
8. Articles such as those reviewed in *Reviews of Infectious Diseases* 8(4) (July/Aug. 1986).
9. Adler, J., et al. The AIDS conflict.

10. Leerhsen, C. Epidemics: A paralyzing effect. *Newsweek*, Sept. 23, 1985, 23.
11. Court decisions: *Brown v. Board of Education*, 347 U.S. 483 (1954); *Scopes v State*, 154 TNN. 105, 289 S.W. 363 (1927); *Engel v. Vittale*, 370 U.S. 421 (1962).
12. Gillam, J. Group seeks ban of "obscene" AIDS material in schools. *Los Angeles Times*, April 22, 1987, Parts 2, 3.
13. Rabbi Steven Robbins. Personal communication, March 1, 1987.
14. *The Harvard Medical School Health Letter* 11(2) AIDS update (Part II). Dec. 1985, 2–5.
15. Friedland, G. H.; Saltzman, B. R.; Rogers, M. F.; Kahl, P. A.; Lesser, M. L.; Mayers, M. M.; Klein, R. S. Lack of transmission of HTLV-III/LAV infection tohousehold contacts of patients with AIDS or AIDS-related complex with oral candidiasis. *New England Journal of Medicine* 314(6):344–349 (Feb. 6, 1986).
16. Sande, M. E. Transmission of AIDS. *New England Journal of Medicine* 314(6):380–382 (Feb. 6, 1986).
17. McAuliffe, K. Health/Medicine. *U.S. News & World Report*, June 30, 1986, 63.
18. Barber, J., and Luckow, D. An epidemic of fear. *Maclean's*, Sept. 23, 1985, 61, 62.
19. Cimons, M. Loved ones latest victims of AIDS discrimination. *Los Angeles Times*, June 2, 1986, Part I, 1, 12, 13.
20. Dobbin, M., and Kyle, C. The youngest victims of AIDS. *U.S. News & World Report*, July 7, 1986, 71–72.
21. Johnson, L. Kindergarten suspends AIDS victim, 4. *Los Angeles Times*, Sept. 11, 1986, Part I, 3, 34.
22. Kirp, D. Commentary: AIDS victim. *San Francisco Examiner*, July 16, 1986, Section A, 11.
23. Mitchell, J. Beverly Hills School Board calls for creation of medical advisory panel to review AIDS cases. *Los Angeles Times*, March 2, 1986, Part W, 1, 13.
24. Overend, W. Judge orders return to class for AIDS boy. *Los Angeles Times*, Nov. 18, 1986, Part I, 1, 22.
25. *Los Angeles Times*. Group raises cash in fight to bar AIDS victim from class. March 3, 1986, Part I, 14.
26. Barber, J. An epidemic of fear.
27. Cimons, M. Loved ones latest victims of AIDS discrimination.
28. Dobbin, M. The youngest victims of AIDS.
29. Kirp, D. Commentary: AIDS victim.
30. Dobbin, M. The youngest victims of AIDS.
31. Ibid.
32. Ibid.
33. Lamers, E. P. The dying child in the classroom. In *Children and Death*, edited by G. Paterson. London, Ont.: King's College Press, 1986.
34. Lamers, W. M., Jr. Helping the child to grieve. In *Children and Death*, edited by G. Paterson. London, Ont.: King's College Press, 1986.
35. Gould, M. S., and Shaffer, D. The impact of suicide in television movies: Evidence of imitation. *New England Journal of Medicine* 315:690–694 (1986). Ostroff, R. B.; Behrends, R. W.; Lee, K.; Oliphant, J. Adolescent suicides modeled after television movie. *American Journal of Psychiatry* 142:989 (1985). Correspondence, *New England Journal of Medicine* 316:876–878 (1987).
36. McDougal, D. Shock radio crackdown jolts industry. *Los Angeles Times*, April 18, 1987, Part 6, 1, 11.

CHAPTER 15

Individual Education Programs for AIDS Control

DEAN F. ECHENBERG

The strategies used to deal with the AIDS epidemic must evolve as our knowledge of the epidemic evolves. We must continually evaluate what we are doing and how we are going to do it. The interventions will be very different depending upon the local situation.

The goal of an AIDS prevention program is to prevent transmission of human immunodeficiency virus (HIV) infections. A broad range of intervention programs will be needed to attain this goal. Programs must be appropriate to the particular circumstances of each community in which they are implemented. Although no single strategy will be successful everywhere, education must be the cornerstone of each effort. Devising the appropriate education program is critical. This education must be focused on targeted groups or individuals, on those who are either infected or at risk of becoming infected.

One factor which will determine how this education is to be applied in any population depends upon the prevalence of the disease in that population. When many are infected, obviously mass education directed to the entire affected population is one of the most important methods. When there are very few infected, additional attempts must be made to locate these individuals and then educate them individually. In San Francisco two strategies have been developed to deal with both a high and low prevalence situation.

The AIDS epidemic has spread with great rapidity in certain areas. The first cases of what came to be diagnosed as AIDS were reported in Los Angeles in June 1981.[1] One month later similar cases that had presented in the previous 30 months were reported from New York and San Francisco.[2] All of these cases had appeared in young homosexual or bisexual men who lived in urban settings. Many of them used drugs and were affected by various infectious agents. Reviews of case reports and hospital records of the previous 10 years in New York and San Francisco revealed almost no cases during that period in men in similar age groups.

In the absence of a reliable test for AIDS, the Centers for Disease Control (CDC) established a working case definition. The definition incorporated two major features: It was a disease at least moderately predictive of a defect in cell-mediated immunity, and it occurred in a person with no known cause for diminished resistance to that disease. Although CDC did not include the full spectrum of disease subsequently known to be caused by the virus, the initial definition provided a useful classification for establishing an intensive surveillance system.

A look at the epidemiology of AIDS in San Francisco reveals how different control strategies evolved. A cohort of homosexual men in San Francisco recruited from the municipal sexually transmitted disease (STD) clinic has been followed since 1978.[3,4] These men were voluntary participants in a hepatitis B study. In 1984 it was learned that many of these men were infected with the AIDS virus. They were subsequently asked to consent to participate in an AIDS study and to agree to an examination of their blood serum saved from 1979 and 1980.

One of the most tragic aspects in this overall tragedy is that by the time the first publication on AIDS appeared in the medical literature in July of 1981, 30–40% of the men in this cohort were already infected.[5] It took another a year before the sexual mode of transmission was more clearly understood, at which time 40–50% of the cohort was infected.

The strategies that evolved in San Francisco in that high prevalence situation were obviously very different than those that would be used where the prevalence is much lower. In addition there is now a blood test to detect seropositivity.

PREVENTION

The goal of an AIDS prevention program is to prevent transmission of and infection with the AIDS virus. Accurate knowledge of the nature and extent of the virus must be the cornerstone for stopping both the AIDS epidemic and hysteria. Other related goals are to reduce morbidity and premature mortality in those who are already infected. The prevalence of infection and disease in each geographical area or group should determine, in part, where the emphasis should be placed in any prevention or education campaign.

In order to effectively prevent transmission one of two basic approaches are used. First, an assumption can be made that everyone in a geographical area or group is infectious through certain actions. Education about prevention of transmission should be aimed at everyone in these areas or groups. This approach is particularly suited if the prevalence is high.

In the initial stages of the epidemic in San Francisco, a strategy was evolved that said, in effect, all people in the classic high risk group should consider themselves infectious through sexual contact. This included not only homosexual and bisexual men, but also included hemophiliacs and intravenous (IV) drug users.

Education targeted to broad population and identity groups has been relatively effective. Mass education has had a great impact in decreasing the frequency of unsafe sexual activities that can transmit the virus.[6] For example, an average of 382 cases of rectal gonorrhea were seen each month during 1982 at the sexually transmitted disease clinic in San Francisco. By the end of 1986 the monthly case totals had decreased to less than 30 per month.[7]

A second generation approach to prevention education program strategy is to target education to individuals who have a high likelihood of being infected. (This will obviously increase the effectiveness of the intervention as well.) This is a classic approach which has been used in the control of a variety of infectious diseases. The smallpox eradication campaign, for instance, use case-finding techniques and sexually transmitted disease programs utilize a contact-tracing strategy. However, for smallpox and most sexually transmitted diseases, interventions are available in the form of either vaccination of contacts or treatment of infected individuals. With AIDS there is no vaccine, nor is there available treatment in the classic sense. Therefore, individuals who are infected with the AIDS virus must be educated and properly counseled as to their risk of transmitting the disease to others in the community. This education will be most effective if it is focused on those individuals known to be infected.

Individual education is especially important in areas where disease prevalence is low, because care providers in the general community might not yet be aware of the salient issues of AIDS prevention. In contrast, when disease prevalence is high, the death rates are also high, and mass education programs can rapidly raise the level of awareness and of concern which likely results in behavioral changes. Where the prevalence is low such changes cannot be expected to occur when mass education programs are applied.

In San Francisco, when it became apparent that cases could also occur in individuals outside of the classically defined "high risk" groups (those in low prevalence groups such as the general heterosexual population), it was realized that other strategies were needed. An estimated 50% of all homosexual men in San Francisco are infected with HIV.[8] In the general heterosexual population, the prevalence of HIV infection is currently less than a fraction of one %. For heterosexuals, the progression of the epidemic may prove more insidious then for homosexuals and bisexuals, because heterosexuals won't suspect or know that they are infected.

The incubation period for AIDS is thought at this point to be as long as seven years, and possibly even longer.[9] An infected individual can unknowingly carry the virus and infect others for the entire incubation period. The immediacy of the epidemic among heterosexuals is very different than it has been among homosexual and bisexual men. Many individuals in the homosexual and bisexual community have become ill and died as a consequence of HIV infection. This widespread morbidity and mortality has not yet occurred in the heterosexual population. Therefore, mass education campaigns designed for the heterosexual population are not likely to result in the dramatic decrease in unsafe sexual activity observed in the homosexual and bisexual community.

Attempts must be made to locate heterosexuals who have been unknowingly exposed. These individuals should be offered risk reduction education and serological testing. San Francisco has established a model for heterosexual contact-tracing.[10] Without contact notification, rivulets of undetected AIDS virus infections will extend unchecked into the general heterosexual population, leading to problems of a much greater magnitude in the future.

A tracing program for heterosexual contacts of HIV-infected persons has been in place in San Francisco since 1985.[11] This program is part of an active surveillance program to locate all cases of AIDS in San Francisco. All individuals who have been diagnosed with AIDS are interviewed and asked to provide the names of their heterosexual partners so they can be contacted and informed of their exposure to HIV infection and its possible consequences. The program employs sensitive, trained investigators with experience in STD control. The investigators get a very high degree of cooperation. The identity of the initial case is never revealed to the contacts. The program is completely voluntary: any individuals who choose to inform their sex partners themselves have that option, or, if in some cases they'd rather not participate directly, that is their prerogative (although such an occurrence has been rare).

In San Francisco these same tracing techniques have been used for over 6000 cases of syphilis and gonorrhea. Although there is no treatment for AIDS as there is for syphilis and gonorrhea, intervention is still possible. People who would not otherwise realize that they might have been infected can be so informed. A major assumption underlying the program is that an individual would not want to infect others unknowingly. Several women who were infected but unaware that they had been exposed to the AIDS virus were located with this program. To date, most of the individuals named as heterosexual partners are women of childbearing age. A contact-tracing program is especially important in preventing perinatal transmission of HIV as well as further transmission through sexual or parenteral means.

Twenty-seven heterosexual contacts have been investigated since the beginning of this program.[12] Seven of these were HIV antibody positive. Almost all of these were women of childbearing age. It is interesting that about half of the women had concerns about being infected even prior to their being contacted by our investigators. They thought they were at risk because of their sexual activities and were greatly relieved when the blood tests proved to be negative. Those who actually were positive did not know they were infected.

It is extremely important for anyone who is contemplating this type of program to understand the necessity for maintaining confidentiality. There must be very strong legal protections to safeguard this information from all subpoenas. In addition, there is a need for a precise, technical approach based on knowledge of HIV transmission along with very sensitive, well-trained investigators.

In addition to contact-tracing of the heterosexual partners of people with AIDS we have begun a similar program of contact-tracing of individuals who have become infected after receiving contaminated blood and for mothers of pediatric AIDS cases. In addition, all HIV-infected persons are encouraged to refer their partners for education, counseling, and testing.

In conjunction with individual contact-tracing and partner referral programs, other components are essential to HIV prevention.

1. *Community education.* In both low and high prevalence situations education on risk reduction must be developed for the entire community. It is important to stress both how the disease is transmitted and who is at risk, as well as how the disease is not transmitted and who is not at risk.
2. *Health provider education.* Education for health care providers about the prevention of AIDS transmission is extremely important. In high and low prevalence areas all health care providers must know who is at risk and who is not. In addition to knowing how to counsel individuals, they must understand when it is appropriate to suggest a test for the HIV antibody. When they find an individual who is infected in a low prevalence situation, the providers must understand the importance of stressing that the patient inform his or her sexual contacts. This is especially important in areas where HIV infection is not reportable and public health officials are not involved in contact-tracing programs.
3. *Risk group education.* Just as any clinical intervention involves a dialogue with the individual patient, a public health intervention involves a dialogue with the affected community. The most effective way to establish this dialogue and develop educational strategies for a community is to involve members of that community. This is especially true in the AIDS epidemic, a tragedy which has been compounded in that it has struck communities that have been historically suppressed. In many places in the United States where AIDS spread rapidly and entire segments of the community were infected, programs were established by the community, in collaboration with local public health departments, to disseminate information rapidly and effectively.

One of the most important aspects of any prevention program is the establishment of strong constraints against the misuse of the information obtained by public health officials. If there is not effective governing legislation that prevents inappropriate disclosure of confidential information, disease control programs based on ascertaining the prevalence of infection in the community are doomed to fail. Without strong protections of individual rights, infected individuals will have cause to stay away from health providers and control programs. This may result in increased spread of the virus within the community.

INAPPROPRIATE INTERVENTION

Precise information must be gathered in order to plan appropriate intervention techniques. Inappropriate interventions can also hasten the spread of this disease. Unlike tuberculosis, AIDS is spread by consensual acts. Except in the case of perinatal transmission it takes two willing individuals to transmit this disease. AIDS cannot be spread by casual contact. If there are good community education programs, an individual will not unknowingly be infected with the AIDS virus—he or she will be aware that he or she is taking a risk. Education programs should ensure that discrimination does not occur with AIDS-infected individuals. It is important that public health officials remain firm in the face of demands for restrictive actions to stem the epidemic; such actions are inappropriate. Actions must be based on scientific information and sound principles of public health.

REFERENCES

1. Gottleib, M. S.; Schanker, H. M.; Fan, P. T., et al. Pneumocystis pneumonia. *Los Angeles, Morbid Mortal Weekly Report,* 30:250–252 (1981).
2. Friedman-Kien, A.; Laubenstein, L.; Marmor, M., et al. Kaposi's sarcoma and pneumocystis pneumonia among heterosexual men. *New York City* and *California, Morbid Mortal Weekly Report* 30:305–308 (1981).
3. Jaffe, H. W.; Feorino, P. M.; Darrow, W. W., et al. Persistent infection with HTLV-III/LAV in apparently healthy homosexual men. *Annals of Internal Medicine* 102:627–628 (1985).
4. Jaffe, H. W.; Darrow, W. W.; Echenberg, D. F., et al. AIDS, AIDS-related conditions, and infection with HTLV-III in a cohort of homosexual men: A 6-year follow-up study. *Annals of Internal Medicine* 103:210–214 (1985).
5. Echenberg, D. F.; Rutherford, G. W.; O'Malley, P., et al. UPDATE—acquired immunodeficiency syndrome in the San Francisco cohort study 1978–1985. *Morbid Mortal Weekly Report* 35 (1985).
6. McKusick, L.; Wiley, J. A.; Coates, T. J., et al. Reported changes in the sexual behavior of men at risk for AIDS, San Francisco 1982–1984: The AIDS behavioral research project. *Public Health Report* 100:622–628 (1985).
7. *San Francisco Epidemiologic Bulletin,* Rectal gonorrhea in San Francisco, Oct. 1984–Sept. 1986. Vol. 2, No. 12 (December 1986).
8. Winkelstein, W.; Lyman, D.; Padian, N., et al. Sexual practices and risk of infection by the human immunodeficiency virus. The San Francisco men's health study. *The Journal of the American Medical Association* 257:321–325 (1987).
9. Jaffe, H. W., et al. AIDS, AIDS-related conditions, and infection with HTLV-III.
10. Echenberg, D. F. A new strategy to prevent the spread of AIDS among heterosexuals. *The Journal of the American Medical Association* 254:2129–2130 (1985).
11. Echenberg, D. F. Education and contact notification for AIDS prevention. *New York State Journal of Medicine* 87:296–298 (1987).
12. Ibid.

CHAPTER 16

The Malignant Metaphor: A Political Thanatology of AIDS

MICHAEL A. SIMPSON

In that country if a man falls into ill health or catches any disorder or fails bodily in any way before he is seventy years old, he is tried before a jury of his countrymen and if convicted is held up to public scorn and sentenced more or less severely as the case may be. But if a man forges a check, or sets his house on fire, or robs with violence from the person, or does any such things as are criminal in our own country, he is either taken to a hospital and most carefully tended at the public expense, or if he is in good circumstances he lets it be known to all his friends that he is suffering from a severe fit of immorality, just as we do when we are ill, and they come and visit them with great solicitude—for bad conduct, though considered no less deplorable than illness with ourselves, and as unquestionably indicating that something is seriously wrong with the individual who misbehaves, is nevertheless held to be the result of either pre-natal or post-natal misfortune.

Samuel Butler was writing in Erewhon,[1] over one hundred years ago, of a mythical land where criminal behavior is seen as sheer bad luck, while illness is wicked and deserves punishment. The tendency to cossett criminals, and to view them as "sick" rather than conceivably ever "bad," has increasingly been built into many legal systems, especially the American. Now the second part of the prophecy is coming true.

AIDS has become the most political of diseases: a contagion within a stigma within a prejudice. Just as OPEC ended the era of cheap energy, AIDS has ended the era of cheap sex.

With this incurably fatal disease doubling its victims every six months, alarmed projections point out that if it continued at such a rate, it would within a decade kill everyone in the USA, and in a further decade would kill everybody on earth ten times over. Since the age of nuclear weaponry and planned megadeath, such projections look less fanciful than they might have, once.

The other image that recurs in recent writing is the medieval Great

Plague. In many historical records, the period of the Black Death, especially from 1348 to 1352, is simply a blank. Monastic chronicles tend to pause at the same point. If any entry appears for the year 1349 it tends to be the same words: *Magna mortalitas*.

Such colorful images are understandably popular in the purple prose[2] that has accumulated in recent years—for sheer vividness they effectively stimulate the sense of *Schadenfreude,* the sheer "isn't it *awful*" titillation enjoyed by those who enjoy the horror of others.

Susan Sontag[3] has written vividly and effectively of the metaphorical uses of illness—and AIDS has the perfect characteristics to make an especially powerful metaphor. It is intractable, incurable, deadly, when Medicine is supposed to be able to cure or control everything. It is insidious, sneaky, implacable, ruthless; the secret agent that lurks within, biding its time before it strikes; a wicked, all-powerful predator.

Such diseases, as Sontag emphasized, "will be felt to be morally, if not literally contagious." How much more powerful the literally contagious disease, so closely identified with morally controversial causes, seen as arising from morally condemned activities, and arising from body parts and actions embarrassing for society to acknowledge! AIDS has followed the course Sontag delineated for such conditions, "awash in significance." The disease becomes identified with "the subjects of deepest dread"—decay, pollution, death, weakness, corruption—and then itself becomes a metaphor. Then it is used as a metaphor, to describe and typify the horror of other matters. "The disease becomes adjectival" in Sontag's fine phrase. "Something is said to be disease-like, meaning that it is disquieting or ugly." So it has been with AIDS —it makes its appearance in bad jokes ("What's the hardest thing about having AIDS? Trying to convince your Mom you're Haitian"); then, literally, in the writing on the wall. Next it is used in popular speech ("Why are you all avoiding him? Anyone would think he had AIDS!"); and finally in literature.

Pollution and stigma are related so much more to some causes of death than to others. AIDS joins a robust heritage of horrors. Tuberculosis used to be thought to be caused by "too much passion, afflicting the reckless and sensual." Others thought that its successor, cancer, was a disease "of insufficient passion," arising in those who are sexually inhibited, repressed, inactive. The tuberculous were sexy, as the Romantics exploited the aesthetics of cruelty, and the beauty of the morbid as Mario Praz[4] so eloquently described. Tuberculosis, however, gave a spiritual, ethereal, redemptive death—even to the morally questionable. Victorian literature is teeming with the tidy, peaceful, good deaths of the tuberculous, especially the pure and pious children. Syphilis, on the other hand, was a morally polluting disease that could give a dirty death even to noblemen.

We have grown unused to the experience of major epidemics not amenable to technological control. In 1983 (oddly ignoring AIDS) William McNeil[5] wrote that a major difference between us and our ancestors, profoundly different from earlier ages, "is the disappearance of epidemic disease as a serious factor in human life. Nowadays, if a few score of people die of an infection, officials declare an epidemic." If the male chauvinist ignores the woman's point of view, here is the voice of the Western chauvinist. Though it accurately reflects a popular point of view in the West, it is inaccurate. In the unheard Third World, what the West would consider epidemics are part of the routine burden of the people. Even in the West, new diseases aren't a novel experience—Burkitt's lymphoma, Legionnaire's disease, Toxic Shock syndrome, Congo Fever, Lassa Fever, O'nyong nyong fever—have all emerged in recent decades. Those most Westernly in their impact, like Toxic Shock syndrome and Legionnaire's disease, were quite rapidly brought to heel. This century has seen a similar scale of afflictions, even in the USA. In 1918, Spanish flu killed 400,000 Americans, with an average age of 33 years. The polio epidemics throughout the fifties struck down large numbers of the young, too, and similarly led to anxious scrutiny of self and loved ones for the stigmata of the peril.

There has often been international political chauvinism in the naming of such afflictions—Spanish Flu, Asian Flu, Mao Flu. The English disease Syphilis has been, in its time, called the French Pox (Morbus gallicus), and the Spanish, Portuguese, Italian, Neapolitan, Burgundian, German, and Polish disease, and so on. AIDS hasn't yet been given a clear nationality. Haiti was damaged by a reputation for harboring it, and African nations have been keen to avoid being blamed for its origins. Black[6] has perceptively pointed out how "Americans take perverse delight in being proud of their flaws; and many in the United States have adopted AIDS as the national disease. If it's a terrible plague, it must be ours." The Russians were reputed to like to think they invented things first (though they have notably failed to lay claim to AIDS); Americans like to think that their version is bigger, better, more awful, more something or other, than anyone else's.

There are marked similarities between the ways in which society responded to previous plagues and pandemics, and the way in which modern society is reacting to AIDS; and much may be learned about potential future social developments by a study of the past. A neglected area of study has been how some epidemics have been clean of metaphorical contamination and moral contagion. Some pandemics—Malaria, Yellow Fever, Diphtheria, Polio—have been relatively unencumbered by such muddling excess baggage. But others have aroused responses familiar to the AIDS crisis.

Plague itself, which became an immortal metaphor for contagion,[7-20] showed three great waves of infection and death—around the sixth century A.D., in the fourteenth century, and in the late nineteenth century through to the Second World War (the latter mainly in China and Asia, though it also became endemic among rodents in the Western USA during that time). The plague's early symptoms—fever, malaise, fatigue, large glands, other infections—were not unlike those of early AIDS, and were similarly perfect material for hypochondriasis and panic—sweats, dry cough, skin blotches—all are easy for almost anyone to perceive and fear that they are infected. Self-scrutiny and monitoring for the fatal stigmata are and were common, just as in the 1950s the child who had "overexerted" himself and had a headache, gave rise to fears of Polio. But Bubonic Plague killed within one to five days, unlike the stealth of AIDS.

The first pandemic, Justinian's plague, led to what contemporary sources and historians including Gibbon considered to be 100 million deaths. Modern historians estimate a lower total—but, still, the death of 20–25% of the population. With accompanying diseases, social disruption, and wars, the population in many parts of Europe fell by 50% between the sixth and eighth century. Arab sources describe major outbreaks in the seventh century. The Moslem religious leaders at the time saw the plague as sent by God as a mercy and martyrdom for the faithful, a direct invitation to Paradise. (For the infidel, it was merely a horrid death with no consequent benefit.)

The second great pandemic, the Black Death, has led to controversy over its origins, similar to that over the roots of AIDS.[21] An early outbreak among Tatars besieging a city illustrated the political uses of infection—they used catapults to lob the corpses of plague victims over the citadel walls, leading to the plague spreading to the Christians within (an early example of the use of germ warfare and of lethal missiles!). Around 25–30% of the population of Europe died; in some cities 50–60%, though the Pope received a curiously exact report that 47,836,486 had died in Europe! There were recurrent outbreaks in succeeding centuries, often (as in the Great Plague of London in 1665) affecting individual cities catastrophically. A Papal Bull of 1348 proclaimed that the Black Death was "the pestilence with which God is afflicting the Christian people" (though medical opinion at the time favored an astrological explanation), a sign of God's displeasure with the extent to which people were ignoring His commandments.

One writer[22] has suggested a connection between social reactions to the Black Death and the emerging hostility towards homosexuality within the Middle Ages. The early history of prejudice is not well documented,[23] but a major historian of this field, Boswell,[24] considers that the homophobic hostility arose well before the fourteenth century plague. Early psychology at times favored the view that suppression of desires was dangerous. Kant, in *Anthropologie* (1798)[25] wrote that "The passions are . . . unfortunate moods that are pregnant with many evils," and that "He who desires but acts not, breeds pestilence." In the late sixteenth and seventeenth centuries it was popularly believed that "the happy man won't get plague." Latterly, it seems, the gay man can.

There certainly was a connection between the Plague and anti-Semitism. As has so routinely been the case in epidemics, "people blamed their enemies for propagating it,"[26] and blamed those marginal in society. Very early in the cycle, lepers had been blamed for poisoning the wells. The lepers blamed the

Jews. From around 1348 in France, a wave of anti-Semitism, with the extermination of Jews in over 350 individual massacres in Europe, spread widely; the waves or ripples of that orgy of anti-Semitism have not yet stilled.

The Black Death led to a useful stress on cleanliness and hygiene, and a social move towards the restraint of passionate excess. There was also a desperate search for wierd and complex treatments. The class bias was opposite to that of AIDS—the well-to-do were less afflicted, being less crowded and more able to avoid infection.

Leprosy was another instructive example.[27] It actually had a relatively low mortality and was not as highly infectious as popularly believed. But its cruel capacity to cripple and disfigure led to a disproportionate degree of horror and social scapegoating.

One explanation for the expulsion by Rameses II of 90,000 Jews from Egypt was that they harbored "a disgraceful disease," probably leprosy. Leprosy, too, was seen as a corruption, the consequence of sin, unclean and wicked. Lepers lost the right to marry, to inherit, to protection, to religious participation. They were segregated to colonies or lazarettos, and had to be marked by special clothing, and to warn others by sounding bells or clacquers. There was the "Leper's Mass"[28] in which the leper was declared "dead among the living," the subject of a form of requiem mass, and symbolically buried alive, while socially dead. Saul Nathaniel Brody wrote eloquently in *The Disease of the Soul*[29] that "The leper was by turns the object of vilification and of sympathy. A physician could assure the leper himself that his disease was a sign that God had chosen to grant his soul salvation, but he might simultaneously include in his diagnosis that his patient was morally corrupt. The Church might similarly decree that leprosy was a gift of God, but its bishops and priests would nonetheless use the disease as a metaphor for spiritual degeneration. The leper was seen as sinful and meritorious, as punished by God and as given special grace by Him.

In fact, the Church seems less simultaneously ambiguous than Brody depicts. The Church appears to have played a leading part in the exclusion and stigmatization of the leper until the Crusades. Once Crusaders began to return with what appeared to be leprosy, contracted in the Holy Land, the Church began to recall Christ's Compassion, and converted leprosy into a holy disease, and the lepers into "Christ's poor." The "Leper's Mass" ceased.

Cholera[30–33] was pandemic in the nineteenth century, and millions died from it. It, too, was seen as the result of the commonness of sin in society. The rich feared the poor, who in turn felt Cholera to be an agent of oppression, even a conspiracy to destroy them. Riots and social turmoil accompanied earlier epidemics, even in Paris, London, and New York.

But before AIDS, no major disease has so richly and obviously linked sex and death and personal behavior as *syphilis* (before antibiotics).[34] Syphilis, too, arrived as a mysterious epidemic, previously unknown, spreading rapidly while physicians could do nothing to cope with it. Wide epidemics were seen

in Europe in 1494–1497. A popular theory claims that the sailors with Co-
lumbus brought it back from the Carribean. Reports of no signs of syphilis in
old world skeletons prior to 1493, but in Amerindian skeletons 500 years
earlier, would support this view. Like AIDS, syphilis may indeed have been a
donation from the Third World to the Old World. As we've seen, the nations
of Europe hastened to name it and blame it on each other. It was, obviously,
seen as a punishment "on the parts of shame" for dissolute excess; and the
Emperor Maximilian I of the Holy Roman Empire declared that it was
Heaven's punishment on blasphemers, reminding us that even where the
sexual connection with the disease was fairly obvious, its moral meanings were
seen as even wider and more serious.

Some writers[35] have claimed that widespread outbreaks of syphilis in Renaissance Europe were an important influence in the rise of Puritanism. The
career of epidemic syphilis, like AIDS, has shown the typical pattern—the
"moral panic," the shift from seeing the unfortunate events as a threat towards stereotyping victims as moral monsters, not worthy of human considerations, leading to an escalation of the perceived threat and to absolutist positions and postures, the popularity of extreme and repressive "solutions," and
the compassionless moral burlesque of cruelty in the name of the compassionate Christ.

Syphilis accumulated a typically heavy accretion of metaphorical
meanings as the grimmest of gifts—yet its uses as metaphor were slightly
limited, as it wasn't seen as especially mysterious. Trotsky spoke of the syphilis
of Stalinism, and there's a grisly harping on syphilis in *Mein Kampf*. The fears
of "bad blood" and contamination have been revived by the risk of AIDS
transmission by blood transfusions. Like the Jews and lepers accused of poisoning the wells, there have been wild rumors of people with AIDS deliberately contaminating blood supplies, and of "call-boys of death" in London,
bitter at their fate, deliberately trying to infect as many people as possible.

The same proud persecuting prejudice has reared up with the AIDS
epidemic as it did among the religious bigots who hunted the lepers, the
plague victims, and the others. A shameful editorial in the *Southern Medical
Journal* wrote with questionable medical ethics of the disease as "a fulfillment
of St. Paul's pronouncement," and of its victims as suffering "the due penalty
of their error." A self-congratulatory fundamentalist has complained of the
spending of tax dollars to "allow these diseased homosexuals to go back to
their perverted practices without any standards of accountability." Popular,
snide jokes are, as ever, highly indicative of the slavering prejudices that un-
derlie them. One refers to the disease as WOGS—the Wrath of God Syndrome. Another says "It affects homosexual men, drug users, Haitians, and
hemophiliacs—thank goodness it hasn't spread to human beings yet." Black[36]
quotes interviews, with one respondent saying "It's having a good effect on
homosexual behaviour, causing them to be—um." (Interviewer: "Less pro-

miscuous?") "No—Dead." And then there are those who say that they hope for a cure—but not too soon.

When one observes the relish with which the pious celebrate the suffering of the impure as divine retribution, one wonders what may be the divine punishment for heartlessness.

It is surely ironical that the perfect Right-Wing virus, with its fortuitous preference for stigmatized victims, made its appearance in the West at a time of Conservative government policies (Reagonomics, Thatcherism). Their support was in part a reaction to the "permissive" trend of the 1960s and 1970s;[37] their policies (slashing health and welfare spending) impaired the ability to respond to the new agent. Society's own "immune system" was impaired. During the search for the causative agent, for instance, biased thinking may have delayed progress. Early victims were identified as homosexuals, rather than according to what their actual behavior was, and a gay drug addict was usually listed as gay rather than as an addict. There is little doubt that had AIDS first become recognized in the USA as a plague exclusively killing Fundamentalist born-again WASPS, the response in terms of research funding and care programs for people with AIDS would have been very different.

Some have emphasized the novelty of the AIDS epidemic in the modern experience (in the West at least) as a cause of the selective death of large numbers of young men without the ideological justifications of war or church. But such a distribution of deaths is not unusual in this century, and Vietnam gave us the experience of a war lacking a consensus of justifying ideology and widely perceived as meaningless. Elliot[38] estimates that there have been some 100 million man-made deaths in the twentieth century. Admittedly, man-made death has tended to replace epidemics as the cause of megadeath. Back in 1972, Elliot commented drily that, "To this day there survives, amongst some of the well fed and cared for, a nostalgia for the slums of disease." That nostalgia has, by now, surely been fully indulged.

AIDS is as yet a long way from matching the carnage of the First World War. In Britain, some 6 million men fought, over half the adult male labor force—and 1 in 8 were killed, a further 1.5 million disabled. The war deaths, too, were concentrated in younger age groups. Of men 20–24 in 1914, 30.58% were dead; of those 13–19, 28.15%.[39] One calculated that if the British Empire's war dead marched four abreast down Whitehall, it would take them three and a half days to pass the Cenotaph that was their memorial. There are relatively few serious studies of the consequences of such patterns of mass death,[40,41] but they are very relevant when we consider the potential impact of AIDS. The war dead included a high proportion of the talented. The birthrate went up immediately afterwards, making good the losses numerically, before returning to its routine rate (an unconscious community healing effect, also seen following disasters like Abervan); but of course the qualitative loss was not so promptly recoverable. Will the AIDS losses prompt some similar increase in the otherwise wide trend towards lower birthrates in the West?

There is also a potential not only, as has already been demonstrated,[42,43] for a change in sexual behavior towards monogamy and more traditional forms of expression, but also towards less loving behaviors, if the projected high death rates occur and last. The historical experience has been that where mortality is high, there is reduced emotional involvement. As Aries said[44] in his study of the history of childhood, "People could not allow themselves to become too attached to something that was regarded as a probable loss." Stone, in a more formal study of the family, sex, and marriage in England 1500–1800[45] noted that "It is fairly clear that the reactive lack of concern for small infants was closely tied to their poor expectation of survival, and that there is on the average a rough secular correlation between high mortality and low gradient affect." Macfarlane[46] has suggested further ways to study this effect.

The First World War was followed, as AIDS was preceded, by a wave of interest in Spiritualism, with great popularity of books like *Life Beyond Death With Evidence*, just like the *Life After Life/Before Life/Between Lives* genre of the 1970s and 1980s which followed the Vietnam experience. The wide range of modes of public acknowledgment of the reality of the deaths and of their scale, was matched by private denial. Before World War I, spiritualism was diffuse and ineffectual. But influential figures like Sir Arthur Conan Doyle and the scientist Sir Oliver Lodge (both of whom had lost sons in the war) encouraged intense "scientific" interest (which was not scientific at all) in parapsychology.

There are other consequences of national consciousness of large-scale losses. After the First World War, detective novels became far more violent, bloody, and murderous—as did movies after Vietnam. Indeed, the extent of such effects of the AIDS pandemic may be less perceptible only because we are still seeing similar effects from Vietnam.

The constant relationship of death and sex shows in other ways, too. It has been argued that the more active sexual freedom of the 1920s was a response to the death of the earlier generation, and part of the drive behind the sexual hedonism of the 1960s to the 1980s may have had similar roots. The "Make Love, Not War" slogan of the Sixties has almost, in the Conservative Eighties, become "Make War, Not Love."

The relationship is an ancient one[47]—that soldiers, the more they feel close to the threat of death, feel driven into sexual activity. Julius Caesar flogged soldiers with symptoms of gonorrhea; Richard III had soldiers with "pox" hung. Promiscuous French soldiers under Louis XIII in Italy in the fifteenth century busily spread the new horror—the French evil, *il morbo Gallico*—syphilis. Wars have always needed busy anti-VD campaigns, stressing the mortal danger of sex. A notable British wartime poster showed a skull wearing a woman's exotic hat and orchid, saying "Coming *my* way?" and adding "The 'easy' girlfriend spreads Syphilis and Gonorrhea which, unless properly treated, may result in blindness, insanity, paralysis, premature death."

Whatever the roots of the Sexy Sixties and Seventies, the Anxious Eighties might engender in some quarters the opposite of the safe monogamy advised just *because* of the very real risk of death. Costello[47] cites a G.I. saying "the typical soldier gives himself up for dead before he ever sees combat . . . so every woman might be his last . . . imagine what its like to make love while assuming that tomorrow you'll be dead." He also quotes a celebrated Madam during the First World War as saying "I've noticed it before, the way the idea of war and dying makes a man raunchy, and wanting to have it as much as he could. It wasn't really pleasure at times, but a kind of nervous breakdown that could only be treated with a girl and a set-to."

The homosexualization of AIDS, and its stigmatization has had an obvious impact in slowing the extent and efficacy of our response to it. The happenchance that it first became noticeable among homosexuals led to an excessive focus on the search for uniquely homosexual causes for it, including what Jacques Leibowitch[48] called the "Sodom and Gonococcal" theory of causation. The overlapping complexities have been ignored: homosexuals who are addicts; the high incidence of prostitution and unsafe sex in addicts; the high incidence of addiction in prostitutes.

Spending on research was niggardly. The Centers for Disease Control (CDC) budget for AIDS in 1982 was $2 million. Yet in 1976, for the ludicrous "Swine Fever" fiasco, $135 million was hurriedly spent in order to fail to prevent a nonexistent epidemic of a very minor disease with a campaign which killed well people! But then Swine Fever was expected to have much more decent and vote-earning victims. The journal *Science*[49] complained petulantly of an "unprecedented spending spree" on AIDS research, due to the power of the U.S. gay community—contriving to be inaccurate, prejudiced, and unscientific, all at once.

As in previous major epidemics, bizarre conspiracy and "plot" theories have arisen, blaming AIDS on a chemical agent sprinkled on bathhouse floors, or added to KY jelly; or to a germ warfare agent that may have gone astray (or may even have achieved its intended purpose). Though obviously farfetched, one doesn't have to travel so far to farfetch something these days. We do now know that for two decades, the U.S. Army did explore the practicality of germ warfare by releasing what they thought to be harmless germs in U.S. cities, airports, and subways.[50]

As with other sexually related studies, there have at times been hints almost of jealousy and awe, as inhibited scientists and epidemiologists encountered the promiscuous and active. The virgin scientist encountering a group with a median of 1160 different sexual partners may have difficulty in comprehending the alternative lifestyle ("When do they have time to get sick?" asked an epidemiologist).

In Russia and Eastern Europe, where AIDS is considered a symptom of Western decay, there has been similar reluctance to admit to the potential extent of the problem. In December 1985, Prof. Victor Zhdanov in Soviet-skaya Kultura admitted to ten cases in the Soviet Union, and an official estimate of 60 cases by the first quarter of 1986 is quested. Sixty cases out of some 400 million people may represent an underestimate. Unofficial reports of AIDS deaths in Czechoslovakia have appeared, and in Hungary, antibody screening of blood donors, homosexuals, and drug addicts seems to have been in operation since January 1986. Again, an isomeric politicization of AIDS, identifying it with foreign decadence, may hamper the response to a biological Chernobyl.

The promiscuous were already well familiar with sexually transmitted diseases and infections—proctitis, urethritis, amoebae, hepatitis, shigella, worms, gonorrhea, syphilis, herpes, even lymphogranuloma venereum were accepted risks. But "For those doing a sexual high-wire act, medicine was a safety-net."[51] Everything was felt to be already or imminently curable. Until AIDS, which rekindled the deadly risk of sex that had haunted them in previous centuries. The age of safe danger had passed.

I have written elsewhere in early work[52,53] towards a feminist thanatology, of the nearly universal and persistent relationship between women, sex, and danger. Over the ages, there was a persistently prejudicial emphasis on Woman as the historic cause of misfortune and mortality, the danger being ascribed to her insatiable, irresistible, but deadly sexuality and guile. Belief in the evil of woman was sustaining to the development of an all-male Establishment, and the long litany of lethal ladies popularly reinforced the message—Eve, Pandora, Salome, Jezebel, Lucrezia Borgia, Lilith, Kali, Astarte, Medea, Messalina, Circe, Delilah, and other grisly girls.

The association between sexual pleasure and danger is new to men (except for the Mors Syphilitica which was always blamed on the women); similarly new is the association between male sexuality and danger to men. Women[54] have long been subject to dangerous sex—the risks of pregnancy, childbirth, abortion, miscarriage, and the puerperium have limited woman's potential across the centuries. Heterosexual AIDS, the form which dominates the picture in Africa, may radically affect attitudes. Gay sex has been more experienced at encompassing dangers, with the risks of violence, police intervention, blackmail, and betrayal having been especially real in earlier decades. As there was some diminution in those risks, almost as if there had been some habituation to the added spice of danger and related condiments, there seems to have been a move towards higher risk sexual forms—promiscuity, physically hazardous acts, fantasized, simulated, or real sadomasochism. The risky and the risqué became blurred.

This sex/death margin remains barely explored. The Victorians, despite public ostentation in the matter of death and grief, had not, so the quieter and more intimate documents of history reveal, successfully come to terms with these eternals in their private lives. Similarly[55,56] they showed public prudishness and private prurience. But the popular view has persisted, as Cannadine has expressed it[57] of the "beguiling and nostalgic progression from obsessive death and forbidden sex in the nineteenth century, to obsessive sex and forbidden death in the twentieth." And just when we contrived in Western society to frankly rediscover death while still freely dealing with sex, what arrives? Lethal sex and sexual death.

The forbidden and dangerous can have a powerful appeal, as Nietzsche noted in the Wanderer and His Shadow[58]: "A prohibition, the reason for which we don't understand or admit, is almost a command not only for the stubborn but also for those who thirst for knowledge: we risk an experiment to find out *why* the prohibition was pronounced." The complex lifestyles of gay sex and of the intravenous drug addict have elaborately evolved, and maybe in some forms they have done so not despite the dangers, but in part because of the danger.

Behaviors that were proscribed and forbidden became politicized as acts of defiance against a resented repression. To some, it seemed important not just to have won the right to behave as one wished, but to exercise that right as frequently as possible, as if the more it was exercised the more free one was. In the original sense *Carnivals* were occasions to celebrate the temporary flesh while it still exists; *carne vale*, "farwell, meat." They could represent, as Black[59] has said, not just the orgy preceding the asceticism of Lent, but "Saturnalia before the endless abstinence of death."

Intravenous addicts have contrived to ignore their high-risk profession as effectively as men who work high on steel scaffolding or high-risk hobbyists like free-fall parachutists. The risk may have become not a barrier to overcome before deciding to take part, but a primary reason for doing so. Gay sex may come to incorporate premature death within the lifestyle, as black ghetto life has led to—for young black males in America, murder or drug overdose have been leading causes of death for some time. Gay culture has long included a powerful interest in eroticism and death—as seen in the works of Thomas Mann, Genet, Mishima, and Fassbinder.

Black[59] quotes a report that some sadomasochists are already eroticizing AIDS, viewing it as "the ultimate S-M trip: the thought that one might be pumping one's 'lovers' full of death . . . is considered 'hot.' " The same respondent claims that medical "scenes" during sex play have increased. So an alternative to abstinence or monogamy for some might become the deliberate seeking of the danger, gaining thrills by copulating on the brink of eternity. Apocalypse Wow!

Clearly, the epidemic will give life to both amateur and professional prejudices. It fits so well with the popular contagion theory of homosexuality and of drug abuse—the idea that social "deviants" somehow "recruit" or infect otherwise straight people, as if homosexuality or addiction were themselves viruses which could be "caught" (premises which the pro-censorship lobby would seem to inhabit).

Just as one saw in the responses to previous plagues and epidemics, there are very serious threats to liberty. In various countries there have been instances of great risk to civil liberties: a man refused treatment unless he listed the people with whom he'd had sex; refusals to serve on a jury because the defendant had AIDS; police objecting to give breathalyser tests; patients being neglected in hospitals. There have been proposals to restrict international travel; to ban people with AIDS from airline flights; to forcibly administer tests for AIDS; enforced isolation of possible carriers; compulsory hospitalization. There's a report[60] that in New South Wales, Australia, it has been made a criminal offense "to knowingly infect someone with HIV."

As Black has said, perceptively,[61] "Draconian laws to control the spread of AIDS, which violate basic civil rights, may be more dangerous to the community than the disease itself." AIDS is being used by many as an excuse for a sexual counterrevolution, to discard not just unsafe behaviors, but as many as possible of the other changes wrought in the sixties (and somewhat overwrought in the seventies). Black sees the issue very clearly. "How one reacts to AIDS is a measure of what one believes about sexual pluralism—and, even more importantly, what one believes about the individual's freedom in all ways, not just sexual, to be different. AIDS tests how a society balances the rights of the few with the good of the many."

There are many similar issues bound up in these affairs. Black is brilliantly incisive in analyzing the Western scene in a rather Americo-centric way. In Africa, AIDS is not a minority problem, not a disease of the "others," of those already marked out for misfortune—it afflicts the majority.

Another issue, intertwined, is that of self-inflicted disease. Some argue that public monies should not be spent on people with AIDS, because "they brought it on themselves," because it is the direct result of something they chose to do, of their own free will. The issue of "free will" in relation to some of the behaviors involved is debatable. But there are entire specialties like Sports Medicine, with expensive facilities, devoted entirely to self-inflicted disease and self-inflicted injury. There has not been any serious protest against the gigantic cost to society of the disease caused by cigarette and tobacco addiction, and little concern with the high costs of alcoholism and recreational drug abuse.

Indeed, there has been a long tradition of allowing people to die in pursuit of fun. America even has a constitutional devotion to protecting life, liberty, and the pursuit of happiness—not the limitation of risk. And *their* pursuit of happiness, even if in ways that wouldn't make me happy, does not threaten my life or liberty. Unless I have sex with them or exchange blood with them, people with AIDS don't endanger me—unlike the smoker who pollutes my lungs and specifically damages my health, or the drunken driver who kills others. Analogous to the principle of informed consent to treatment or research, it would be preferable that people could make informed dissent, to make a behavioral choice fully informed as to the risks (especially when the benefit may be immediately obvious, and the risks late and hidden).

It is odd that societies that encourage the sale and promotion of death on the installment plan in cigarettes and alcohol, and prefer the sale of cars that operate most efficiently at illegal and dangerous speeds, should be so selectively interested in controlling other people's sexuality, whether or not it may limit a risk to themselves or others. Smokers know exactly what risk they are taking; people with AIDS are generally suffering the results of a risk undertaken when no one knew that the risk existed.

A Director of the National Institute for Human Sexuality in South Africa, Dr. L. I. Robertson, has reported an increasing number of inappropriate referrals from psychologists and physicians suggesting aversion therapy to "convert" homosexuals to heterosexuals, to "save them" from the risk of AIDS. To propose that people should fundamentally alter their sexual behavior is a far more major undertaking than giving up smoking or drinking. If one doubts that, it may be a homophobe response, assuming that an "abnormal" sexual identity is easy to give up, especially if its good for one to do so. If a heterosexual finds (as many in Africa have) that this form of sex life is dangerous, how quickly and easily could they adapt to life as a homosexual? or a celibate? or switch to zoophilia? When syphilis made heterosexuality dangerous, very few people gave it up.

In fact, a surprising degree of adaptation seems to be taking place, with dramatic changes in sexual behavior recorded. As early as 1983 there were reports of a sharp decline in the number of partners and in the incidence of high-risk activities, and in the incidence of VD in various cities. In the 1960s a humorous magazine set a competition to define a new erogenous zone—and there wasn't a single response. Yet recently there have been trends towards nongenital stimulation, and an eroticization of nipples, massage, and condoms. Masturbation is showing a rising popularity and is less abused. The large U.S. sex industry seems to have shown some responsibility towards encouraging safer practices—certainly it has shown far more social responsibility than the tobacco industry has ever shown, anywhere.

Quite apart from civil liberties issues, there is the question of whether drastic legal responses actually help to control disease. Throughout history, governments have tended to fight epidemics with legislation and information.[62] Quarantine tactics across Europe did help to control the bubonic plague, from Medieval times. As recently as the turn of the century in San Francisco, a detention center was set up for plague victims, and there was talk of isolating or even burning Chinatown.[63] During the Cholera pandemics of the nineteenth century, emergency laws allowed for the compulsory isolation of victims and controlled burials, despite protests about the erosion of personal liberty. Compulsory admission to hospitals was enacted for infectious diseases. Some of the laws are still unrepealed in many states.

The Contagious Diseases Acts in mid-Victorian Britain (trying to avoid a defeat of the British Army by VD) allowed the authorities to detain any woman suspected of prostitution, and allowed compulsory medical examination and enforced treatment. But apart from their obvious appeal to those who like to feel that complex social problems can be forcibly solved, such measures have not been effective. It perverts the doctor-patient relationship when doctors must become informers and enforcers. It drove those most in need of help (for everyone's benefit) to avoid it rather than seek it. The Contagious Diseases Acts were a failure, and had to be repealed.[64] As Porter[65] has written in a wise summary of the experience of medical history, "If we begin to treat victims like criminals we alienate those whose co-operation is most needed and encourage them to behave like criminals; not least, we risk turning doctors into gaolers."

There is even room for an elegantly unpleasant interplay between the stress of a population being discriminated against, and the likelihood of contracting an infection and of succumbing to it. As I have shown in my review of behavioral microbiology[66] stress, especially if poorly coped with, can lead to changes in immunity, increased vulnerability to infection, and a potentially worse outcome of the disease. These effects are clearly demonstrated chemically and at a cellular level. It is still not clear why some people exposed to the virus develop an infection and others do not; or why only some of those infected by the HTLV-III virus develop AIDS. It is expected that numerous co-factors will be identified as contributing to the development of AIDS infection. Early studies of people with AIDS are beginning to suggest that they may indeed have suffered particularly stressful life events in the year before diagnosis and may express more guilt and unease about their sexual behavior (though it is far from clear that the latter is not an effect of the diagnosis, rather than its cause).

Clearly AIDS is likely to change the way we look at life. A generation or two had the easy illusion of safe sex. The general impression was that there were drugs to cure syphilis and gonorrhea, and Herpes didn't kill; the Pill seemed to be a safe way to avoid pregnancy. Drugs could be thought of as brave ways to explore one's inner self, and their risks due only to bad luck or carelessness. Though each of these beliefs were only partly true and often dangerously untrue, the drive towards finding completion in some substance or somebody external to oneself, was powerful. There was something as heady as any drug in the sharing of sex; something sexual in the insertion of shared needles. But the searches for completion now, more clearly than ever, can lead to dissolution and disaster instead.

As Porter has said:[67] "In contrast to smallpox, it takes two consenting partners to spread AIDS. The days of sex without responsibility are over. Responsible sex infringes no person's liberty. It is our only practical option."

REFERENCES

1. Butler, S. *Erewhon.* Harmondsworth: Penguin, 1970.
2. Britton, A. AIDS—Apocalyptic metaphor. *New Statesman*, March 15, 1985.
3. Sontag, S. *Illness as Metaphor.* New York: Farrar, Straus & Giroux, 1978.
4. Praz, M. *The Romantic Agony.* 2d ed. New York: Oxford University Press, 1951.

5. McNeil, W. *The Plague of Plagues.* The New York Review of Books, July 21, 1983.
6. Black, D. *The Plague Years: A Chronicle of AIDS, the Epidemic of Our Times.* London: Pan Books, 1986.
7. Webster, C., Ed. *Health, Medicine & Mortality in the Sixteenth Century.* Cambridge: Cambridge University Press, 1979.
8. Slack, P. Mortality Crises and Epidemic Disease in England, 1485–1610. In *Health, Medicine & Mortality in the Sixteenth Century,* edited by C. Webster. Cambridge: Cambridge University Press, 1979.
9. Gottfried, R. S. *Epidemic Disease in Fifteenth Century England: The Medical Response and the Demographic Consequences.* Rutgers, NJ: Rutgers University Press, 1978.
10. Rosebury, T. *Microbes and Morals.* New York: Viking, 1971.
11. Slack, P. *The Impact of Plague in Tudor and Stuart England.* London: Routledge & Kegan Paul, 1985.
12. Alexander, J. T. *The Bubonic Plague in Early Modern Russia: Public Health and Urban Disaster.* Baltimore: Johns Hopkins University Press, 1980.
13. Dols, M. W. *The Black Death in the Middle East.* Princeton, NJ: Princeton University Press, 1976.
14. Gottfried, R. S. *The Black Death: Natural and Human Disaster in Medieval Europe.* New York: Free Press, 1983.
15. Pollitzer, R. *Plague.* Geneva: World Health Organization, 1984.
16. Ziegler, P. *The Black Death.* New York: Harper & Row, 1971.
17. Williman, D., Ed. *The Black Death: The Impact of the Fourteenth-Century Plague.* New York: Medieval & Renaissance, 1982.
18. Mullett, C. F. *The Bubonic Plague and England: An Essay in the History of Preventive Medicine.* Philadelphia: Porcupine Press, 1977.
19. Dyer, A. D. The influence of the bubonic plague in England. *Journal of the History of Medicine and Allied Sciences* July 1978, 308–376.
20. Schrewsbury, J. F. D. *A History of Bubonic Plague in the British Isles.* Cambridge: Cambridge University Press, 1971.
21. Norriss, J. East or West? The Geographic origin of the Black Death. *Bulletin of the History of Medicine* 51:1 (1977).
22. Lancaster, R. What AIDS is doing to us. Christopher Street (New York), 1983, no. 75.
23. Gerard, K., and Hekina G., eds. *The Pursuit of Sodomy in Early Modern Europe: Male Homosexuality from the Renaissance through the Enlightenment.* New York: Haworth Press, 1986.
24. Boswell, J. *Christianity, Social Intolerance and Homosexuality.* Chicago: University of Chicago Press, 1980.
25. Kant, I. *Anthropolgie.* In *Kant Werke: Akademie Textausgabe Preussiche Akademie der Wissenschaft.* Hawthorne, NY: De Gruyter, 1986.
26. McGrew, R. E. *Encyclopedia of Medical History.* London: Macmillan Press, 1985.
27. Dols, M. W. Leprosy in Medieval Arabic medicine. *Journal of the History of Medicine and Allied Sciences* 34:314–333 (July 1979).
28. Simpson, M. A. Thanatology, Death & the Middle Ages. Keynote address, Durban Conference, Medieval Society of South Africa, July 7, 1986.
29. Brody, S. N. *The Disease of the Soul.* Ithaca, NY: Barker, 1974.
30. McGrew, R. E. *Russia and the Cholera, 1823–1832.* Madison, WI: University of Wisconsin Press, 1965.
31. Pollitzer, R. *Cholera.* Geneva: World Health Organization, 1959.
32. Morris, R. J. *Cholera: Eighteen Thirty-Seven.* New York: Holmes & Meier, 1976.
33. Delaporte, F. *Disease and Civilization: The Cholera in Paris, 1832.* Cambridge, MA: MIT Press, 1986.
34. Crosby, A. W. *The Columbian Exchange. Biological and Cultural Consequences of 1492.* Westport, CT: Greenwood Press, 1972.
35. Lancaster, R. *What AIDS Is Doing to Us.*

36. Black, D. *The Plague Years.*
37. Moorcock, M. *The Retreat from Liberty: The Erosion of Democracy in Today's Britain.* London: Zomba Books, 1983.
38. Elliot, G. *The Twentieth-Century Book of the Dead.* London: Allen Lane, 1972.
39. Winter J. M. Some aspects of the demographic consequences of the First World War in Britain. *Population Studies* XXX:541 (1976).
40. Winter, J. M. Britain's 'Lost Generation' of the First World War. *Population Studies* XXXI:450 (1977).
41. Cannadine, D. "War and Death, Grief and Mourning in Modern Britain." In Whaley, J. (Ed.) *Mirrors of Mortality: Studies in the Social History of Death,* edited by J. Whaley. London: Europa Publications, 1981.
42. Burton, S. W.; Burn, S. B.; Harvey, D. et al. AIDS information in Scotland. *Lancet* 2:1040–1041 (1986).
43. Judson, F. N. Fear of AIDS and gonorrhoea rates in homosexual men. *Lancet* (1983).
44. Aries, P. *Centuries of Childhood.* New York: A. A. Knopf, 1962.
45. Stone, L. *The Family, Sex and Marriage in England, 1500–1800.* London: Weidenfeld & Nicholson, 1977.
46. Macfarlane A. "Death and the Demographic Transition: A note on English Evidence on Death, 1500–1750." In *Mortality and Immortality: The Anthropology and Archaeology of Death,* edited by S. C. Humphreys and H. King. New York: Academic Press, 1981.
47. Costello, J. *Love, Sex and War, 1939–1945.* London: Pan Books, 1986.
48. Leibowitch, J. *Un Virus Efrange Venu Diailleurs.* Paris: Grasset, 1983.
49. Kolata, G. Congress, NIH open coffers for AIDS. *Science* July 29, 1983, 436.
50. *Washington Monthly,* July-August 1985. Cited by Black, D. *The Plague Years.* London: Pan Books, 1986, pp. 174–175.
51. Altman, D. *AIDS and the New Puritanism.* London: Pluto Press, 1986; Altman, D. *AIDS in the Mind of America.* New York: Anchor Press/Doubleday, 1986.
52. Simpson, M. A. Death and Ideology: Political Thanatology and the "Femme Fatale" Syndrome. Monograph, Seminar in Contemporary Cultural Studies, 6-CCSU, University of Natal, Durban, South Africa, October 1985. (ISBN 0-86980-474-X).
53. Simpson, M. A. *Femme Fatale.* London: Quartet. 1988, in press.
54. Shotter, E. *A History of Women's Bodies.* London: Allen Lane, 1983.
55. Harrison, B. Understanding the Victorians. *Victorian Studies* X:239–262 (1966–1967).
56. Pearsall, R. *The Worm in the Bud: The World of Victorian Sexuality.* London: Penguin, 1983.
57. Cannadine, D. War and death, grief and mourning in modern Britain.
58. Nietzsche, F. "The Wanderer and His Shadow." In *Complete Works,* by F. Nietzsche. New York: Gordon Press, 1974.
59. Blade, D. *The Plague Years.*
60. Porter, R. History says no to the policeman's response to AIDS. *British Medical Journal* 293:1589–1590 (1986).
61. Blade, D. *The Plague Years.*
62. Porter, R. History says no to the policeman's response to AIDS.
63. Trauner, J. The Chinese as medical scapegoats in San Francisco, 1870–1905. *California History,* Spring, 1972.
64. McHugh, P. *Prostitution and Victorian Social Reform.* London: CROOM-HELM, 1980.
65. Porter, R. History says no to the policeman's response to AIDS.
66. Simpson, M. A. Stress and Infection—Towards a Behaviorial Microbiology. *Infection Control,* August 1986, pp. 8–9.
67. Porter, R. History says no to the policeman's response to AIDS.

CHAPTER 17

Impact of the AIDS Epidemic on the Gay Political Agenda

JIM FOSTER

Within the gay community the AIDS epidemic is pervasive. It is impossible to avoid it. You cannot go to any gay community meeting without hearing of yet another death or another friend's recent diagnosis.

Five years or ten years ago, no one would have believed that we would attend so many funerals. No one believed that we would worry over every skin blemish, every cough, every headache. No one believed that the simple phrase, "How ya doing" would take on a new and much deeper meaning or that so many of us would be devoting our spare hours to caring for those unfortunate enough to be stricken with the disease.

Five years ago life was wonderful. Life was full of gay bars and bathhouses. Life was a disco party full of beautiful men, all of whom seemed available, if not tonight then tomorrow. Life was psychedelics and other recreational drugs and everyone believed in Peter Pan: I'll never get old. I'll never get sick. I'll never die. The party will last forever.

No matter where you went—San Francisco, New York, Los Angeles, Houston—the party was in full swing and not just in those cities which were known as "gay meccas," but in Atlanta, Philadelphia, Boston, Chicago, Phoenix, Denver, Charleston, Seattle. You could even find a party in Reno, Lubbock, Sioux Falls, or Dubuque, if you knew where to go or whom to ask.

After all, why shouldn't there be a party? Hadn't the sexual revolution of the sixties and seventies freed everyone from the old constraints? In fact, it was healthy to throw your inhibitions away and experiment with new expressions and new people—lots of new expressions and lots of new people. There were, of course, a few bothersome matters that needed to be dealt with such as Anita Bryant's campaign in Florida to overturn the gay rights ordinance and the Brigg's Initiative in California which would have prohibited gay people from teaching in the schools. The fundamentalists were organizing and using the burgeoning gay rights movement as a focal point; Ronald Reagan's election to the presidency indicated an end to political gains being made at the federal level. Some of us had heard about a strange form of cancer and an unusual pneumonia that seemed to affect only gay men, but no one we knew had it. These were no more than sprinkles on the parade.

Larry Bush, a gay journalist and legislative aide suggests that the role model for gay people prior to the epidemic was the medieval troubadour. An itinerant artist in "glad rags" of lace and codpiece, spontaneous, full of life, and unfettered by convention. The troubadour represented a spirit of individuality and lived in a free zone outside everyday life. His was an individual, not a collective mind-set. There was nothing of yesterday about him. He was not a part of the continuum of history. Indeed, history began the day he was born and everyday he was born anew. His was not a case of "Today being the first day of the rest of your life." Today was the only day of his life. Although the troubadour might recognize fellow gay travelers on the road, he recognized them with a wink and a nod as kindred spirits. He was out there doing his own thing and expected everyone else to be doing theirs.

The dynamic of the gay rights political movement reflected the troubadour as a role model, both in its activity and philosophy. The dynamic, simply stated, was: get government off our backs and let us be ourselves.

The decade of the seventies created dramatic improvements in the lives of gay people whether they were self-acknowledged or not. The Stonewall Riot of 1969 changed our lives forever. Gay people had challenged the ability of the police (as guardians of the public morality) to regulate our existence, and what's more, gay people had won. From that moment on, arrests for being gay or being seen in a gay establishment would be fought in court. There was renewed interest in challenging state laws that regulated consensual sexual behavior and in California and several other states those laws were overturned. Cities across the country passed nondiscrimination ordinances. Gay business people successfully challenged city codes and ordinances which had been used in the past to deny them opportunity. Gay people ran for public office and sometimes won. Other gay people were appointed to positions on city commissions and boards. New organizations of gay people sprang up like mushrooms after a rain and although some of them were formed for specific political purposes, such as the Alice B. Toklas Memorial Democratic Club, many more were formed around specific, mutual interests. Groups of lawyers, doctors, insurance agents, social workers, baseball players, bowlers, stamp collectors, Mormons, and Roman Catholics were organized.

In San Francisco, Jon Sims noticed that a Gay Freedom Day Parade had no music. He put up hand-lettered posters on telephone poles in the Castro, Polk, and Folsom Street areas of San Francisco asking people who had experience in marching bands to call him. Within a week he had over 800 phone calls and out of these responses he formed the San Francisco Gay Freedom Day Marching Band, Tap Troupe, and Twirling Corps. Soon there were marching bands in a dozen other cities. The bands were quickly followed by choruses of lesbians and gay men. In short, gay people were discovering themselves and each other and the more discovery that took place, the larger and more diverse the organizations became. Self-help groups were formed to assist gay alcoholics and drug abusers. The Metropolitan Community Church, a Christian body with a special outreach to gay people, became international. The general media began treating gay issues seriously and gay media developed in nearly every major city in America. In San Francisco a group of lesbians in business formed a professional organization which now numbers over a 1000 members. Medical clinics were created and staffed by gay medical professionals for gay men and women. Parades to celebrate the victory at Stonewall were held annually in major cities across America. The San Francisco parade attracts a quarter of a million people.

All of this activity had the effect of creating the beginnings of a sense of social community; in addition it brought gay people together as gay people within the larger community. It wasn't possible for a gay politician, for instance, to function alone. He or she had to interact with politicians as a group. A gay lawyer had to interact with the rest of the legal profession and a gay doctor had to deal with the California Medical Association or the American Medical Association. In those places where gay people had organized there was an increasing amount of interaction with other communities. This, in turn, led to putting a human face on homosexuality. Friendships and respect developed, myths and stereotypes were destroyed.

If I were asked the day the party stopped for me, I would have to respond that it was the day that Larry Kramer's open letter to the gay community appeared in *The New York Native* and was later reprinted in many gay newspapers across the country. I suspect it was the day the party stopped for a lot of others as well.

Kramer, who later wrote *The Normal Heart,* one of the first plays to deal with AIDS and the political and social implications of the epidemic, wrote a scathing denunciation of the gay community's denial of a growing epidemic and the indifference of not only the media and the political establishment, but of gay leaders themselves to what was clearly the most dangerous situation we had ever faced. The letter, entitled "1,112 and Counting,"[1] referred to the number of AIDS cases and deaths at that time. Kramer's letter was a clarion call to action and a prophesy of the future. His letter and the production of *The Normal Heart* became the manifesto of a new, gay political dynamic. In the process, a new role model was created—the historical Jew of the holocaust. I do not use the term "holocaust" to mean a specific, historic event which took place in Western Europe in the 1930s and 1940s. I mean it to encompass the Jewish experience.

The new role model is diametrically opposed to the old. If the troubadour sees himself as fundamentally individualistic, the Jew sees himself as a part of the collective. He is a link in a chain from the past which runs through him to the future. He only survives if the community survives. If any part of the organism survives, they all survive. The historical Jew of the holocaust believes that Christian tolerance has before and will again turn against him. The only way to survive in a seemingly hostile world is by adopting the ultimate defensive posture—investing in each other.

In 1982 the Gay Men's Health Crisis published a declaration for survival in *The New York Native*.[2] The advertisement bluntly stated that a crisis existed in the health of gay men and no one would help us except ourselves. We could expect nothing but indifference from the media, the political establishment, and the medical profession. Even the institutions developed in our own community were not prepared or equipped to deal with AIDS. We could expect nothing for education, or research, or the care and treatment of those already afflicted. Therefore, we needed to create a new structure and a new ethic. This was to be our one and only task. The declaration was in effect both an appeal for survival and the method by which it was to be achieved. Apolitical gay people must come together to defend themselves. We must invest in each other because there was no one but ourselves who would do this for us.

In a scene from *The Normal Heart*, Dr. Emma Brookner says to Ned Weeks, a thinly disguised Larry Kramer,

> Health is a political issue. Everyone's entitled to good medical care. If you're not getting it, you've got to fight for it. Do you know that this is the only country in the industrialized world besides South Africa that doesn't guarantee health care for everyone? One of my staff told me that you were well known in the gay world and not afraid to say what you think. Is that true? I can't find any gay leaders. I tried calling several gay organizations. No one ever calls me back. Is anyone out there?"

To which Ned Weeks responds,

> There aren't any organizations strong enough to be useful, no. Dr. Brookner, no one with a brain gets involved in gay politics. It's filled with the great unwashed radicals of any counterculture. That's why there aren't any leaders the majority will follow.[3]

The pre-epidemic troubadour was able to avoid involvement in the political agenda of the gay rights movement if he so chose—and many did choose noninvolvement. In fact, it is safe to say that the vast majority of gay people had either a peripheral interest in or completely ignored the political agenda. For instance, during the Dade County, Florida campaign to overturn the local gay rights ordinance, many gay people voted against the ordinance which would have granted them some measure of protection. They felt that the people pressing the issue were "rocking the boat." They agreed with the worst arguments of Anita Bryant that somehow or other the ordinance would allow men in dresses to teach in the public schools. They were resentful that the little secret of their homosexuality might be exposed if there was too much political freedom before there was sufficient social acceptance. Differences of opinion existed about exactly how much freedom was desirable. Many felt that extending rights to those who wore drag or leather was going too far and were uncomfortable being grouped with what the media, in its search for the most extreme and bizarre examples of behavior, characterized as "gay."

Most homosexuals in America today are hidden or "closeted" and until the epidemic, most were able to succeed in their double life. Many are married with families and live in the suburbs of America. Their only communication with the organized gay community is an occasional night out at a bathhouse or a drink at a gay bar after work. According to a recent and unpublished study, 80% of wives of bisexual men in their sample were ignorant of their husband's gay activity.

Much of this bears some resemblance to the experience of the immigrant Jew in this country. There was, for instance, much discrimination among the various groups of Jews themselves. French and German Jews were embarrassed by what they viewed as the excesses of Hasidic Jews from Poland and Russia. Wealthy and middle-class Jews looked askance at the poverty of the Lower East Side in New York and did not wish to be identified with it. Many submerged themselves in the new culture, denied their heritage, and changed their names and religion. Like the early gay rights organizations, Jewish institutions fought to convince Jews to take pride in being Jewish. They ought not hide, change their names, nor their religion.

That their efforts were successful is proven by the phenomenal strength of Jewish benevolent institutions and their political ability to protect the state of Israel as the symbol of their community. The Holocaust in Western Europe during the 1930s and 1940s brought the Jewish people back to the perspective of the historical holocaust and the investment in each other as the ultimate defensive posture. Just as Hitler's S.S. and Gestapo did not differentiate among Jews, the HIV virus does not differentiate among gay men. The S.S. did not care whether you were a French Jew or a Polish Jew. They did not care whether you were a rich merchant or a poor peasant nor did they care if you were an Orthodox, Conservative, or Reform Jew. Indeed, they did not care whether you were a practicing Jew or a Lutheran or Roman Catholic convert.

The HIV virus doesn't discriminate either. It doesn't care whether you wear drag or leather or a three-piece suit. It doesn't care whether you are a famous actor or entertainer or a bartender or department store clerk. It doesn't care whether you live in a gay ghetto or with your wife and family in the suburbs. In short, gay men cannot hide anymore than could the Jews of Europe. They are no longer protected by their wealth, position, or their anonymity. This is having a profound effect on the evolving gay political agenda.

In addition to the growing awareness that the existing gay institutions are not equipped to seek the resources necessary to fund the needs of AIDS patients, a debate has developed over what many gay political activists see as the very basis of the gay political movement—a permissive view of sexual behavior, both in and out of relationships.

Dennis Altman, in his book *AIDS in the Mind of America,* wrote,[4] "The growth of gay assertion and a commercial gay world meant an affirmation of sex outside of relationships as a positive good, a means of expressing both sensuality and community." Altman goes on to say, "I do not think it is too fanciful to see in our preoccupation with public sex both an affirmation of sexuality and a yearning for community, which may be one of the ways we can devise for coming to terms with a violent and severely disturbed society."

By 1982 the need for gay men to significantly change their sexual behavior was being forcefully debated in the gay press. Altman admitted that his former views had caused him some embarrassment as it became clear that the virus was sexually transmitted and that certain sexual acts commonly practiced by gay men carried the greatest risk of transmission.

In an article in *The New York Native* entitled, "Sexual Manners," Neil A. Marks wrote, "The one connection that has made us the unique community that we are leads to the one attack that we all respond to: the attack against life itself."[5]

Later in 1982, Michael Callen and Richard Berkowitz wrote an article for *The New York Native* entitled, "We Know Who We Are." They said, "Disease has changed the definition of promiscuity. What ten years ago was viewed as a healthy reaction to a sex negative culture now threatens to destroy the very fabric of urban gay male life. What we have in the 1980s is a positive political force tied to a dangerous lifestyle. We must recognize the self-hating short-sightedness involved in knowingly or half knowingly infecting our sexual partners with disease, only to have that disease returned to us in exponential form."[6]

Clearly, a major shift was occurring. The debate in the gay press was followed by debates in several cities over the closing of bathhouses and other commercial establishments where sex occurred. These debates pitted gay political activists who for a variety of reasons sincerely believed it was necessary to close down establishments which encouraged multiple, anonymous, high risk sexual encounters, against other gay political activists who just as sincerely believed that closing the bathhouses constituted a grave violation of civil liberties which could ultimately lead to complete reversals of all the small gains we had won.

Another change was taking place among many leaders of the gay political movement. They were leaving their positions in the old institutions and moving into positions in government and the larger community where they felt they could make a greater contribution to the growing demands of the epidemic. Virginia Apuzzo left as Executive Director of the National Lesbian and Gay Task Force and joined the staff of Governor Mario Cuomo of New York. Larry Bush, a noted gay journalist, joined the staff of Assemblyman Art Agnos of California where he is able to influence state legislation on AIDS. Bill Bogan, a former president of the Gertrude Stein Democratic Club of Washington, D.C., is now a Commissioner of D.C. General Hospital and Vice President of COSMO, an Hispanic health organization. Many others have taken positions with local AIDS organizations where their contacts and political skills have been useful to the fledgling institutions.

Much has been written about the model program for AIDS management in San Francisco and how that came about because of the political clout of the gay community. There is no question that many politicians feel that the gay vote in San Francisco is an important vote and they are careful not to offend a large block of voters, but that isn't the entire story.

The Mayor of San Francisco and most of the Board of Supervisors have very close friends and advisers who are gay. For them, the AIDS epidemic is not something that only affects a minority of people in their city. AIDS is killing their friends. Assemblyman Art Agnos, who represents that portion of San Francisco that includes the Castro district and has the highest number of gay residents in the city, has been the leading legislator in the state capitol for gay rights and AIDS. Agnos is married and the father of two children. He has lost several of his closest friends to the epidemic. His commitment to these issues makes good political sense, but the loss of good friends gives him personal reasons as well for involvement. The mayor and members of the Board of Supervisors also are frequently seen at funerals of people who have died of AIDS or visiting those who are still alive at home or in the hospital. What is remarkable is that 15 or 20 years ago that would not have happened, even in San Francisco. Politicians would not have admitted that they knew any openly gay people and there would not have been any open gay people advising politicians. Indeed, in many parts of the country this is still the case.

In those cities across America where one can find a flourishing gay social life, there has been a discernible decrease in social activity. It would be a mistake, however, to assume that the decrease in social activity indicates a setback in the gay political agenda.

Rick Pacurar, president of the Harvey Milk Democratic Club in San Francisco, sees fewer people attending general meetings, but more people volunteering for specific tasks. Pacurar says there are more and more people saying, "give me something to do." He observes, "We appear to be more united politically than ever before and the AIDS epidemic has strengthened our resolve."

Gay people may have decreased their attendance at bars and bathhouses, but they certainly have not stopped volunteering for work at the various AIDS organizations across the country. They constitute the vast majority of the people who are performing patient services and educating the public about the disease. This is as true in Boston and Atlanta as it is in New York and San Francisco. AIDS organizations such as the Shanti Project and Coming Home Hospice in San Francisco, the Health Crisis Network in Miami, AID/Atlanta to name a very few, were created, staffed, and funded by gay people. Five years later, most of them are still staffed and funded by gay people.

The Gay Men's Health Crisis (GMHC) in New York City has become the

largest and wealthiest organization in the country with the word "gay" in its
name. GMHC provides education and other services for persons with AIDS
in New York. Ironically, although it was founded by Larry Kramer and others
to lobby for a political agenda among other things, Kramer has written a
scathing denunciation of current GMHC priorities and lack of political action.
Kramer accuses the GMHC board of hiding behind their 501(C)(3) tax ex-
emption status as a reason for not engaging both the local and federal governments. In another call to action he writes, "Get off your self-satisfied asses
and fight! That's what you were put there for. You continue to deny the
political realities of this epidemic. There is nothing in this whole AIDS mess
that is not political."

Later in the same letter he returns to the theme of the new role model.
"There is no one to do anything, but ourselves. If the Board of GMHC have
been cowardly, we have allowed it to become so. If GMHC is on the wrong
course, we have allowed it to drift. If Reagan has not uttered the word
"AIDS," we have abetted this." He then goes on to link the new role model to
a political agenda. "GMHC cannot hope to provide patient services for the
dying at the rate they are dying, or preventive education for the potentially
infected at the rate they are becoming infected. The only way to force the
system to provide these services across the board is by political pressure.

"Our only salvation lies in aggressive scientific research. This will come
only from political pressure. Every dime for research that we've had has come
from hard political fighting.

"Thus all our solutions can only be achieved through political action. All
the kindness in the world will not stem this epidemic. Only political action can
change the course of events."[7]

Kramer's second "Call to Arms" will not fall on deaf ears. Across the
country, most AIDS organizations are dominated by gay people and their
leadership in the epidemic will continue for at least another five or ten years.
There is a growing recognition that the epidemic is political. Indeed, there
has never been a more political epidemic in the history of this country. The
organizations realize that they must develop a more aggressive and sophisti-
cated political structure in order to achieve a partnership with government.

The change taking place between pre- and post-epidemic gay role
models is not one that can occur overnight. Indeed, what we are seeing now is
the gradual evolution of change. The sort of political activity necessary for
success in the face of the epidemic represents a complete reversal from previous political activity. In those pre-epidemic days the major theme of political
action was to get government off our backs. Today, the theme is to make
government a partner in solving the research, education, and care and treatment issues raised by the epidemic. Yesterday, the movement needed people
who could organize marches, rallies, and voter registration drives. Today, in
addition to those people, we need grant writers, cost study analysts, and
skilled lobbyists who can convince legislators and administrators that it is in

the best interests of the county, state, or federal governments to form partnerships with us to find the resources necessary to save lives.

Although there are some areas of the country where this change in
theme has occurred—San Francisco comes immediately to mind—most areas
have yet to develop the necessary skills to address a new political agenda and
strategy. It should be noted also that most other parts of the country have not
made as many resources available to their AIDS organizations as is the case in
San Francisco.

It is impossible, however, to observe the work done by these AIDS organizations without developing a profound respect for their commitment, dedication, and sacrifice. Often they achieve minor and major miracles in home
support services, housing programs, and community education with little or
no support from local governmental bodies. Small volunteer groups are
coping far beyond their means with death and dying and are hanging by their
financial fingernails while doing so. Housing programs for people with AIDS
who have lost all their financial resources are minimal, if they exist at all.
Local health departments, themselves struggling with reduced funding,
throw a little money at some volunteer agency and expect them to educate the
entire city or county.

Drastically needed cost analysis studies and strategic planning which
could help in the development of government priorities are not being developed in most sections of the country. Small, poorly funded volunteer organizations, composed primarily of gay people, are valiantly attempting to deal
with the most severe health crisis this nation has ever seen. Is it any wonder,
then, that until they can get some help from their state and local governments
there will be no resources available to put into the kind of massive political
efforts called for by the new agenda. These groups feel caught in a classic
"catch 22" situation. The demands on their time and abilities continue to
grow as the epidemic grows, and the daily demands of the epidemic leave no
time or resources to deal effectively with the newly emerging political realities. The resources that are needed to hire effective lobbyists, or conduct cost
studies, or do strategic planning are more desperately needed to provide the
day-to-day needs of AIDS patients.

This situation cannot, of course, go on. Even as this chapter is being
written there is considerable movement at the federal level which would indicate that there are preparations being made to assume responsibility for many
aspects of the epidemic which small, local, volunteer agencies have been handling. Since becoming chairman of the Labor and Human Resources Committee of the U.S. Senate, Senator Edward Kennedy has strongly indicated
that he intends to make AIDS a major priority. Congresspersons Henry
Waxman, Ted Weiss, Barbara Boxer, Ed Roybal, and William S. Natcher (to
name just a few) have consistently moved an AIDS agenda in the U.S. House
of Representatives. The introduction of the Bowen Bill and the amendments
which will be made to it, will greatly increase our ability to deal with the care

and treatment issues of people with AIDS. It seems likely that there will be tremendous pressure in the 100th Congress to overcome the inertia of the Reagan administration and add much greater funding than the administration has been willing to spend thus far. Significantly, more funds will be made available for education and for care and treatment, the two areas most seriously underfinanced in the past and in which volunteer groups have attempted to fill the gaps. As the epidemic grows, state and local governments will also need to spend more money on education and care and treatment.

During the last California election, I asked a friend of mine, a prominent gay Republican if he intended to vote for George Deukmajian's reelection. He told me that although he did not want to be quoted by name, he felt very certain that no gay Republican would vote for Deukmajian because of the governor's atrocious record on AIDS funding. He went on to say that although Deukmajian, who is widely believed to have national aspirations, would easily win reelection in California, his sorry record on AIDS funding would hurt him badly among gay Republicans in a national contest.

Certainly the growing numbers of people with AIDS have had an enormous impact on government, but so too have the efforts made by those who have attempted to implement the new gay political agenda. It is no accident that those in public office on the federal level mentioned previously have been the leaders in the effort to secure AIDS funding. They are also representatives that gay people know well and with whom gays have long, established relationships. There is another group which has been quietly working behind the scenes to ensure a new governmental partnership: gay people who work as congressional aides. To date, they are the ones who have done the most effective lobbying, who have prepared the cost studies, who have worked up the budget figures, and who have fought hard and tenaciously for adequate funding.

The epidemic has created strong allies for gay people in the parents, friends, and loved ones of those who have died and are dying of this disease. While this alliance is being forged at a terrible cost, it nevertheless is taking place. Just as it is impossible to observe our institutional response to the epidemic without developing a tremendous respect, so too it is not possible to observe the courage of people with AIDS and their friends and lovers who are caring for them, without developing a great respect. This is having a profound impact on parents and relatives who frequently had no previous knowledge of or relationship with gay people. The respect has frequently grown into love and support. I strongly suspect that for every horror story one hears about parents disowning their gay children, there are ten stories of healing and reconciliation.

It would appear that the epidemic has changed the gay political agenda but has not weakened nor destroyed the determination of gay people to seek a guarantee for their place in American life. We have been forced to examine fundamental issues about the nature of being gay and have realized that being gay is as much as a sense of identity and connection to other people as it is an expression of our sexuality. Out of this realization is growing a powerful sense of community and a powerful new direction for the gay political agenda.

NOTES

1. Kramer, Larry. "1,112 and Counting." *The New York Native,* March 14, 1983.
2. *The New York Native,* 1982.
3. Kramer, Larry. *The Normal Heart.* New York: New American Library, 1985.
4. Altman, Dennis. *Aids in the Mind of America.* New York: Anchor Press/Doubleday, 1986.
5. Ibid.
6. Ibid.
7. Kramer, Larry. "Dear Richard." *The New York Native,* January 26, 1987.

CHAPTER 18

Creative Acceptance: An Ethics for AIDS

REV. BERNARD BROWN

Current ethical principles seem to be inadequate for the problems associated with AIDS. Perhaps a simple, new structure of hope is needed—an ethic in which the person with AIDS creatively accepts himself[1] as still growing; moreover, the larger community actualizes its integrity and its bonding by accepting and supporting the persons with AIDS. Searching the past Christian experience in providing hospitals for the dying, the new ethics described here proposes two points of acceptance useful for all people willing to move beyond denial and to spark concrete ethical progress.

TWO ETHICAL PRINCIPLES OF ACCEPTANCE: PATIENTS ACCEPT DEATH; OTHERS ACCEPT THE PATIENT

This twofold acceptance is a key to enriched ethical action in the AIDS crisis. The principle that the AIDS patient realistically admit his condition requires true acceptance of self as the patient really is: sick and certain to die too soon, but accepting this dying as a process of moving toward a completion of one's life. The patient simultaneously knows and accepts himself as living, growing, worthy, with more love yet to expend, and hopeful of available holistic support.

The second principle is that the larger society grow to become so creative in its thinking that it can accept with new insight these brothers and sisters who need our care. Our growth through the challenge of their presence requires of us true acceptance of our AIDS-infected neighbors as they really are: not essentially different from the rest of us who will also face death; still growing creatively in their human virtues, but lonely and needing whatever physical, emotional, or spiritual hope we can give.

Two Christian Culture Points Facilitate Acceptance

An ethics for AIDS is best based on an actual working *ethos,* a successful cultural pattern that for 20 centuries has helped millions in their sufferings. Such a Christian *ethos* has been a successful ethics model both in earlier plague and leprosy times and for modern AIDS. Just as the denial problems coalesce around the patient and society, the acceptance reasoning will follow two corresponding basic points of Christian vision: (1) The terminal patient's actions and decisions can create maximum fullness of personality development and some will envisage graduating into a new and better life-after-death, with consequent new hope and nobility, and (2) society recognizes our bonding as brothers and sisters forming one organism which Christians, echoing Paul, call "the Body of Christ." This is but an escalation of the Jewish heightened consciousness of the clan and our shared fate within it.

A Mystical Examination. These two roots flowered to produce new insights in Christianity. The mystic kernel of these tenets—that the patient who accepts dying grows into eternal life, and that society grows by accepting brotherhood with the sick—unfolds as follows.

Graduating into the Community of Eternal Life. "De subitanea et improvisa morte, libera nos, Domine." This supplication, chanted through some 15 centuries of Christian prayer in the Litany of the Saints, "From a sudden and unprovided death, do deliver us, O Lord," expresses a considered and stable value with which Christians have preferred to approach death—as a final occasion of personality growth with time enough to prepare themselves. Until a medical cure is available, most persons with AIDS know that they face death—all too soon, but with time to prepare. Where some see in this imminent death cause for despair, deeper Christians among them see a boon and a blessing: growth time to prepare for the most important event of conscious life. Such is the vision of achieving final affirmation of one's basic inner goodness and worth, then moving on gracefully, with the hope of eternal life. The Christian model of a good death includes dignity and the peace of mutual forgiveness, love, and support.

The dying patient's assurance of eternal life after death makes a difference in his present life and in his ethical decisions and actions. Countless dying people have found that the hope of continuity into eternal life validates efforts toward personal development, since one's unique personality will be forever dynamic and operative among all the others in the community of heaven. This New Testament-based vision[2] guarantees the promise of the last wrapping-up moments of one's life and helps avoid the suicide of despair by showing that in the period of suffering one's personality growth is finally forged.

Motivation for Compassionate AIDS Outreach. The first Jewish Christians envisaged themselves as a people together who formed a fabric, a moral entity, a community here on earth which *is* the divine reality called "Christ"— the "mystical body of Christ." Jesus, who had explicitly identified with the poor, the suffering, the sick, the imprisoned, the leper, the outcast, the dying, said that in reaching out compassionately to such persons, his followers would find and be kind to *him.* Today one enacts this Christic love in caring for the person with AIDS. This collective human moral action is identified as the "corporate Christ"; it *is* the salvific *reality,* for it constitutes the Christ-reality of the twentieth century.

Acceptance in History

Hospitals and Nursing: Dedicated Healers. Precisely in such compassion for the poor and for persons with AIDS is the collective salvation, that is, the corporate health and nobility of the whole people. If a culture is judged by how it cares for its weakest members, the Western culture of early Christian Europe up through the Middle Ages gradually grew to find its soul and its success as a human society. Historically, it has been those formally dedicated to following Christ—the monks and nuns of the 10 centuries after the fall of the Roman Empire—who out of their vision of Christic love pioneered working in the contagion of the charnel houses. Perhaps the most glorious (because both visionary and successful) chapter in history is that of the religious origins of today's Western hospital and nursing system. The vision, Christ-seen-in-the-poor, was translated into the reality of ethical action also in times of plague and leprosy. This was the successful vision in which both the healthy helpers and the poor and sick found their nobility; from such a powerful principle of ethics their actions and decisions flowed—to the benefit of all around them.

Leprosy: A Parallel in Denial and Acceptance. For centuries, leprosy was more persistent and feared than any of the plagues in Europe. It established a pattern of how Christian people acting as the corporate Christ would respond to plagues like the Black Death. Some good did come from the tragedy of leprosy: there were heroes among civilized Christians who learned not to run away from leprosy in denial, but to accept lepers as part of the body of Christ.

An important question from the leprosy experience that applies to the AIDS crisis is, how did pre-Medieval Christian Europe act? First, with great psychological distancing and denial (just as we do). They echoed the Jewish biblical precepts of thorough precaution before contagion of all sorts. But in Europe, caution led to such extreme measures as ostracizing lepers from towns, even from roadways. Some "Dark Age" Christians were even known to perform the complete funeral service over a leper, stand him in a grave, and take all his property because he was declared "dead" and probably was being punished by God. The healthy ritualized the lepers' banishment from human society as much as possible. Harbinger of our hospital warning signs, a rattle was given to the leper to forewarn all of his tainted presence. In just such a milieu, however, some of these same people found their Christic roots and provided care for the lepers. In spite of all the stories about decadent clergy in the Dark Ages,

> the fact remains that it was through the brave and unceasing labors of the priesthood that leprosy was finally stamped out in Europe. At a date when the ominous sound of a leper's rattle sent most scurrying, the early monks rallied together and converted their houses into leper hospitals and lazar houses. In France, during the thirteenth century, it is recorded that no less than *two thousand* of these institutions existed and in England at the same period there were two hundred founded, of which the majority were controlled by the ecclesiastics.
>
> "All guests who come shall be received as though they were Christ" was the rule of the lazar houses and it was a rule that was faithfully observed. Nobody, in those times of famine and pestilence, cruelty and persecution, was ever turned away and the same hearty welcome and treatment was accorded all, regardless of rank. . . . For the first time in history consideration was shown the leper; he was well fed . . . a roof was over his head and his spiritual needs were attended.[3]

A major strength of Christianity throughout history has always been its slow but eventual ability to identify unerringly the principle of Christ in the outcast.

NEW ETHICAL PRINCIPLES APPLIED TO THE PERSON AND SOCIETY

Now that we have seen the Christic motivation that can spark acceptance, how might it open to all people some of the helpful ethical possibilities based on the twofold vision of acceptance of growing-towards-death and acceptance of the neighbor?

Actions of the Person Accepting Self as Dying

Telling Others. For persons with AIDS courageously to decide to be honest with others who might be endangered by continued high risk behavior involves a basic acceptance-versus-denial issue; it requires one to accept the truth of one's own predicament. The experienced counselor appreciates the difficulty with which personal acceptance of the AIDS diagnosis is achieved, the necessary first step before being able to tell others. One man came home from the doctor and showered for hours, as if he wanted to scrub out that damned spot of archetypal uncleanness. All libido is said to be immediately lost in certain people upon learning of their AIDS diagnosis. This further weakens a self-image that will have to be stronger than ever, for courage before the community posits a new challenge to one's honesty in self-revelation.

Should a person with AIDS tell friends? Why should they know if there is no danger to them? After all, does he not have a right to the privacy of his own body? Not in an absolute sense. The collectivity of the community in this situation is even more important, even holy. Both an ethics of acceptance and honest, mature relationships help the person with AIDS and friends and family members to face the facts. They might all learn to live more truthfully and interact more openly through the difficult process of knowing, accepting, and dealing with such a threat to their friendship.

Should the person who has AIDS tell his employer when the danger to others is little or none? Suppose he knows the employer would summarily fire him? With mounting medical bills, the AIDS victim cannot afford to lose his job and health insurance. For the sake of both dignity and finances, he needs to work and should be allowed to do so. An ethics of acceptance finds it vitally important for these people to keep their jobs, for reasons of human dignity, productiveness, and sense of community. Some AIDS counselors list workplace continuance as the number one priority both in chronology and in importance.

Personal Desires versus Public Safety. The San Francisco *cause célèbre* of gay bathhouse closings is an excellent example of the conflict of personal desires and the common well-being.[4] In this case there were indeed personal rights at stake which the gay community was loathe to surrender, but such rights do not constitute an absolute in ethics, where personal rights often must be relinquished to maximize public safety. Disregard for others' health has no defensible ethical position in our responsible acceptance of each other. On metaphysical grounds, the collective health of the corporate group comes much closer to being an absolute compared to individual rights; the health of the whole might be called holy. In Christian language, when there is true conflict the corporate Christ formed is more important than the desires of the individual.

Suicide: Denial of Life or Acceptance of Death? Suicide by terminal AIDS patients is a serious problem.[5] This phenomenon reflects the cumulative sense of suffering from pain, of being a burden to others, of having no future, as well as the shame that society heaps upon both the homosexual and the intravenous drug user with AIDS. In addition, the strain of repeated hospital stays and multiple treatment regimens, none of which produce a cure, adds to the stress. The patient may know that there is organic brain damage with consequent dementia that will worsen. All these factors contribute to a questioning of life and death. Even the standard Christian counseling that encourages personal growth and nobility right to the natural end may seem pointless in the face of dementia or coma (which restrict any growth)—and many persons with AIDS are certain of that prognosis. With such a future, those who had enjoyed higher self-esteem, but who now lack the adaptation techniques gained from earlier suffering, and who lack strong systems of support, are more likely to commit suicide.[6]

Passive suicide is more common than active suicide in this population.[6] One medical doctor who had AIDS-related violent diarrhea and vomiting deliberately did not seek help. Evicted from his former residence for "health reasons," he did not even unpack his boxes in his new apartment, but expressly let himself go into extreme dehydration and death. Beyond questions of responsibility to the community, the main ethical issues of autonomy were freedom of choice and personal control over one's destiny. To other persons with AIDS with such dismal medical prognoses, theoretical distinctions between active and passive means to achieve the end (death) more quickly are viewed as invisible boundaries. Did this doctor exhibit a stoic acceptance of what life had to offer? Was the giving up positive or negative? Did he have a further vision that made letting go a constructive act?

During times of crisis there is an increased need to not sidestep the life/death issues but to make those difficult decisions and make them in a more practical way than past ethical theories anticipated. With the increase of older sick people, this society was already heading toward a moral crisis over the permissibility of voluntary euthanasia and assisted suicide. But suddenly AIDS appeared and exacerbated the need to examine the question of the right to choose the timing of one's own death.

For many people, norms for suicide often mean "permission," as they might wish to seek some assurance of freedom from guilt. A patient-centered practical conclusion, drawn from many larger systematic philosophies of death and suicide,[7] finds the real impetus against suicide is actually love of life, not the classic theoretical textbook *reasons* prohibiting suicide which may be inapplicable or meaningless in many cases. No doubt most involved in caring for the seriously ill at the bedside day and night agree that in certain grievous cases there is no persuasive reason which would convince the person to go on living. But as recent cases in the Netherlands and Florida show, a major ethical problem exists: no one seems to know how to formulate any generalized rule against suicide, valid for all cases, which would also allow greater understanding of the extreme sufferer needing unusual compassionate "permission" (to assure freedom from guilt) for going against this rule about suicide. Society's hesitancy here stems both from fear of slippery-slope misuse (by which society begins to slip into letting the single exceptional suicide become the norm), and from the fact that in such an intimate area every case is unique and must be handled individually. The harsh realities call more for society's helpful care than for suicide guidelines. From a patient-centered practical viewpoint, the following ideas are important in an ethics of acceptance.

Peace of Mind and Freedom from Guilt. As hospital chaplains and counselors of the dying can attest, both ethics and religion are truly concerned about norms for achieving peace of mind and for freeing from guilt. If some norms steer one away from certain types of actions (suicide), it is societal wisdom which speaks for one's emotional peace and freedom from future guilt, both of which are crucial not only for the patient, but also for the survivors. A classic example is that guilt-reducing staple of death-and-dying ethics, voiced yet again in the official assurance of Pope Pius XII:[8] don't feel guilty about not using extraordinary means to keep someone alive; be at peace, it's okay for them to die when nature's timing has come. While everything about death is touched by ambiguity ("it could have been different") and even by the mystery of eternity, the clearest possible assurances and norms are necessary because so many people do feel a vague spontaneous guilt before the mystery of death.

There are three groups of people to be considered in a suicide: the survivors (be they family or friends), the possible facilitator of an assisted suicide, and, most importantly, the patient near death contemplating the necessity to end the pain. For the survivors, understanding the uniqueness of another's pain and limitations and why the suicide happened, is the necessary first step before consolation and healing can develop in the grief process. So much of grief is love unfinished, and one often has cause to feel guilty about that incompleteness. An important and creative antidote, good for Christians and so many others, is that the love is so dynamic that it *will* go on for all eternity, that one can look forward to rejoining the beloved in that community of perfect love where there is no more pain nor prejudice.

The surviving family will, for their own peace of mind, grasp at the thought that the suicide victim saw no other viable alternative. A criterion from the lore of the moralists is helpful for an ethics of suicide: When dealing with a genuine dilemma, the most important question is, What is the *viable* alternative? This brings us to the awareness that real dilemmas are not a choice between good and evil, between what to do and not to do on the basis of what is good, but rather are usually a reluctant choice between the lesser of two relative evils, one of which must be humanely chosen. Suicide is always an evil when evaluated against personal and community love and growth issues, but it is sometimes perceived as the lesser of two evils by those involved when compared with dementia or such great pain that one can neither grow with it nor profit from human contact. On the other hand, the surviving family may feel that there clearly would be more peace and less guilt if the patient had persevered in giving to and receiving from others the growth and love still available in the unfinished business of life.

The assistants in a potential suicide may take their first ethical cue from the person dying, who may insist that suicide is a better or necessary choice. However, if they truly want to be helpful in a work of charity and comfort, this question must be considered: Can they not find yet new ways to make this life not only endurable but worthwhile for their friend? If the dying one sees suicide as ethical and necessary, the potential facilitator, with different ideals, may or may not be ethically able to assist in good conscience. Because most ethical people are so oriented toward the positive, they will normally stand against suicide. The danger when persons with AIDS "accept death" by contemplating suicide is that their "acceptance" can go too far and disguise a despairing life-rejection which aborts the available hope and growth life still has to offer.

But what about voluntary euthanasia by the patient near death who views his living in pain or dementia as futile or even impossible? Can the proposed suicidal action of a living person be construed as constructive and consistent with the life values for which this person and this life have stood or have yet to stand? For we do presuppose that a certain common level of aspiring to be constructive and to make a good impression is true of human nature. Is suicide a disappointing undoing of those very values within that individual?

How then do we deal with the pressures pushing some persons with AIDS toward suicide? Our clear norm in the face of suicide is to accept life and growth for all they are worth.

Making Life Worth Living. The underlying acceptance and valuing of life, seen by some as a gift from God, is no doubt the fundamental reason for opposing suicide. If this is so, then society must realistically raise the quality of life for its weaker members instead of simply rejecting the concept of suicide. Too often it is as if we hear society and the court telling the Elizabeth Bouvias[9] of the world, other sufferers in intractable pain, and persons with AIDS alike, "We the healthy find life worth living, or at least we can accept our relatively comfortable lot in life; therefore thou shalt also accept thine."

Rev. Harold Burris,[6] who arranges housing and care for homeless AIDS patients in Washington, D.C., said that none of his charges have committed suicide. His network, which provides companionship, recreation, all types of caring, even feeding for those who cannot feed themselves, and a clean and dignified place to live, seems to make the difference between hope and despair. This practical example of the ethics of helping the neediest of the sick and, therefore, of accepting the other is so successful that the stickier questions of suicide are obviated.

The real issue then for the counselor helping the patient to grow is how to make hope accessible. If the patient can be energized to pursue inner growth even through pain and suffering in the final days and to surmount the temptation to despairing suicide, a sense of personal dignity will surely follow. More important, such personal internal growth and its consequent ethical sense also contribute to the whole community's goodness and peace.

The natural fruition of human nature is to approach death in its natural biological timing, perhaps because one loves this life, this growth, these people, enough to stay here as extensively and as intensively as humanly possible. The principle of acceptance keeps even sick and weak patients accepting more life and growth here and now, doing something positive and creative with life's darker moments.

Actions of Others Accepting the AIDS Patient

Medical and Religious Idealism and Denial. Many doctors and nurses, clearly overburdened, are doing all they possibly can for AIDS patients; they are genuinely courageous and dedicated to improving the quality of individual life.[10] After the families and the medical community, the religious community is perhaps the next most vitally interested and caring group—witness Mother Teresa's newest home for homeless terminally ill AIDS patients in Washington, D.C. And yet, in the psychodynamics of denial and acceptance, because acceptance is so difficult to attain, these three groups (families, medical, and religious communities) with most at stake are, not surprisingly, also the first *loci* of predictable denial.

Institutional idealism (we see a ready example in the church) by its very nature will predictably deny the individuals ill with AIDS in its own ranks—idealistically they don't exist. Perhaps more surprising than the natural first stage of institutional denial is the often unfounded presumption that the dedication and idealism of caregivers (clerics or physicians, for example) should make them immune to the deviations from monogamy or celibacy that increase the risk of AIDS. In the real-life contradictions that exist, there is a logical and necessary distinction between the universal *ideal* with the limitations in its stance and its language on the one hand, and the individual members, some of whom will engage in less than ideal behavior on the other hand. It is helpful to see the moral failings behind personal cover-ups or denials of AIDS that occasionally occur among doctors or clergy for what they are: personal failures to live up to an ideal and not therefore an issue of ethics, assuming that this individual is not infecting or influencing others. In every individual case known to this writer and his sources, personal affliction renders that doctor or cleric more compassionate and helpful, a better ethical person who reaches out to help others.

Public Policy and Sex Education: Acceptance of Basic Realities. Taking the truth—and the facts of life and death—in stride seems not yet possible in our puritanical society that is not mature enough to deal openly with the sexual education of its youth. How, then, will society deal with the challenge presented by Surgeon General Koop who proposes,[11] among other things, a more frank and thorough sexual education of school youth to help prevent the further spread of AIDS? What value is to be put upon the personal prudishness and reluctance to speak of such sexual facts to one's children when

society is faced with a deadly unchecked epidemic? Embarrassment or squea-
mishness about the *education* regarding sexual *facts* and practices has little religious standing or moral valence when measured against the "principle of the
common good," the overwhelming religious imperatives of charity and
courage involved in protecting a population from a deadly virus. But lest the
specter of sex (including use of condoms) education in public schools loom
too large on the horizon as the only means necessary to reach the Surgeon
General's health goals, there must also be opportunities for, as well as respect
for, the classic involvement of parents in instilling their personal values which
foster abstinence and monogamy. Both public and parental education are
types of acceptance (as opposed to denial) of sexual truth; an acceptance into
which this society has yet to grow. By comparison, children of many other
cultures, in past and present history, sleep in one room with parents, witness
childbirthing, and know more about the facts of life and death and, consequently, cope more naturally and healthily with these realities than American
youngsters. Future generations might well credit the AIDS epidemic with finally ending the puritanical period of this country in this one regard.

Families and Churches. Families sometimes dispossess their own members
because of AIDS. Counselors find an interesting pattern among family
members of male homosexuals with AIDS. Blood sisters of persons with
AIDS are the all-time winners for loyalty in visiting their sick brothers. Next,
it is the lovers and friends who remain steadfast. In the middle range are the
patients' mothers. Male family members have the most severe reactions
against homosexually transmitted AIDS; the fathers and, least supportive of
all, the blood brothers are too often found to be most devoid of sympathy and
understanding.

Churches are like families in their idealistic rejection patterns. One interpretation says that those Christian churches with a history of rejection or
fear of sex outside its traditional place in marriage have been the slowest to
come forward in activating their theories of Christian charity. It is no paradox
that their rigid human morality inhibits their human charity. To their shame,
Christian churches still drag their feet today in proportion to the sexual connotations associated with AIDS. An ethics of acceptance would rise above any
putative sexual origins of AIDS (which in any event is not true for increasing
numbers of cases of infected needle, blood transfusion, or perinatal transmission). Why or how someone became sick is completely beside the point of
their needing care. Assuming punishment and guilt as an explanation of misfortune is a throwback to a theology outmoded by the Book of Job; it is misguided and found incorrect by Jesus (John IX, 3). Especially in a Christian
system proclaiming brotherhood, only compassion and holistic healing are to
the point.

Schoolchildren seem to be in less danger from infected children than is
indicated by the intense response of emotional parents ignorant of the med-

ical facts about AIDS. The very atmosphere and purpose of a school is precisely for absorbing basics of science and ethics and learning how to cope wisely and successfully with the realities of life, which may include such serious medical (and other) difficulties. An ethics of acceptance envisions a society, beginning in our elementary schools, that is wisely aware of AIDS and how to avoid its dangers; a society that is helpful, holistic, and hospitable; a society that insists on accepting reality by living and coping, facing and mastering it.

"But I might catch it!" We who are the "others," the caretakers, fear becoming the newest persons with AIDS; hence our hesitancy in working with or accepting these sick individuals into our lives. An ethics of acceptance has a two-pronged response: information and inspiration.

First, to allay fear, one will seek wisdom and information. Media reports about AIDS are usually our most frequent sources of information (or misinformation) about this epidemic. Ethical problems immediately arise since the very nature of much of the media seeks sensationalism. We, the public, should be aware both of the media's shortcomings and of accurate medical facts. With an ethics of acceptance, we want the whole truth.[12]

Second, as a people valuing this gift of struggling humanity, we remind each other of one of our culture's true heroic stories. Exactly one century ago Damien de Veuster, the Belgian priest who volunteered to live forever with the lepers of Molokai (Hawaii), began his famous sermon with "We lepers . . ." He was stricken with leprosy only after some 20 years of serving in utter poverty, lacking even simple hygiene. Sister Marianne and her followers who continued Damien's work determined that they would take hygienic precautions; not one of them ever caught leprosy even though they served as nurses for decades. Damien remains for both the medical and the religious communities, an outstanding historical and psychological study of creative acceptance leading to personal peace and dignity.

AN ETHICS OF ACCEPTANCE: A SUMMARY

WHAT to do? Ethics is, in part, about actions—thoughtfully chosen, value-laden actions that we *do.* For a terminal patient, there is the serious work of acceptance—or preparing for death—by coming to peace with oneself and one's family and friends. For society, there is holistic healing to be done and loving care to be given to the sick and dying patients. A nonmoralizing stance is essential for communication between the person with AIDS and the caregiver. Both can then become more creative, exploring a vision for filling the time remaining. Thus patient and society can strive together to maximize the peace, love, and hope in each other. While these endeavors have been often based in visionary ideals found in religious models, the actual implementation is in reality, as always in ethics, going to admit of a yet broader range of thoughtful ethical choices.

WHOM to care for? Those who see themselves committed to new personal and societal growth through such an ethics of acceptance would care, in whatever ways needed, for *everyone,* no illness excluded. To put it more strongly: We reach out to care, not in spite of the nature of AIDS, but precisely because the very need attracts such caretakers. Since religions are institutions of idealisms, the "official church position" on how one views AIDS patients is known more accurately from its charter documents and its macro-history than from any individual deviants. Thus any classical Christianity—and certainly its ancient Catholic core (occasional uninformed or insecure bishops and priests notwithstanding)—firmly repudiates the recent fundamentalist cant of looking down on the homosexual as having incurred a punishment from God in the form of AIDS. Although a large group of sincere Christians do espouse this "punishment" explanation of AIDS, the most basic law of universal charity and their own scriptures make an even more fundamental demand: "Do not judge lest you be judged." Another older Christian approach drew a distinction between the sin (to be rejected) and the sinner and his sickness (to be accepted and cared for). An even more basic distinction is shown in the adage, "Love the sinner but hate the sin." Doing this demands some creative growth in society, and will lead to the necessary distinction whereby one can choose to reject the homosexual lifestyle, neither encouraging nor condoning it, and at the same time mercifully accept and tend to the sick person.

Priests and ministers have expressed fears of status loss if they even mention AIDS from the pulpit in any compassionate way. They fear for their jobs and their respect, as if they might be thought to "condone the sinner," when they really mean to encourage imitating the mercy of Jesus the Healer.

Christianity has sometimes been called a study in the history of heresies, better known for its aberrations from its idealism than for its excellent fulfillment. Perhaps the AIDS crisis shows society's latest insecurity (before both the gay lifestyle and the disease), an imbalance that results in harsh treatment of the sick. To better buttress ourselves in the Christic courage to care for all the sick, it should be remembered that Jesus was harsh on only one type of sinner—the Pharisee who in his righteousness was harsh on others. Preferring mercy, Jesus refused to be led into conversing about any individual's sin as he always denied any consequent punishment by calamity,[13] unlike so many of his followers who become eloquent about the sins of others and conclude by punishing them.

Those of good will who may have hesitated to reach out in caring to the homosexual person with AIDS should be reassured by the knowledge that Jesus (see John IX, 3) rejected the claim that misfortune (of the blind man in this case) is punishment for sin, saying that such infirmity is there "so that the glory of God might be revealed," which occurs whenever we step in with healing and compassion to create new hope and new life.

WHO does the caring? Everyone who can does the caring, as the recent hospice movement of putting patients back into the homes also shows. Within Christian ethics, when patience grows thin and there is temptation to give up, the caring person ideally is transfused with a renewed awareness and motivation of vitally functioning in the community of the corporate Christ. At this moment of weakness, some are strengthened by identifying themselves as Christic caretakers, doing what Jesus would do, thereby etching out further delineations of their own heaven-bound personalities.

WHY? Why does one accept the AIDS patient and do so with such a creative acceptance that leads to caring? In Christian traditions there are three reasons: (1) self-transcendence in (2) an archetypal truth and (3) a great history proving the first two. Throughout history, religious motivation has proved to have a very firm constancy and resolve. For centuries, thousands of hospital nuns consistently kept at their loving care when few others would, creating the first international system of hospices, and giving witness to what a powerful ethic human nature can indeed achieve. Small wonder that mainly those with heroic or supernatural motivation would do this work, for the nature of the medieval contagions often meant that the caretaker had to be ready to die with her patient. Their self-transcendence was two-fold: it's worth it to die because there is heaven beyond death and because this patient here before me participates in being not just a mere individual, but is bonded to that vital organism which achieves its heights in the "body of Christ." Both caretaker (facing possible infection and death altruistically) and patient fit into the archetype of Christ on the cross. Patients frequently approach death with the perennial question, "Why must one go through this?" They are helped to transcendence by an archetypal model ("Christ showed that the normal way to glory is through such suffering"). This simple vision sparked tremendous creative growth in self and in caring for the neighbor: the truth and work of the universal Crucifixion goes on day by day—that is, the ongoing necessity to help others (and self) live and die well on the way to eternal life with God and community.

CONCLUSION: A CONSCIOUSNESS OF COMPASSION

Acceptance is a concrete structure of hope. What we have experienced with AIDS is only the tip of the iceberg—not just in the quantity of cases, but also in the nature of the challenges facing hospitals and hospices, the caring and acceptance structures in the future. A qualitatively different energy based in greater love, humanity's strongest point, will be asked of all members of human society.

What can we hope for? An ethics of acceptance gives a consciousness of compassion that can always transcend the fear of communicability of disease. Like Elisabeth Kübler-Ross struggling to care for AIDS children today, so too were Damien of Molokai and Mother Teresa moved by a qualitatively different love, an I–Thou energy of caring which inspired each with a vision whereby nothing could be more important than compassionate solidarity with the afflicted. They lived out an ethics, a principled thoughtfulness guiding their actions, tapping a deeper energy that changes the world.

Persons with AIDS rely on this compassionate energy. This spiritual energy becomes an ethical principle from which creative actions flow. Acceptance is the first step in actualizing our vision, the ground of our being who we most deeply are. Holistic healing of both patient and society is then the goal of an ethical principle of acceptance.

Ethics, as well as the whole human race, will have failed in its ideals if science alone vanquishes AIDS while strong and healthy persons ostracize and neglect their weak and ill fellow beings. There is every hope that, with an ethics inspiring so many caretakers to stay by the bedsides, the sick, in their hour of growth and of need, will find us truly brothers and sisters, truly ethical and creatively accepting.

NOTES

1. Our focus here, unlike the empathic *Newsweek* article cited in 10., which centered on a lovable, innocent female social worker and mother with AIDS, will be primarily on the more typical AIDS patient whom society blatantly rejects on the basis of homosexuality. Although this writer subscribes to nonsexist language, since virtually all AIDS patients referred to in this chapter are male, it will be both accurate and efficient to refer to them with masculine pronouns. We will also be focusing on the United States.
2. Cf. Hellwig, Monika. *What Are They Saying About Death and Christian Hope?* NY: Paulist, 1978 and Teilhard de Chardin, S. J., on how a mystic views his own death in *The Divine Milieu.* NY: Harper & Row, pp. 89–90. See also Karl Rahner, S. J. *On the Theology of Death.* NY: Herder, 1961.
3. Farrow, J. *Damien the Leper.* NY: Doubleday Image, 1954, pp. 97–98.
4. Fitzgerald, F. "A Reporter at Large: The Castro-II" *The New Yorker,* July 28, 1968, pp. 44–63.
5. Conference with Joseph Izzo, M.S.W., Whitman Walker Clinic, Washington, D.C.
6. Conference with Rev. Harold Burris, Whitman Walker Clinic, Washington, D.C.
7. Beauchamp, T., and Perlin, S. *Ethical Issues in Death and Dying.* Englewood Cliffs, NJ: Prentice Hall, 1978; Hellwig, M. *What Are They Saying about Death and Christian Hope?* NY: Paulist, 1978; Maguire, D. *Death by Choice.* NY: Doubleday, 1974; Lebacqz, K., and Englehardt, H. T. "Suicide and the Patient's Right to Reject Medical Treatment." In *Death, Dying, and Euthanasia,* edited by Horan, D., and Mall, D. Frederick, M. D.: University Publications of America, 1980, pp. 669–705.
8. *Acta Apostolicae Sedis* 49 (1957), pp. 1031–1032.
9. Elizabeth Bouvia is the name of the quadriplegic woman in southern California who peti-

tioned the courts (at first unsuccessfully) to discontinue her forced feeding and to allow her to die of the natural consequences of her MS by which she could not feed herself.

10. See the inspiring story by Goldman, P., and Beachy, L. "The AIDS Doctor." *Newsweek,* July 21, 1986, pp. 38–50.
11. *Journal of the American Medical Association* 256 (Nov. 28, 1986), pp. 2784–2789.
12. The broader range of journalistic ethics is well described in Check, W. "Public Education on AIDS: Not Only the Media's Responsibility." *Hastings Center Report,* August 1985, Special AIDS Supplement, pp. 27–31.
13. John VIII, 6; John IX, 3; Luke VII, 39; Luke XV, 32; Luke XIX, 7.

CHAPTER 19

AIDS: Seventh Rank Absolute

ROBERT FULTON
GREG OWEN

INTRODUCTION

Images of what threatens to be a major human catastrophe were presented to the American public in 1986 in the form of a two hour PBS "Frontline" documentary entitled, "AIDS." It featured a *cinema verité* presentation of the life of an afflicted black, male, homosexual prostitute—Fabian Bridges. The program offered the viewer a microcosm of the world within which Fabian found himself, that is, a medical establishment confronted with a new, lethal disease for which there is no known cure or vaccine; a public health service threatened with being overwhelmed by AIDS patients; legislators pulled in different ways by their constituents to respond to the epidemic; and an embattled homosexual community aware that its members currently represent more than two-thirds of all AIDS patients.

Following the film, a panel of medical experts, a legislator, a public health official, and representatives of several gay rights organizations were asked to comment on the scenes of Fabian moving about the city of Houston, making contacts with men and engaging in sexual acts. The general confusion and unpreparedness of civic authorities to deal with the disease or the civil rights issues it raised were highlighted by the inability of public officials to prevent Fabian's behavior or remove him from the street. While the program recognized that the AIDS virus was indifferent to race, sex, income, or age, and that others (IV drug users and transfused individuals) were also afflicted with the disease, the film footage and the discussion focused primarily on the

In the game of chess, when a player places a rook on an opponent's seventh rank, thereby severely limiting the mobility of the opponent's king and threatening checkmate, the positioning of the rook is called the seventh rank absolute. Similarly it could be said that AIDS has positioned itself on humankind's seventh rank, for it not only severely limits our options as to what we can do, it also possesses the potential for checkmate.

male homosexual. Some panel members expressed deep concern that the film depicting Fabian's life would merely serve to exacerbate homophobia across the country and intensify the hysteria that has surfaced in reaction to this still largely unknown disease. They objected to what they perceived to be a distorted vision of the behaviors of persons with AIDS and felt the film did not reflect actions typical of gay men in the community.

The authorities' treatment of Fabian following his arrest for simple theft reflects several concerns. He was kept in solitary confinement; the materials that he handled (paper, pen, cutlery, etc.) were destroyed; he was not physically touched by any of the police or court officers; and to make certain that he did not constitute a threat to the local community of Houston, the charges against him were dropped and the police department purchased one-way airfare for him to Cleveland where he had relatives. To ensure Fabian's departure, the presiding judge personally contributed $20 towards the fare.

BACKGROUND

In 1981 the initial report of Pneumocystis carinii pneumonia (PCP) among five male homosexuals in Los Angeles marked the recognition of what has come to be known as AIDS. In 1984 a human retrovirus, HTLV-III/LAV (human T-cell lymphotropic virus type III/lymphadenopathy-associated virus) now called HIV (human immunodeficiency virus) was determined to be the etiologic agent of AIDS, and in 1985 serologic tests for antibodies to the virus were developed and made available.[1]

Over this relatively short period of time, AIDS cases have been reported in all 50 states, the District of Columbia, and four territories. It is estimated that there are upwards of 2 million Americans infected with HIV, and that 20–30% of them are expected to develop the disease within five years. By the end of 1991 it is projected that the cumulative cases of AIDS in the United States meeting the Centers for Disease Control (CDC) surveillance definition will total more than 270,000 cases. During 1991 alone, more than 145,000 individuals will require medical attention for AIDS and it is expected that of this number, 54,000 will die. The CDC cautions, however, that the empirical model upon which these estimates are based may underestimate the morbidity and mortality attributable to AIDS by as much as 20% in the United States.[2]

In the last half decade, AIDS has reached pandemic proportions. More than 85 countries report the presence of the disease, with some European countries such as Belgium and France reporting a threefold increase in the incidence of the disease annually.[3] It is estimated that in Africa about 5 million persons are presently infected with the virus.

SOCIAL RESPONSES

When the mode of transmission was initially identified with the particular sexual practices and reported promiscuity of homosexuals, many persons viewed AIDS as a consequence of immoral and self-destructive behaviors by a socially disreputable group; the same attitude was held with respect to the intravenous drug user. Religious attitudes toward homosexuality and the social and legal disapproval of drugs also helped to define the AIDS epidemic in its early stages as a disease that was essentially self-inflicted. The historical condemnation of homosexuality and its designation as a felony in over 25 states in this country also permitted many persons to disregard the illness and its consequences.

The interpretation of illness as a punishment for immoral behavior, as well as the impulse to blame the victim, has a very long history in Western culture. Susan Sontag, in her book *Illness as Metaphor,* describes illness as the "night side of life."[4] She reminds us that throughout history, disease has frequently been taken as metaphor, that it has often been represented as supernatural punishment or demonic possession. Death among the Greeks, for instance, was often seen as a consequence of personal fault or as a result of an ancestor's wrongdoing. With the ushering in of Christianity, the association of disease with divine judgment became even more specific and illness came to be seen as appropriate and just punishment. This is most vividly illustrated in the general response to the Bubonic Plague of the fourteenth century. Reactions took two separate directions. First, the plague was treated as an act of God, as a judgment upon sinners in the way Sodom and Gomorrah were reported to have been destroyed as a result of God's displeasure. In response to such a belief, groups of flagellants appeared in different parts of Europe and beat themselves and others bloody in acts of propitiation and atonement. Anti-Semitism also flared up and Jews were attacked and killed, because of the belief that they were responsible for spreading the pestilence. On the other hand, there were those who reacted to the plague passively. The death and misery associated with the plague were seen as the very quintessence of order and control. The view taken was that while illness was indeed a punishment God inflicted on whom He willed, He granted clemency to the faithful.[5]

In *Shoah,* a recent documentary on the Nazi Holocaust, one hears repeated these ancient ideas that have reverberated down through history. In the film, the annihilation of the Jews is justified by some of those interviewed as a consequence of divine judgment: they were killed as a result of their moral corruption and their adamantine refusal to accept Jesus as the Messiah.

So, too, the idea of God's justice is presently heard in the United States in relation to the AIDS epidemic. Throughout the country, particularly among fundamentalist Christians, the disease called AIDS is presented as God's scourge levied against homosexuals, drug users, and prostitutes. Various references to the Old Testament are made to support this view:

> If a man also lie with mankind, as he lieth with a woman, both of them have committed an abomination: they shall surely be put to death; their blood shall be upon them. (Leviticus 20:13)[6]

> Neither shalt thou bring an abomination into thine house, lest thou be a cursed thing like it, but thou shalt utterly detest it, and thou shalt utterly abhor it; for it is a cursed thing. (Deuteronomy 7:26)[7]

Theological judgment with respect to AIDS is also related to the traditional prohibitions against fornication and abortion. From the point of view of certain religious communities, abortion clinics, family planning, and sex education programs are essentially all of a piece. They are viewed as a falling away from God's ordinances concerning the sanctity of marriage and procreation. Responsibility for, and guidance in, the moral and ethical education of children belongs solely to the parents and not to the government of other agencies. Even educational programs that attempt to check the spread of AIDS are seen not only as an assault on parental rights with respect to the moral education of a child, but also as introducing libertarian views and inducements for immoral behavior.

American society is currently challenged to strike a balance between the community's responsibility to prevent the spread of illness through various educational and public health measures, and the rights of parents to decide how and in what form their children will receive sex education. Despite the Surgeon General's recent national television appearance recommending that children from the earliest grades be informed about the risks associated with sexual intercourse and that they be fully instructed to ensure the maximum safety for themselves and their sexual partners, many religious groups in the country not only are failing to respond to the issue of AIDS, but also are attempting to terminate such sex education programs as do exist.[8]

While it is clear that AIDS is a sexually transmitted disease, sex education alone is not sufficient to change the customs and mores associated with sexual behavior or the extent to which various precautions will or will not be observed. Research has shown, for example, that otherwise sexually knowledgeable young women will avoid birth control measures in order not to be perceived as promiscuous by their sexual partners.[9] Moreover, for some men and women, engaging in sex without birth control is a way of both expressing and calling forth commitment.

The struggle to direct the minds and the sexual behavior of the young is fraught with other difficulties as well. Of significance is the fear among some blacks that sex education and family planning programs may constitute a conspiracy on the part of the white community to perpetrate genocide against them. The first author encountered this largely unspoken concern when, as a guest speaker at Dr. Martin Luther King's alma mater, Morehouse College, in Atlanta some years ago, he had occasion to address a group of pre-seminary students on the topic of death and dying. He was challenged by several students who questioned him sharply about the white community's efforts to restrict black population growth. In any program dealing with sex education in the schools, this issue must be addressed if black support for AIDS education is to be successful.

While we have observed that the black community fears that family planning organizations have hidden agendas, it must also be recognized that this fear is present in a somewhat different form among white groups. There is a concern that blacks, Hispanics, Orientals, and Catholics have greater birthrates than white Protestants, and that promotion of birth control can only aggravate a situation in which particular white groups see their numbers overwhelmed by growing minority populations.

Containment of the epidemic, however, is not the only challenge that AIDS presents to American society. The role of professional caregivers is also brought into question. Because of the relative newness of the disease, few health care professionals have had prior training or experience in treating AIDS patients. Information and technologies concerning the disease increase at a rapid rate and professional caregivers are often hard-pressed to keep current. Moreover, the psychological, neuropsychiatric, and broader psycho-social aspects of AIDS are still emerging. In the face of the fact that over 70% of AIDS patients develop psychiatric or neuropsychiatric signs and symptoms, lack of appropriate therapies often diminishes the professional caregivers' sense of efficacy. As a consequence, many are expressing a growing unease about the AIDS epidemic.[10] This has led, in turn, to a refusal in some instances to accept acutely ill AIDS patients, a reluctance to carry out invasive procedures and autopsies, or a refusal to admit a seropositive person for medical treatment.[11]

Studies are also beginning to show that caregivers are becoming less tolerant of AIDS patients, particularly homosexuals. In one study, three-quarters of the respondents felt that special units for AIDS patients would provide better care than that available in ordinary hospitals, but only 11% said they would be willing to work in such units.[12]

FEAR OF AIDS

The general public, too, displays increased fear and anxiety in the face of the specter of AIDS. Almost daily the news media report incidents or issues involving the disease. The frequency of these reports is in response to the public's growing awareness and concern. These concerns include: the risk which children afflicted with AIDS pose to their schoolmates; the advertisement of condoms on television; the distribution of free needles to drug addicts; and the legal and civil propriety of identifying seropositive persons in official records. Still other reports and new stories tell of persons with AIDS who have lost their jobs, their homes, their medical insurance, or the support of their families and friends.

Individuals from all groups and classes of people seem to fear the disease. Dr. Elisabeth Kübler-Ross, the noted psychiatrist who is recognized worldwide for her work among the dying, was forced to end a presentation early when her largely sympathetic and middle-class audience in Virginia demonstratively opposed her suggestion that the community establish a hospital for the care of abandoned children afflicted with AIDS.[13]

It is ironic that AIDS has appeared at a time in history when American youth, who are much more sexually aware and liberated than their forebears, are to a great extent insulated from the immediate experience of death. The present cohort of young men and women often referred to as the "baby boom generation" have, for the most part, experienced death at a distance. Life expectancy for these persons is beyond 70 years. This generation has received the maximum benefits of an urbanized and technologically advanced existence, while modern health care institutions have protected them from general exposure to illness and disease. For them death has been invisible and abstract. In fact, this is the first generation in history in which there has been only a 5% chance that an immediate family member would die before a member of the "baby boom generation" reached adulthood.[14] While death today can be said to be an experience of the aged, the advent of AIDS threatens to effect a profound change in the mortality rates of the young.

In contrast to Sontag's thesis that illness has historically been viewed as supernatural punishment, this age group would explain the AIDS epidemic as a result of failure to practice proper hygienic measures with respect to both sex and drug use. As in so many other aspects of our culture, the "baby boom generation" thinks of illness as something that can be controlled by the individual or prevented, if not cured, by medical science. Such an attitude, however, fails to recognize the extent to which our collective well-being is often dependent upon the good will of strangers. Surgical patients, for instance, must rely on the generosity of those who regularly volunteer their blood and, as sociologist Richard Titmuss has pointed out in his prescient monograph, *The Gift Relationship,* they have traditionally been assured the greatest margin of safety when the blood they received was donated rather than purchased.[15]

Recently, however, the American Medical Association (AMA) has come out in favor of a system of private blood banking, that is the storing of the patient's own previously donated blood, so that persons anticipating the need for surgery may eliminate the risk of receiving contaminated blood from an anonymous donor. While this may be useful in certain cases where a limited amount of blood will be needed, and where the scheduling of the operation can be both planned and controlled, it poses serious limitations in other circumstances. Some of these limitations are: the shelf life of whole blood is only six to eight weeks; an individual is limited in the amount of blood that can be safely withdrawn over a 12-month period; blood must be stored within a reasonable proximity to the patient in the event of immediate need; at least one and one-half hours are required for blood to be thawed; and, finally, the cost of such a program may be prohibitive for many.

Over and above these considerations, however, the AMA's recommendation evokes a specter of a new mind-set for the American people: a world of the future in which one donates only to oneself or to immediate family members, who in turn must show evidence of being AIDS-free in order to reciprocate in kind. The proposal offers the prospect of a new definition of community, one characterized not by civic responsibility and neighborliness, but by a dramatic shift toward self-preservation and "lifeboat" ethics and measured in terms of blood purity.

Titmuss's study of blood donation reminds us of the importance of the voluntary act, especially the gift of blood. Such donations, he argues, serve not only to bind a society together, but also to identify it. When we recall the blood philosophy and policies of the Nazi regime, as well as the American public's own attitudes toward race and blood (until 1942 the American Red Cross identified and kept separate white and black blood), the prospect of such a program threatens to assault the sense of community, as well as militate against the tradition of altruism and volunteerism.

Community is, at best, a fragile thing. Research shows both its strengths and its weaknesses; its substance and its volatility. Extensive studies have shown that communities will respond quickly, vigorously, and sympathetically to victims of accidents, as well as to victims of natural disasters such as floods, hurricanes, or earthquakes.[16]

On the one hand, people who are sick or injured are not blamed for their illnesses, particularly if they act in ways that indicate their desire to get well. Rather, they are described as victims of or as suffering from diseases over which they have no control. On the other hand, persons who contract a disease such as AIDS and who are perceived to have brought their illness on themselves by their lifestyles are generally held responsible for contracting the disease not only by the public, but also by health care personnel. This opprobrium is in sharp contrast to the concern manifested for athletes who incur injuries in the course of "play". This comparison clarifies that it is the taboo sexual behavior or intravenous drug use which are anathema and not merely the involvement in the development of the disease or injury. Were it simply the latter, individuals who develop lung cancer following years of smoking would be treated with the same degree of disrespect. The negative evaluations of AIDS patients not only result in ostracism, but as research has indicated, also threaten abandonment by their caregivers.[17]

The challenge of care, given the psychosocial and neurological aspects of the disease, presents a configuration of problems and tasks that caregivers have difficulty confronting. In addition to the fears and apprehensions caregivers may harbor, the patients themselves can display a spectrum of problems ranging from irritability and noncompliant behavior, to anger and depression. Furthermore, the patient may also manifest such neurological symptoms as aphasia, seizures, blindness, and dementia, which create further problems in patient-caregiver relationships.

At a recent meeting of the American Academy of Arts and Sciences, Paul Volberding, director of the AIDS program at San Francisco Hospital, cautioned his audience that the health care system in San Francisco is showing severe signs of stress.[18] While the rest of the nation has come to look upon San Francisco as a model for coping with the AIDS crisis, Volberding is concerned that the burnout of health care workers, the ever-increasing number of AIDS cases, the competing needs of other patients, as well as the lack of coordinated long-range planning, may overwhelm San Francisco's health care system. Part of the problem is the sheer burden of caring for this group of patients given the increasing numbers of patients and limited resources, as well as the severe emotional stress upon caregivers of watching so many young persons die. While he notes that the most pressing current problem is one of chronic care, the situation will inevitably worsen, Volberding predicts, as the number of AIDS patients increases, making both the acute and the chronic care systems "hopelessly inadequate". In the face of these and other considerations, the moral and ethical cement that has traditionally bound caregivers to patients threatens to crumble.

HISTORICAL PERSPECTIVE

History records the challenges that plagues and pestilences have presented to humankind. In his study, *Plagues and People,* William McNeill cites the many instances of death-dealing epidemics among human populations.[19] He notes that one advantage the West had over the East in the face of deadly epidemics was the role of caring for the sick, which among Christians was a recognized religious duty. As he observes, elementary nursing care, even when all normal services broke down, greatly reduced mortality. The simple provision of food and water by the caregivers allowed many persons to survive who would otherwise have perished from starvation. Moreover, the effect of a prolonged epidemic more often than not strengthened the church when other social institutions were discredited for not providing needed services. McNeill further observes that the teachings of the Christian gospel made life meaningful, even in the immediate face of death: not only could survivors find spiritual consolation in the vision of heavenly reunion with their dead relatives or friends, but God's hand was also seen in the work of the life-risking caregivers.[20]

The United States, too, has had its share of plagues and epidemics, one of the most notable of which was the outbreak of Yellow Fever in Philadelphia in 1793. During the course of that long summer and fall, thousands of citizens of the Capitol city perished. William Powell, in his currently relevant book, *Bring Out Your Dead* (1965), vividly describes the scene Philadelphia presented at that time: the dying were abandoned, the dead left unburied, orphaned children and the elderly wandered the streets in search of food and shelter. Nearly all who could fled the city, including the president, leaving the victims of the Fever to their fate. Among those who remained, however, were Dr. Benjamin Rush, a cosigner of the Declaration of Independence, the mayor, a handful of medical colleagues and their assistants, and an appreciable number of clergy. With the help of a small, but redoubtable group of ordinary laborers and craftsmen, they undertook the enormous tasks of maintaining law and order, providing medical care, food, and shelter to the sick and helpless, as well as gathering up and burying the dead.[21]

From reading Dr. Rush's diary and voluminous correspondence written during the time of the epidemic, Powell was able to report that what kept Dr. Rush and the others at their posts, even though many of them were made ill by the fever and some died, was their overriding sense of professional obligation, along with a conviction inspired by the precepts of the New Testament.[22] Unlike the Old Testament with its stern and unforgiving ordinances presently being called upon to validate a punitive or passive reaction to the AIDS epidemic, the New Testatment calls forth a different view of illness and a different vision of the sick. For example:

> Blessed are the merciful, for they shall obtain mercy. (Matthew 5:9)[23]

> . . . Jesus went about all Galilee, teaching in their synagogues, and preaching the gospel of the kingdom, and healing all manner of sickness and all manner of disease among the people. And his fame went throughout all Syria; and they brought unto him all sick people that were taken with diverse disease and torments, and those who were possessed with demons and those who were epileptics, and those who had the palsy; and he healed them. (Matthew 4:23–24)[24]

But even this vision, shared by Christians for centuries, which distinguished sickness from sin and which, along with a sense of professional commitment, permitted Dr. Rush and his fellow Philadelphians to risk their lives in the care of victims of Yellow Fever, may not be sufficient to persuade contemporary caregivers to stay at their posts. The "baby boom generation," well-educated, highly secular, and self-oriented, has learned to blame AIDS on groups whom the society defines as deviant and on the fringes of the community—homosexuals and drug users. There is a very strong likelihood, therefore, that today's young health care practitioner may turn away from those perceived as underserving of care, despite the fact that a 1981 Gallup Poll of the religious beliefs and practices of 14 countries shows that the United States leads the world, not only in church membership, but also in voluntary service.[25]

The situation is made problematic by the fact that professional caregivers perform their duties by reason of the ethics and standards of their professions, beyond whatever religious or moral commitments they may embrace. Moreover, as more is understood about the transmission of AIDS, personal health risk to the caregiver and subsequent fear of contracting the disease are reduced. Other considerations, however, conflict with the traditional code for professional conduct. In addition to holding homosexuals and IV drug users responsible for the problem of AIDS, caregivers are beginning to see them as self-seeking, imprudent, and acting without regard for the condition or well-being of others. Concern for the health of one's family members, as well as the anxiety felt by family and friends for the AIDS caregiver, also threaten to diminish the caregiver's commitment to the task of serving persons with AIDS. Finally, moderate and enlightened Christian caregivers who subscribe to the ethic of grace and compassion are again challenged in their distinction between the "sickness and the sin" by the New Testament theology proclaimed by Paul:

> ... and likewise also the men, leaving the natural use of the woman, burned in their lust one toward another, men with men working unseemliness, and receiving in themselves that recompense of their error which was due. (Romans 1:27)[26]

Given such a perspective, acts of altruism can become strained and may cease to be offered.

A singular challenge in this regard is the problem of AIDS among incarcerated populations where homosexual behavior is extensive and where a substantial number of prison inmates fall within identified high risk groups for AIDS. As with society at large, AIDS within a prison is more than a simple health problem. Decisions concerning prevention, education, identification, and treatment, as well as legal and ethical issues related to medical care and its costs, are but some of the problems that confront the correctional administrator.[27]

As of January 1987, there have been 646 confirmed cases of AIDS reported in the prisons of New York, New Jersey, and Florida alone.[28] A recent *New York Times* article reports that in New York State AIDS is now the leading cause of death among all prisoners.[29] The threat of AIDS has raised a multiplicity of problems that would have been unimaginable just a few years ago. For example, some defendants report being deprived of their civil rights because court officers refuse to go near them or even take them into court, while other defendants are released or the charges against them dismissed, because they are dying of AIDS. In fact, judges and parole boards are beginning to question whether persons with AIDS should even be prosecuted and whether dying inmates should not be released.

At Rikers Island correctional facility in New York State, it was estimated in 1986 that of the 50,000 inmates who were sentenced or were pending indictment, between 11,000 and 12,000 were infected with the AIDS virus. Nevertheless, despite the call by correctional officers for the screening of all prisoners for AIDS, state and city policies prohibit such testing. The result is that infected inmates with no confirmed diagnosis are housed with the general prison population. The significance of this policy becomes clear when examined in light of the National Institute of Justice Report on AIDS in correctional facilities which estimated that prior to the advent of AIDS, 30% of all inmates engaged in homosexual activity, while 10–20% of the overall prison population are subject to rape or other involuntary sexual acts.[30] Unless these behaviors are modified, the prospect of AIDS continuing to spread among prison populations is great, and with it an increase in fear among prison staff and administrators.

General concern, moreover, is heightened by the fact that blacks and Hispanics, who make up 39% of all persons identified with AIDS in the United States, are also overrepresented in prison populations. This awareness has sparked some minority leaders to demand greater resources to educate minority communities.

ROLE OF SOCIAL SCIENCE

In the face of this burgeoning pandemic for which there is currently no vaccine for prevention or medication for cure, the question before us is what can social science contribute to the understanding and mitigation of the wide range of social and psychological, as well as clinical problems associated with AIDS?

If education is one of our major lines of defense against this lethal disease, it is our challenge as professionals and as community members to determine what the major social issues are and to bring to them the knowledge requisite to increased understanding and hopefully resolution.

Sociologists have already begun to address the challenge of AIDS, both as educators and as researchers. An organization known as the Sociologist AIDS Network (SAN) has been formed and an agenda drawn up that includes the development of a bibliography on the social dimensions of AIDS, the publication of a newsletter, and the compilation of a directory of sociologists working in the area.[31]

Karolynn Siegel directs sociological research on AIDS at Memorial Sloan-Kettering Cancer Center in New York City and is presently studying the sexual behavior of gay men. Siegel and others have also made a content analysis of AIDS information brochures published around the country. It is their judgment that many brochures fail either to inform successfully or to motivate for change. In order to effect a change in behavior, they conclude, anxiety levels must be high enough to promote change, but not so high that they trigger denial.[32]

Albert Chabot, a medical sociologist whose area of specialty is the sociology of death, has established a program called "Wellness" that provides training for volunteers who offer personal attention to individuals with AIDS. The program also provides them with information about relevant medical and social resources in the Detroit community.[33]

Jill Joseph, an epidemiologist, with her colleagues at the University of

Michigan School of Public Health, is studying 1000 sexually active gay men from the Chicago area. The study is designed to determine to what extent gay men are changing or modifying their attitudes and behaviors in response to the perceived risk of AIDS. Preliminary findings indicate that about 80% of the subjects have changed their behavior in some way to reduce the risk of contracting AIDS.[34]

Levi Kamel, a former director of AIDS services in California, designs AIDS education programs. He works in small towns where gay populations are largely invisible. By drawing upon his skills in qualitative research methods, he is able to estimate the size of the gay community and its level of consciousness about the epidemic.[35] Such ethnographic research makes it possible to design and estimate the costs associated with proposed educational programs.

Samuel Friedman, of Narcotic and Drug Research, Inc., is conducting research on the potential for organizing education and self-help programs among IV drug users. There are several strong inhibitors to self-organization among this population. On the one hand, the illegality of the activity makes organization dangerous, while on the other hand, time, money, and attention to their addiction leave few resources for other activities.[36]

Medical and sociological research teams have made significant progress since 1981. Over this brief period of time the etiologic agent of AIDS has been identified, serologic tests to check the blood supply have been developed, and recommendations for the prevention of AIDS have been published. Sociologic understanding came first, however. It was the early research of William Darrow, a research sociologist at the Centers for Disease Control, and others that enabled the development of sociograms (i.e., a diagrammatic display of social linkages) of sexual contacts which linked AIDS patients in different cities. By questioning these homosexual men, specific behaviors and sexual practices were uncovered which allowed for greater understanding of the manner in which AIDS was transmitted. This information was critical and continues to be of the utmost importance for AIDS education and prevention programs.[37]

Social scientists actively involved in AIDS education and research programs have expressed concern, however, that neither public policy makers nor behavioral scientists are responding appropriately to this social problem.[38] The National Academy of Sciences recently went on record, stating that AIDS is the greatest catastrophe of the twentieth century.[39]

In the face of this devastating disease and the absence of an effective cure, our only recourse to limit the spread of AIDS is effective educational programs directed toward prevention of the transmission of the virus. Even if these programs are successful, other programs will be needed which focus on the mitigation of the many social and psychological problems that follow in the wake of an AIDS diagnosis. Given our current knowledge it will be a test of our professional skills and our human capacity to respond to this challenge that will determine whether or not AIDS will put our society in "check" and thereby change it irretrievably.

NOTES

1. *Public Health Reports.* July–August 1986. Vol. 101, No. 4. Washington, D.C.: U.S. Government Printing Office, 341–342.
2. Ibid., 342.
3. Serrill, Michael. "In the Grip of the Scourge." *Time,* February 16, 1987, 58–59.
4. Sontag, Susan. *Illness as Metaphor.* New York: Farrar, Straus and Giroux, 1977, 3.
5. Ibid.
6. *Holy Bible,* Authorized King James Version, New Scofield Reference Edition. New York: Oxford University Press, 1967, 153.
7. Ibid., 227.
8. *Minneapolis Star and Tribune,* November 28, 1986.
9. Thorton, Arland, and Marlene Studor. "Adolescent Religiosity and Contraceptive Usage." *Journal of Marriage and the Family,* February 1987, 117–128.
10. Mckusick, Leon. *What To Do About AIDS: Physicians and Mental Health Professionals Discuss the Issues.* Berkeley, University of California Press, 1986.
11. "Odyssey of AIDS Victims Ends in Death." *American Medical News,* November 4, 1983, 3. (See also T. C. Gayle and D. G. Ostrow, "Psychiatric and Ethical Issues Pertinent to the Design and Evaluation of AIDS Health Care Programs." *Quality Review Bulletin. In press.*)
12. Douglas, C. J. and T. Kalam. "Homophobia Among Physicians and Nurses: An Empirical Study." *Hospital and Community Psychiatry* 36:1309–1311 (1985).
13. Engel, Wayne. "AIDS: Dealing with the Hysteria." *Virginia Medical* 113:222 (April 1986).
14. Fulton, Robert, and Greg Owen. "Death and Society." *Omega,* 1987 (in press).
15. Titmuss, Richard. *The Gift Relationship.* New York: Vintage Books, 1971, 22.
16. Pijawka, K. David, Beverly Cuthbertson, and Richard S. Olson. "Towards An Understanding of Human Adaptation to Extreme Events: Emerging Themes in Natural and Technological Disaster Research." *Omega,* 1987 (in press).
17. Gayle, T. C. and Ostrow, D. G. op. cit.
18. Deborah Barnes. "AIDS Stresses Health Care in San Francisco." *Science* 235:964 (February 27, 1987).
19. McNeill, William H. *Plagues and Peoples.* Garden City: Anchor Press, 1976.
20. Ibid., 108.
21. Powell, J. H. *Bring Out Your Dead.* New York: Times, Inc., 1965.
22. Ibid., passim
23. *Holy Bible,* op. cit., 998.
24. Ibid., 997.
25. Analytica, Oxford. *America in Perspective.* Boston: Houghton Miffin, 1986, 121–124.
26. *Holy Bible,* op. cit., 1211.
27. National Institute of Justice. *AIDS in Correctional Facilities: Issues and Options.* Washington, D.C., Department of Justice, U.S. Government Printing Office, 1986, 10–13.
28. Loc. cit.
29. *The New York Times,* March 5, 1987.
30. National Institute of Justice, op. cit., 15.
31. Berg, Ellen. "Sociological Perspectives on AIDS." *Footnotes,* American Sociological Association: 14(9):8 (December 1986).
32. Loc. cit.
33. Loc. cit.
34. *ISR Newsletter,* Autumn 1986, 3.
35. Berg, op. cit., 8.
36. Ibid., 9.
37. Ibid., 8.
38. Loc. cit.
39. *The New York Times,* November 1986.

Index